# Long Term Care

## for Activity and Social Service Professionals

## Second Edition

Elizabeth Best Martini, MS, CTRS, ACC
Mary Anne Weeks, MPH, SSC
Priscilla Wirth, MS, RRA

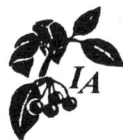

*Idyll Arbor, Inc.*

Published and distributed by

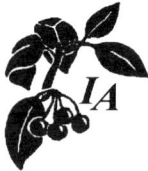

Idyll Arbor, Inc.

PO Box 720, Ravensdale, WA 98051 (206) 432-3231

ISBN 1-882883-28-4

# Contents

# Table of Forms

# Index of Activities

# Acknowledgments

This book was created from the many years of combined direct clinical experiences, teaching and consulting expertise of the three authors. It was not only these experiences that melded together in the philosophy of the work, but much more important — the people whom we each have worked with who inspired us and taught us about what one needs to live a life with meaning and purpose.

There are many familiar faces of friends and family throughout these years who have left an imprint on my life and work and I wish to acknowledge them in this book: Amy Barricklo who first taught me what it was like to see 100 years of age and still look forward to tomorrow with a smile and Charles Vontagen who was admitted to my facility in 1977 in a coma at the age of 20 and today is a member of my Living History Class in a day program, proving that we never can say "no potential for recovery" as he is both articulate, humorous and joyful to be alive.

In addition, Ann Nathan, CTRS, who taught me the importance of our profession through her work and resiliency and compassion through her life; Mary Anne and Priscilla for their expertise; all of the Activity Professionals I have had the honor of teaching and working with; *each* of my family members for their individual beliefs and support of this work and book and most of all me; joan and Tom (our editors) for seeing the potential of this book; and special thanks and love to my treasured husband John who makes each day a gift which I in turn can share with others.

**— Elizabeth Best Martini, MS, CTRS, ACC**

I've always considered myself to be lucky; and now, with the opportunity to write this book, I once again need to say "Thank You." All of my life experiences have led me up to this point and I hope that I have done justice to the world full of people who have inspired me along the way. Some have left their vision with me, some only a word in passing, I am the sum of all that.

Thank you to all the residents and their families over the last 12 years who have taught me my job and given a special meaning to my life; thank you to Betsy and Priscilla: it's been fun; thank you to joan and Tom for having faith in us and thank you always to my family — from the beginning in Holley, New York to the present in Sonoma, California. Thanks, Mom and Dad; thanks Nick, Nick and Lucia.

**— Mary Anne Weeks, MPH, SSD**

I have been most influenced by the countless staff members in many nursing facilities who constantly remind me that health records reflect peoples' lives and that documentation is much more than recording vital signs. I wish to acknowledge Brenda Huntsinger, ART, who first introduced me to long term care consulting; Sharon Carrier, RN, ART, who made it real and fun; my parents who encourage me always; my husband Tom; and all of the medical records directors who teach me new ways of looking at things every day. My thanks to Elizabeth Best Martini for envisioning this book and asking me to contribute and to joan burlingame and Tom Blaschko for pulling it all together.

**— Priscilla Wirth, MS, RRA**

# **Purpose**

*Long Term Care* is a programming and documentation manual for Activity and Social Service Professionals in long term care settings. The book is designed to be a "how to" guide which will discuss the people we serve in long term care, the environment we are working in, programs that we can provide for our residents, work descriptions for an Activity Professional and a Social Service Professional as members of the health care team, documentation of our programs and management issues for the positions, including dealing with federal regulations.

All of the authors have been working in the field of long term care since the late 1970's. It has been a time of great change and progress in the provision of services to long term care residents. One of the greatest changes of all has been the redirection of priority services within a long term care setting. No longer is health care provided only by nursing. Now the focus is much more holistic. In order for an individual to progress, to heal or to accept a new lifestyle with limitations, all services must work together as a team and blend their perspectives and treatment goals. The individual benefits from the diversity of outlooks and develops new strategies for coping both within and outside of the long term care setting.

Because of this new focus, Activity and Social Service Professionals need to have a greater understanding of diagnosis, assessment and team approach. In order to be a vital part of the interdisciplinary team, they need to be both articulate and assertive along with being skilled in documentation and federal and state regulations. They also need to be versed in the varied levels of programming required by their residents, from the resident who is very alert and independent to the resident who is profoundly regressed.

This book is the joint effort of a Certified Therapeutic Recreation Specialist, a Social Service Coordinator with a Masters in Public Health and a Registered Health Information Consultant who is a Registered Records Administrator.

Our hope is that this book will assist you to interpret the many federal, state and facility regulations better and inspire quality programming with new techniques and ideas.

We dedicate this book to the many individuals who have inspired us with their resilience and wisdom. We also dedicate it to you the reader in the hopes of bringing continued inspiration so that your work improves quality of life for others.

**Publisher's Note:**

We have promoted the development and publishing of this book because we feel that those who live in long term care facilities deserve the best of care. This book was written for Activity Professionals, Recreational Therapists (CTRS), Social Service Professionals, Social Workers (MSW and LCSW), Occupational Therapists and Occupational Therapy Assistants.

To the best of our knowledge, the procedures and recommendations of this book reflect currently accepted practice. Nevertheless, they cannot be considered absolute and universal. For individual application, recommendations for therapy for a particular individual must be considered in light of the individual's needs and condition. The authors and publisher disclaim responsibility for any adverse effects resulting directly or indirectly from the suggested procedures, from any undetected errors or from the reader's misunderstanding of the text.

# 1. Introduction

The professional opportunities to care for the growing number of people who will use the supportive assistance offered in long term care are expanding faster than professionals can be trained. These positions can be rewarding, challenging and fulfilling — if the individual feels that s/he is competent because of his/her training and is able to feel like an accepted member of the health care team. The purpose of this book is to help you achieve the status of being an Activity or Social Service Professional.

As of October 1990, all long term care facilities in the United States were required to comply with the new federal regulations known as OBRA (Omnibus Budget Reconciliation Act). These regulations signaled a shift in federal policy from emphasizing the quality of nursing care to a realization that the quality of every aspect of the resident's life was important.

In July, 1995, the "Final Rule" of OBRA was implemented. This modification to the federal regulations changed some of the terminology and F-Tags within the regulations. The most significant change has been to the survey process and the interpretation of the regulations.

These new regulations put the emphasis on the individual and how we provide him/her with personal respect, a homelike environment and care so that s/he may "attain or maintain the highest practicable physical, mental and psychosocial well being.[1]" Significant changes in the work of Activity and Social Service Professionals have resulted from the new OBRA regulations.

---

[1] Omnibus Budget Reconciliation Act, Tag F309.

# The New Approach

Well into the twenty-first century we will build onto the approach to quality of life and quality of care from the Holistic Model — looking at all the elements that create "a life worth living." Here are some of the changes:

## Surveys

Surveys are used by the federal and state governments and other accrediting agencies to assure that the individuals living in institutional settings are being provided with all aspects of quality care. The survey process used to focus primarily on how the facility documented the services provided. Now the focus is on the outcome of the service. How well do we, as a team, provide for the needs and interests of each person residing in our facility? We, as staff, are held much more accountable for each person's well being. If there is a problem in any one area of care, all staff members need to be a part of the solution.

## Resident Rights

The residents have more power in making decisions concerning various types of treatment and schedules. They will be asked to be a part of the team approach in care conferences, resident council, the survey process and much more. The Resident Bill of Rights will be at the forefront of quality of life.

## Ombudsman

The Ombudsman is a state position established to review resident complaints. The role of the Ombudsman has grown in importance into an integral part of the survey process. With the implementation of the Final Rule of OBRA, the Department of Health, Licensing and Certification now contacts the Ombudsman's office to alert them to upcoming surveys in facilities so that they can not only be a part of this process from the entry visit to the exit meeting, but in addition can inform the survey team about any complaints or concerns registered with and or by the Ombudsman office. It is very important for the Activity Professional and Social Service Professional to develop a good line of communication with the Ombudsman.

## Activity and Social Service Departments

The activity and social service departments have been given a new role as advocates for the resident's Quality of Life. They are responsible for making sure that each resident has meaningful things to experience and do and a place to live which enhances capabilities and individual potential.

The environment that one lives in has a profound impact on mood, creativity, healing, accessibility, motivation and growth. For the person with multiple cognitive and sensory losses, the need for a stimulating, accepting environment is of the utmost importance. Each staff member is responsible for ensuring that the resident's environment is a positive, healthy one.

Frequently other staff members look toward the Activity and Social Service Professionals to define what a "good" environment is for each resident.

Activity and Social Service Professionals need to address issues pertaining to the provision of quality interactions, appropriate and motivating environments and programs designed to meet individual needs by providing varied opportunities for the spectrum of lives that they work with.

The Activity Professional should conduct each group experience paying close attention to the environment and how it can enhance involvement and a sense of well being. The Social Service Professional assists in helping to create a warm, homelike environment for each resident's room.

# Long Term Care

In years past, the skilled nursing setting was almost always a facility which provided services to frail elderly people in need of 24 hour nursing attention. This was what defined a skilled nursing facility/long term care facility. Today, this setting is referred to as a long term care facility or a Nursing Facility (NF) according to the OBRA regulations. The people or residents of a nursing setting today vary in age from teenagers to people over 100. There is no "typical" resident.

The need to be admitted is identified not according to age, but instead according to acuity level in relationship to the comprehensive assessment process. Many facilities also have a "special care unit" which functions as an individual unit providing specialized services and programs to residents with Alzheimer's Disease and related dementia disorders. There is a separate activity program designed to meet these special needs. These units are becoming prevalent enough that the Joint Commission on Accreditation of Healthcare Organizations (JCAHO) has created guidelines and intent statements for Special Care Unit standards and criteria for accreditation in the new 1996 **JCAHO Long Term Care Manual**.

The nursing facility can also be found as a special unit within the framework of an acute care hospital. This may be called a Transitional Care Unit, Subacute Unit, Medicare Unit or Extended Care Unit. In an acute care hospital, a patient can be transferred from the acute to subacute unit while remaining in the same hospital. This unit provides the patient with continued coverage of services until they are discharged. This unit financially benefits the hospital because the Medicare coverage continues. It benefits the patient because they do not have to go through another transfer or the transitional trauma associated with many moves while trying to recuperate. Because of these factors, many acute care hospitals are reorganizing their beds to create a nursing facility unit.

This unit is under the same licensure as a nursing facility. It must comply with both federal and state regulations. The activity and social service programs are required as a service within the bed rate. The uniqueness of the setting and the high level of acuity of these residents creates quite a challenge, especially within the context of regulations which were created before the setting was! Most of the residents (who prefer to be called patients as they are focused on short term stay) are too ill and frail to be out of bed and in groups. In a unit such as this the resident may also be dependent on machines and equipment which are new to the Activity and Social Service Professional. The majority of therapeutic activities are provided on a very specialized, one-on-one basis. The greater the acuity level, the more specialized the activity.

As health care reform continues to affect each of us individually in terms of coverage and special services, it also will play a role in determining which professional services will be provided and covered within a managed care system. The long term care facility is required by law to provide an activity program. Because of this, activity programs in this setting (whether it be a separate long term care facility or a transitional care setting) are protected and will become more important as both a service and as a marketing tool. The Activity and Social Service Professionals need to be vocal, goal oriented and clear as to how they play a significant role in the interdisciplinary approach to health care.

# What's in this Book

This book is intended to help you meet the challenges of your profession:
- to work with your residents at their current level of functioning,
- to see how you fit into the larger health care picture,
- to deal with government regulations,
- to provide a safe and stimulating environment for your residents and
- to deal with all of the details of your work (surveys, laws, budgets, quality assurance, time management) without going completely crazy.

The book is divided into chapters which focus on the various aspects of you work:

**Chapter 2. People We Serve** describes the people who are often seen in long term care facilities. No longer (if ever) are these places where old people are left to die. Understanding the variety of residents with their range of skills is an important aspect of understanding how to help them lead the best possible lives they can.

**Chapter 3. Work Descriptions** describes the work involved with being an Activity or Social Service Professional. This is an overview of these positions. Many of the details of the work are described in later chapters.

**Chapter 4. Environment** describes the environment in long term care facilities as it exists for the residents, their families and the health care team.

**Chapter 5. Programs for Your Facility** has information about taking your residents' requirements for care and devising a program for your facility which meets all of your residents' needs and satisfies OBRA regulations.

**Chapter 6. Activity and Social Service Groups** gives you a set of activities and group topics which are appropriate for residents with various functional abilities. We will also talk about the concept of a leisure room where the activities can be easily stored and used.

**Chapter 7. Documentation** discusses the legal requirements for documenting the care you are giving each resident. It includes information about assessments, care plans and monitoring the care plan.

**Chapter 8. Resident Care** talks about writing a care plan from the assessment information, updating the care plan at appropriate (and legally required) intervals, planning a program based on resident's needs and preparing discharge summaries for residents who are leaving the facility.

**Chapter 9. Councils** discusses the OBRA requirement that you give residents (or their guardians) control over their lives, in general and through the specific use of resident and family councils.

**Chapter 10. Volunteers** talks about using volunteers in your programs.

**Chapter 11. Quality Assurance, Safety and Risk Management** deals with being part of the quality assurance program at your facility, being sure that your environment and your activities are safe (and meet the government regulations for safety) and explaining the basic elements of risk management.

**Chapter 12. Management** gives you help understanding resident rights (especially the right to be free of restraints), writing policies and procedures, complying with laws, dealing constructively with surveys, developing a budget and other topics.

**Appendix A. Glossary** provides you with the definitions for many of the terms found in this book and other terms used in health care settings. Understanding what the rest of your treatment team is talking about is vital for being a contributing member of your team.

**Appendix B. MDS and RAPs** shows you examples of the Minimum Data Set (MDS 2.0) and Resident Assessment Protocols (RAPs).

**Appendix C. References and Further Reading** gives you places to learn more about long term care.

# Terminology

We have chosen to use the terms Activity Professional, Social Service Professional and Resident in this book to describe you and the people you are providing services for.

## Activity Professional

An Activity Professional is a person who is responsible for designing and running activity programs for residents of a long term care facility. Most of the book is appropriate for all of you who are responsible for programs. In the particular cases where we discuss the Activity Professional who is responsible for the administration of the Activity Department, we use the term Activity Director.

## Social Service Professional

A Social Service Professional is a person who is responsible for ensuring that the social, psychological and physical needs of each resident in a long term care facility are being met. Most of the book is appropriate for all of you who are responsible for making sure these needs are being met. In the particular cases where we discuss the Social Service Professional who is responsible for the administration of the Social Service Department, we use the term Social Service Director.

## Resident

The government has ruled that we must refer to all those who live in long term care facilities as residents. However, it is difficult for some of us who have come from hospital settings to stop referring to these people as patients. Add to this "old habit" the following idea and we think you will agree that some question about the appropriate name does exist.

If you are employed in a facility which has an active rehabilitation department and, consequently, discharges to lesser levels of care are not uncommon, you are dealing, at that time and in those circumstances, with patients. These individuals are to be considered as they would be in an acute care setting: short-term patients who are ill/injured/disabled and have come to the long term care facility to take advantage of what we can offer on their way to being "healed." It is unlikely that they would be called residents in an acute care setting; it seems equally inappropriate (and disconcerting for most) to be called residents in a rehab center because of the implication that this is a permanent situation.

Then there are residents: those who by nature of illness and family/home circumstances require the 24 hour skilled care best provided in a long term care facility. Although some may be admitted initially as patients, an evaluation of care needs sooner or later reveals that the patient must, of necessity, become a long term resident. Hence the emphasis on environment (which predated OBRA); not so much for the patient who will soon be gone, but mostly for the resident whose options have been exercised and whose choices are limited.

There is also a third category. This is the person (or his/her family) who has had and may always have, difficulty accepting the finality of placement. In this case, being called a patient is more acceptable than being called a resident. Even after many months of care and adjustment, the person may never make the emotional conversion to resident, preferring to hold on to the hope that all will someday work out so that s/he may return home.

The law requires us to call all of these people "residents" in long term care facilities. The fact remains, however, that they are not all the same; it will remain for us to know and to respect, the differences in them. For this book we will consistently use the term resident, in accordance with the laws.

# 2. People We Serve

The long term care setting has no "profile" resident. The type of individuals who find themselves living either for a short time or a long time in a long term care setting span the categories of age, disability, socioeconomic status and diagnosis. An 82 year old man with a fractured hip may share a room with a 19 year old man suffering from a head injury sustained in a motorcycle accident. In the next room, a 17 year old woman who is comatose from an overdose of crack cocaine may have as her roommate a 74 year old woman who is incontinent, suffers from short term memory loss and is blind.

Many people over 65 will spend some time in a long term care facility. Some will live out the rest of their lives there. A much larger percentage of the residents will be admitted for a short period to deal with an acute problem. After their stay they will return to a lesser level of care.

It is important to address the diversity and its consequent impact on programming needs.

This chapter will talk about the residents of long term care facilities and some of their important issues. We will look at the expectations of the residents and their families, the kinds of physical and cognitive disabilities that the residents may have and opportunities for continuing a meaningful lifestyle in a long term care setting.

## Theories of Aging

Philosophy helps us come to terms with so many of life's uncertainties. As life and times have changed, so have theories about aging. It is important to be familiar with theories of aging so that you can develop your own philosophy on the importance of, not only your own life, but also the lives of the residents for whom you work. The following descriptions are taken from **Aging and Leisure Vitality in Later Life**[2].

---

[2] MacNeil, Richard D. and Michael L. Teague, 1987, **Aging and Leisure Vitality in Later Life,** Prentice Hall, Englewood Cliffs, NJ.

*Disengagement Theory on Aging:*

This theory gained popularity in the 1950's. The premise of disengagement was that as an individual ages, s/he begins the slow but sure process of social and psychological withdrawal from others in the social system. It was looked on as a time when older people prepare to say good-bye and withdraw towards death. It did not take into account that many people were living longer and finding not only great adjustment to the aging process but also enjoyment with life and their involvement.

*Activity Theory on Aging:*

The activity theory was developed in the 1960's. The basic premise of the activity theory is that as individuals age, they make a choice not to turn inward and be self-absorbed, but instead keep about the work of their lives and remain an active participant in all that brings importance to them. The activity theory suggests that just because a person ages, it does not mean that they change in terms of their emotional and social needs. This theory did not take into account the individuals who never were active and always held few interests.

*Personality Theory:*

The personality theory establishes that who you are today is the same personality and person who you will be in later years. This theory states that all the "behavior patterns, inner traits, cognitive structures, dispositions, habits and needs"[3] form the personality. If you have a strong sense of humor, ability to problem solve, work with others, accept criticism, enjoy yourself, etc., these will follow you through the course of your life. And on the other hand, if you are lacking some of these traits and skills, you will handle life when you are old the same way you did at a younger age. The personality theory brings all people together in a common experience. Age is not the common denominator; life experience itself is. This theory does not promote ageism. The other positive result of this theory is that you can always change. If you look at yourself now and want to see something different, work on those changes and they will enhance your quality of life throughout your life span.

# Finding Purpose and Meaning In Later Years

The popular theory on aging in the 1940's and 50' was called the Disengagement Theory. At that time it was generally believed that older people began to "disengage" from society in order to turn the work over to the young and to prepare for eventual death. This theory began to outlive its credibility for a variety of reasons.

First, it devalued life after a specific chronological age. Secondly, people began to live longer, work longer and still enjoyed all the same things that were always important to them regardless of chronological age.

People began to question why they should retire at 65 if they were still able and interested in their work. Also, why should an individual cease to be a social being with interests outside of the home and family? Why should an older person be expected to "disengage" when they have many more years to live and feel the "rapture of being alive?"[4]

---

[3] MacNeil, Richard D. and Michael L. Teague, 1987, **Aging and Leisure Vitality in Later Life,** page 120, Prentice Hall, Englewood Cliffs, NJ.

[4] Campbell, Joseph with Bill Moyer, 1988, **The Power of Myth**, p. 3, Doubleday, New York, NY.

From these questions evolved a more recent theory on aging called the Personality Theory. This theory takes into account all of the components which make us individual and special. Who you are at 30 suggests who you will be at 90.

Involvement and purpose are at the heart of quality of life. We need to focus on the abilities. We adapt to the disabilities. Programs need to be offered with special needs in mind to avoid the concept of aging as a disease.

We need to reemphasize the concept of community. The world is too connected for being independent from one another. We need to promote interdependence so we work together and help one another.

Just as we reach outside of our homes and personal lives to make new acquaintances and experience new things, so too does an individual who lives in a retirement home or long term care setting desire involvement with others. The Senior Center plays this role in the community. It provides a social environment in which to mingle and meet others and also offers a variety of recreational leisure opportunities in which to rediscover oneself.

George Washington University carried out a research project on an intergenerational exchange program, focusing on an adult day health center and a children's center. Two findings are especially relevant:[5]
1.  "Some predictors of life satisfaction include perceived health, close friendships and purposeful activities."
2.  The purpose of activity and involvement for the older adult is to "provide as many choices as possible in a non-threatening environment, with appropriate social support, so that older adults may rediscover themselves and thereby complete the important job of life review in the process."

The residents of long term care facilities may be able to continue their life's work or even find a new purpose for their lives. We must provide them the opportunities to do what they can do and the encouragement to do as much as possible.

# Dealing with Now

People change as they go through their lives. When people move into long term care settings, they are different in some way than they were before. They may have slowly become less capable of taking care of themselves as a result of aging or there may have been a sudden event which drastically changed their lives such as a motorcycle accident. We need to understand that **how** they came to be in long term care is a significant aspect of their future expectations. We also need to understand that other people who knew a resident before s/he came into the facility may react very strongly to the change they see in the person.

Often a family member or friend cannot relate to their loved one because s/he has changed so much from what s/he was before. But for us, whenever we meet an individual, that is how we will know that person.

As a staff member, you meet residents as the person they are today. You may not have a complete understanding of who they were, but you can form a realistic vision of what their needs are now. You can see them without their past, which allows you to see a different present and future for them.

The difference in expectations is not always obvious, but there are some general trends. Typically a sudden event leaves the family and friends with strong memories of the person before the event. Consequently,

---

[5] Campanelli, Linda and Dan Leviton, "Intergenerational health promotion and rehabilitation: The adult health and development program model," **Topics in Geriatric Rehab** 1989; 4(3) 61-69, Aspen Publishing, Inc.

they often unrealistically hope for a complete recovery. You will need to deal with the reality of the situation and develop a program which takes the changes into account.

In a gradual process, the family and friends may see the move into a long term care facility as a final step after which they have no further expectations for the person. In those cases you may expect more from the person when those who knew them before harbor fewer expectations and hopes.

> *Helen is a good example. She was a regal woman of 82 years. Married twice, both times to high ranking Navy Officers, she had lived in exotic lands and treasured her possessions that reminded her of adventures and interesting people from those trips. As a widow, Helen had decided to rent out the rooms of her spacious home to artists and musicians so that she could enjoy their company and talents and continue entertaining as she always had.*

> *As Helen became less able to continue this lifestyle with all of its responsibilities, she found herself depending on family more. Her only family was a niece who lived close by. The niece encouraged Helen to seek the care that she felt was needed and to enter a long term care facility. Helen was still fiercely independent, accustomed to attention, good conversation, good books and three shots of whiskey daily. Within a short time at the facility, Helen was experiencing frustration, anger and depression. Her physical strength began to diminish and her memory began to fade. The books that had brought her such joy sat unopened by her bed.*

> *Helen and I still recited her favorite poems and verses during our frequent visits. She shared with me many intimacies, one of which was her unhappiness with her present life. Helen was a frail woman now, but still with the capacity for relationships and friendship.*

> *When Helen died, her niece invited me to attend her memorial service. I found myself alone in a church full of friends and some distant family members, all of whom were wondering how I fit into Helen's life. No one could understand how Helen in her "obvious state" could have developed a friendship with someone. It is understandable, because she was not the woman whom they had known. But I had never known that Helen and I never established expectations of what she could or could not accomplish. Still, I was her friend.*

We share this story because of the lesson learned. No one is to blame. The lesson is that at any age and at any specific time in our lives, we may encounter someone whom we do not completely understand. At these times we need to pay close attention to what is happening now. We should expect as much as we can, anticipate change and look for miracles — because one person can make a difference.

The individuals that we are working with are who they are in the present because of the sum total of many rich and varied experiences. We need to help them get in touch with the good feelings associated with pleasurable experiences, sensory experiences, companionship, exercise and success in doing and being alive. At the same time, we need to be sensitive to the fact that they have limits to what they can do and we should not push them beyond those limits. We need to work with the people who are with us now.

# Reactions to Illness

People react in different ways to their disabilities and illnesses. And depending on events in their lives, the way they react may change. It may help to be able to identify the manner in which the resident is reacting to the illness or disability before determining a treatment plan. (If the resident is denying that s/he will need to live in a long term care facility the rest of his/her life, having a goal of adjusting to living in the long term care facility will probably not be very well received.) You will usually see one of these five identifiable responses:

2. People We Serve

1. The "I Can Live With It" attitude. These people accept their disability or illness and are in the process of going on with their lives in the best way possible. Chances are they will cooperate with therapy as long as it has a meaningful, positive impact on their well being.

2. The "How Do I Get Out of Here?" attitude. These people are being limited in their ability to express who they are and to do what they have enjoyed in the past because of their disability or illness (e.g., multiple sclerosis (MS) which limits mobility, chronic obstructive pulmonary disease (COPD) which limits the activity level and early dementia which limits the choice of behavior). These individuals may have unrealistic goals for improvement, waver between anger/depression (about situation) and bargaining/liability (over hoped changes), making a consistent performance during therapy difficult.

3. The "I'm Not Really That Sick" attitude. These people are not able to accept their disability or illness and are therefore denying the severity of their limitations. Engaging these individuals in therapy may be difficult as they may not recognize that they need to work to improve function.

4. The "Is There Really Any Other Way to Live?" attitude. These individual define their role in life as being "sick" and must have others take care of them and to feel sorry for them. Some people define themselves by this role for their entire lives, while others ease into it. In either case, it's the assumption that one has the *right* to be and act ill. These individuals tend to want treatment to be done to them, not to initiate and be self-guided in treatment.

5. "Unable to Comprehend." The last category is not associated with an attitude, but the reality that due to the severity of the illness or disability the person is not able to engage in meaningful thought about his/her problems. This is especially true for residents with advanced dementia, severe head injuries or other significant insults to the brain. These individuals will tend to be guided by the stimulation (noxious or pleasant) in the environment and by internally felt impulses.

When we define care plans for residents in long term care facilities, we need to take into account how each resident is reacting to being in the facility.

Along with the reaction to his/her illness, there is one reaction which we see in almost every resident: the need to be in control. The need to control one's life is one of our greatest needs. From the robust to the frail, feeling like we are in control of what happens to us is important.

The Resident Bill of Rights goes a long way toward guaranteeing this control. We must use good judgment, however, when we offer choices to our residents. We must take into account the previous life style, current abilities and the person's health status when deciding how to offer the choices.

# Residents and Their Families

One of the most common myths of long term care facility lore — perpetrated far and wide — is that the typical long term care facility resident is dumped into an institution by society or by an uncaring family. In truth, it is the rare resident who has *no one* to care for him/her. This fact actually extends who we serve and requires that we consider not only the needs of the resident but also the needs of his/her family.

As a response to loss of function or declining health with the need for placement in a long term care facility, we find some very complicated, yet common, responses by both the resident and the family. Reactions to placement and the progression of feelings are actually the same as we see in any situation where loss is involved:

1. Denial that the loss of independence has occurred and that the need for placement really exists;
2. Anger/Hostility about/toward the placement;
3. Searching for alternatives and bargaining to try to change the situation;
4. Sadness/Depression in response to the loss;
5. Acceptance of the loss of independence and the need for placement.

The question is "What do we do with all of these feelings and the actions and interactions that result from them?" They will all be there and we need to deal with them effectively.

Any satisfactory placement depends on appropriate staff interventions related to these feelings, actions and interactions. We will analyze them to help you prepare to interpret them and work through them when you see them in your facility.

At any given moment, any of these responses may be occurring between one or another resident and family because the facility is dynamic, with new admissions, new adjustments and continuing attempts to cope with the circumstances of placement.

From your side, you will see the same set of problems played out many times. Remember, though, this may be the first time for the resident and the family. Even though you have seen the situation many times, each situation will be different. There will be a difference in the intensity of each reaction depending on what has come before. For example, the family that has had previous admissions resulting in discharge to a lesser level of care will have had the opportunity to think about this (re)placement and will come in with a different set of emotions/reactions based on already having worked through the progression of reactions to loss. Others will need every opportunity to interpret this new set of life circumstances and will then progress naturally from 1 through 5.

What to do? We suggest that you trust your basic instincts. Ask yourself the questions: "What might I need in this (these) situation(s)? How might I wish to be treated if this were my family?"

We do not pretend to know all of the answers, but there are a few things that all of us can do to bring some comfort and reassurance. No matter what else you say or do, be sincere. Your words may not be remembered but your reactions, the way you act, have the potential of forming a lasting impression and may set the tone for further helpful interactions.

Hear anger and hostility without reacting defensively; offer to seek answers to questions and concerns and then follow up. In any case, genuine warmth and compassion mean the world at times of loss and transition.

In the next five sections, we will identify expected feelings and suggest interventions that will help the resident and his/her family progress from one response to the next.

# Denial

"There's no place like home." Who hasn't felt the comfort of returning home after being away for any length of time? How can home, that place where we most belong in the world, become one day a place that is no longer physically or emotionally nurturing? In fact, how can it represent potential harm for us?

The loss of home, warmth and comfort underlie the residents' denial, especially for people who have been admitted to a long term care facility for the first time. It is unimaginable to most to give up the place where one not only belongs, but is also independent and safe.

**Typical Timing**: Admission to two months

| Person | Feelings/Thoughts | Interactions |
|---|---|---|
| **Resident** | "I'm really not as ill/needy as everyone is saying; if you let me leave, I will be able to take care of myself." | "My home is so well organized for me; I have a routine there which allows me to function." <br><br> "Everyone is counting on my leaving, so I have to." |
| **Family** | "This is really only a temporary placement; soon, Mom/Dad will be out of bed doing just what s/he has always been able to." | "I wonder if this might be a permanent placement. I hate to bring the subject up because I don't want to discourage Mom/Dad from making progress so I will continue to speak about his/her discharge as a given." |

**Intervention**

We feel that false hope is worse than the truth and only postpones facing the facts. But, arriving at the truth is an evolutionary process. For example, 1. ask both the resident and the family to describe actual functioning level and then 2. ask them to describe what level of function is necessary, especially related to the return to the previous environment (usually home). This process takes time; the two steps we recommend are not easily or truthfully answered upon admission. We find, in fact, that a resident is not usually ready to admit that placement may be long term for at least two months from the time of admission. By that time, a sense of security may have set in and, with support from staff and family, the realization that care is required. (We are, of course, speaking only of these needing long term placement.)

We feel that involving the resident, continually asking him/her to assess and reassess the reality of his/her level of function will remove the pressure from the family. It is a tremendous burden for the family to feel they are making this decision against someone's will. The decision is seldom crystal clear. All available resources, including the physician and staff, should be called upon to paint the picture of what is and what isn't possible, what can and what can't be.

# Anger

We will preface this reaction by saying that this is often the most difficult reaction to deal with because of its intensity. Most of us shrink from anger and are frightened by it (in ourselves or in others). As a result, we tend to deny its existence or negate its necessity. By becoming aware of this common human frailty, you can be more compassionate, looking beyond the words and actions to find the motivating pain.

**Typical Timing**: 2 weeks to 2 months

| Person | Feelings/Thoughts | Interactions |
|---|---|---|
| **Resident** | "You've put me here; you're dumping me and leaving me to die. I hate this place and I hate these people. I am not like them." <br><br> "I am terribly disappointed in what you have done to me." | **to staff:** <br> "Everything I eat tastes the same! Why?" <br><br> "Last night instead of helping me, the aide turned my light off. That's no way to treat me!" <br><br> **to family:** <br> "When will you take me out of here?" <br><br> "You've rested enough. How can you leave me here?" |
| **Family** | "Everything is topsy-turvy in my life now; not only has my parent been taken from me, but you don't know how to take care of him/her the way I do. The food doesn't suit him/her, no one comes when s/he calls." | "I know I come early in the morning, but I like to see that Mom/Dad eats breakfast, has his/her dentures cleaned properly and is dressed warmly. That's the way we did it at home and I want to continue doing it that way." |

**Intervention**

The family's frustrations often are seen as anger toward the staff of the long term care facility. They need our help to understand what has happened and where they need to go from here.

Think about what makes a family angry. It may be caused by a lack of control over what is happening to both the resident and the family. It may be guilt about making the placement, the inconvenience of visiting during perceived visiting hours, stress of needing to deal with others who have different cultural values. It may be that at home everything was always neatly in place and easy to find while now the resident can't even be sure that his/her socks will get back from the laundry. We need to look at the possibility that the anger is justified and deal as best we can with concrete and correctable complaints.

In addition to problems that can be fixed, we also need to consider whether the role reversal — parent to child, child to parent — doesn't somehow produce a tremendous sense of responsibility, which shows up as an increase in anger related to expected levels of care. That is, the idea of becoming the parent to our parent may be so threatening emotionally that we feel fear or grief which manifests itself as anger. How can we ever adequately parent the person who gave us life? How can we ever do enough? And will we ever be old enough to outgrow the need for being parented ourselves?

These are all issues we must learn to deal with. They are important because those of us who work in facilities often greet the mad/angry face. If we return anger, it is a significant deterrent to warm relationships between family and staff. If we can wade through some of this emotion, interpret it to the staff and help the family see ways of getting beyond their fears and anger, we will be further along in meeting resident and family needs.

Allow for healing time so that trust can be developed. Time is needed for both the resident and the family. We are entrusted with a great responsibility and it is appropriate that our systems will be closely scrutinized. Do your best to not return anger by realizing that the family's and resident's anger is an attack against the situation, not an attack against *you*.

Advise and inform all concerned about what can be expected of the facility. Guide them in the choice/style of visiting and encourage families to trust the facility resources and to pursue their own, sometimes abandoned, lives.

Establishing trust in communication is most effective in dissipating anger. Become a familiar, reliable source of information and comfort.

# Searching for Alternatives

As a result of recognizing and acting on the anger surrounding the placement, the resident may prevail upon the family to get him/her "out of here." Likewise, the family may respond to their own feelings by shopping around in hope of finding a facility which will be more suitable. Sometimes there is a clear need to change facilities to find one that is more compatible with their needs. Other times simply altering the location of the placement (even if there are only subtle differences in care) will allow the resident and the family to regain some of their lost control. Most of the time, the search for alternatives does not result in the resident leaving the facility, but it is still necessary for both the family and the resident to know that they have done their best to make the situation as ideal as it possibly can be. When they are sure that the situation can't be improved, they can move on toward accepting the situation.

**Typical Timing**: 6 weeks to 3 months

| Person | Feelings/Thoughts | Interactions |
|---|---|---|
| **Resident** | "I feel abandoned and isolated. I just don't think this is the best place." | "I think I can walk as well as I did before. You won't have to lift me at home." |
| | "If I could just go home, I know it would be so much better." | "I'll work very hard in therapy so I get well enough to go home." |
| | "There must be a better place than this." | "Please, please, find a some place else. I just don't fit in here." |
| **Family** | "I heard of a place that really is good about getting people back on their feet. I think I should check it out." | **to resident**: "We're looking for a better place. They are not that easy to find, though." |
| | "There must be some way we can take care of him/her at home." | **to staff**: "We're trying to find a way to take care of Mom/Dad at home. Do you know of any resources that can help?" |
| | "There must be a better place than this." | |

**Intervention**

Remember that there is a chance (even a good chance) that the family and the resident will find a better alternative. Support them in their search, especially by helping them find resources in the community which will make it possible for the resident to return home or to a lesser care setting. Try to remain open to, and applaud, the possibility that the resident would be better suited somewhere else and is actively pursuing this goal.

Some families never reach the point where they feel they have found the best alternative and this can be hard on everyone. For many the weight of responsibility is tremendous; spouses especially may feel guilty whenever they are enjoying themselves and the resident can't share it. We find this to be especially true for spouses of residents with Alzheimer's. They have to watch the person slowly dying and feel neither married nor widowed — in limbo as it were — and guilty for thinking of fun or normalcy in life. If you really feel that the current situation is appropriate, help the resident and family to accept the situation, too.

Support groups help both resident and family to resolve many of the issues of searching for alternatives. It helps to see how others have dealt with feelings and restructured their lives. Residents may need to redefine their lives within the confines of a smaller community (the care facility) and family members must re-enter the community at large with a different identity. Advise the residents and their significant others about support groups and use your experience to assist in reshaping roles and responsibilities.

# Sadness/Depression

Sadness and depression are very individual responses. The depth and length of this period depend on the person's philosophy of life, the support available from family and staff and the medical problems the resident is experiencing. (Some medical problems, such as a stroke, may cause an organically induced depression lasting months.)

**Typical Timing**: 6 weeks to 1 year

| Person | Feelings/thoughts | Interactions |
|---|---|---|
| **Resident** | "There is nothing, absolutely nothing that appeals to me here."<br><br>"I really don't feel like getting up and I certainly don't want to do anything as silly as having my hair done." | Sitting, doing nothing, not interacting with staff or other residents.<br><br>"I'm sorry. I really don't feel like doing that now."<br><br>"I suppose we can talk, but this whole thing just makes me want to cry." |
| **Family** | "I miss him/her. It just isn't the same at home any more."<br><br>"I hate to visit — it makes me feel badly when I come in feeling happy with news from home." | "I cry a lot when I'm home; the only time I'm happy is when I'm here with you."<br><br>"I just can't visit. It makes me too sad."<br><br>"It's always good to talk with you about how I feel. It just makes me feel better." |

**Intervention**

Once again, time, opportunity to experience control and security of placement will contribute to a change in mood away from sadness. It is essential, however, to acknowledge the feelings, never trying to negate or "soft pedal" sorrow.

In order to encourage ongoing family visiting and to make it a positive experience for everyone involved, you might give some of your favorite ideas for visiting[6]:
1.  Come during a meal when you will be assured of having something to focus on; use the meal's beginning (or end) as the beginning (or end) of your visit, a natural breaking point;
2.  Come just before the resident's normal bed time to offer pleasant good night wishes;
3.  Bring in a special treat — a milk shake, a spring bouquet from your garden or some homemade soup;
4.  Bring in a special friend or a new great-grandchild; encourage friends to visit, even for a moment;
5.  Personalize the room with a picture from home, family pictures, a favorite vase. Not only will this trigger happy memories, but these objects will be icebreakers for conservation when facility staff are in the room.

The important thing is to work toward accepting the sadness at the loss of independence and to start looking for the good things that are still possible in the new situation.

---

[6] An excellent reference on visiting someone in a long term care facility is available, Gayle Allen-Burket, 1988, **Time Well-Spent: A Manual for Visiting Older Adults**, BiFolkal Productions, Inc., Madison, WI.

# Acceptance

There are those who appear to acknowledge the need for placement from the time of admission — immediate acceptance, you feel. Don't be fooled!! Almost everyone who starts out seeming to accept the placement will still go through the previously described reactions. Even a person who is being readmitted is back again because something has changed (and probably something has been lost).

We have seen almost everyone work their way through all four of the previous stages. Once those stages have been experienced, you can look for true acceptance.

**Typical Timing**: may start at 2 months

| Person | Feelings/Thoughts | Interactions |
|---|---|---|
| **Resident** | "I am enjoying the activities here, especially cards and BINGO. I have chosen Saturday for one of my shower days so that I can feel good about myself for church on Sunday. My room looks so comfy with my TV and chair and all those family photos. Best of all my son goes to the bank and tends to all of my affairs for me." | You will observe relaxed body language and warm relationships with others.<br><br>"I've made so many friends here, residents and staff. I trust that they do care about me, maybe not as much as my family, but I can still complain and express my true feelings without worrying about what will happen. I know you can't really make me get a lot better, but I certainly appreciate your help making me comfortable." |
| **Family** | "I enjoy visiting a lot more now. It's so nice to see Mom/Dad smiling again. It's fun to bring in flowers from the garden for the room and for the staff. It's nice to have Mom/Dad in a place where s/he feels comfortable. It's nice to be able to get out of the house and do things without worrying all the time if Mom/Dad is all right." | You will see an easygoing relationship with staff; warm and friendly attitude; freely seeking to resolve grievances as they occur.<br><br>"Everyone is friendly here. You are always willing to listen when I have a concern and you usually take care of them right away." |

**Intervention**

Acceptance comes after much hard work and usually some emotional stress. It is welcome as a time for appreciating relationships and enjoying the time left.

At this point, everyone involved (resident, family, staff) is visibly satisfied with the quality and quantity of interactions. An easy camaraderie exists between resident and family and the feeling generates goodwill with the staff. There is usually free give and take and consistent involvement in all aspects of resident care. During this period, you may find residents and families needing more encouragement to attend resident care conferences because they will say, "We're here so often."; "We speak with you regularly."; "I trust you to phone if there is a new problem."; "I know you take good care of me."

**A final note**: The five reactions we have described here are a continuum and people generally go through them step by step. However, residents and families will often seem to drop back several levels. When this happens, look for some additional loss that has occurred. We go through the stages with each loss and there is no guarantee that it gets any easier with time. But our struggles and our eventual acceptance show the lifelong potential for growth and change that all of us carry within ourselves.

# Diagnosis

Diagnosis refers to the reason or reasons why the individual is in a long term care setting and needs 24 hour nursing care. A diagnosis is important to you for two reasons. It helps identify known risk factors during activities (what you can expect of the resident now). It gives you some indication of prognosis (what you can expect of the resident in the future). There are other factors which interact with the diagnosed condition to affect what the resident is capable of doing. The two most significant factors are the acuity of the condition and the excess disability resulting from the resident's environment.

Acuity refers to the severity or the level of intensity of the diagnosed illness or condition at the present time. Perhaps this condition represents a crisis (acute) situation as opposed to a chronic condition that is more stable and long lasting. Residents in an intensive care unit represent a higher level of acuity than an individual who is recuperating from a broken leg. The acuity of the condition can have a significant influence on the types of activity that the resident can successfully participate in. Knowing the level of acuity also helps Activity and Social Service Professionals know how quickly they can expect a change in the resident.

Excess Disability refers to a "decline of functional abilities, alertness, cognitive status, orientation, communication, physical status and socialization attributed to the environment and not specifically attributable to a disease process."[7] This decline is greater than, or in excess of, the decline expected from the illness or disability. Something besides the illness or disability is making the resident worse than expected. One of the jobs of the professional is to help identify what this "something" is.

This term refers to all potential factors that can impact an individual's cognitive and functional level more profoundly than their diagnosis. One set of reasons for this excess disability come from the environment: the physical environment, social issues and attitudes exhibited by staff and family. Other reasons for excess disability are found in individual beliefs and attitudes including problem solving skills, life skills and the ability to be resilient during stressful experiences. Many of these factors causing excess disability can be improved by the Activity or Social Service Professional through changes in the facility environment, group activities and one-on-one interactions between the professional and the resident or family. One other contributing factor is medication which may be increasing memory loss, depression, lethargy and balance problems. The Activity and Social Service Professional can provide information to the health care team about effects of medication that may not be obvious in other settings.

The Activity or Social Service Professional is often the member of the interdisciplinary team who assesses how a person's diagnosis, acuity and excess disability influence his/her leisure needs and interests as a resident. Goals need to specifically correlate to the resident's present functional level. Federal law (OBRA) mandates that the facility provide quality of life experiences to all individuals residing in a long term care setting. (When the quality of life component is out of compliance, the facility is deemed to be in substandard compliance.) As with other determinants, the Activity and Social Service Professional should understand all of the limitations a resident is experiencing related to his/her diagnosis and use that knowledge to find and focus on abilities, rather than disabilities, a holistic rather than medical model approach for planning the activity program.

---

[7] Katsinas, René, 1995, *Excess Disability: Recognizing the Hidden Problem in Long Term Care*, presented at the American Therapeutic Recreation Association Conference, October, 1995.

# The Therapeutic Intervention Grid

This Therapeutic Intervention Grid was designed to provide Activity and Social Service Professionals with a quick overview of specific disorders that may affect individuals in their resident populations. It also summarizes what the individual may be experiencing and the consequent implications for programming and communications for those individuals.

The Therapeutic Intervention Grid is a quick reference to diagnostic groups and corresponding therapeutic programming needs and psychosocial needs. The Activity and Social Service Professionals need to work with the Recreational Therapist for more specific guidelines and treatment plans. In addition, the other rehab therapists have much to offer in terms of continued training and understanding of the residents in long term care.

This form cannot cover all residents or all situations, but it will help explain many of the diagnoses seen in long term care facilities. It is also useful as a training tool and has been successfully shared with staff and volunteers alike who work with the Activity and Social Service Professionals. After becoming acquainted with this chart and its underlying ideas, they will better understand how and why specific activities are designed to meet specific needs.

## How to use the Therapeutic Intervention Grid:

The grid is designed to give you important information about specific disorders and what this individual may be experiencing. After you have met and begun your assessment of the resident, use this grid as a reference to determine what type of activity may be both appropriate and therapeutic for the resident.

**Health Issue (Column One):**
This column defines some of the categories and health issues that may be found in a long term care setting.

**Health Implications (Column Two):**
This column describes some of the implications of the health issues found in column one. A review of these issues will help the professional understand the disorder more clearly by observing common effects and responses.

**Psychosocial Implication (Column Three):**
This column deals with the psychosocial aspects that may be related to the health issue. Some of these may be perceptions of a resident's condition that his/her family members and other visitors may also experience. In order to better understand the diagnosis and current needs of the resident, you must be sensitive to all of the emotional and psychological aspects that affect not only the resident but his/her significant others' ability to cope with the diagnosis or illness and suggested interventions.

**Programming Ideas (Column Four):**
This column suggests a variety of therapeutic programming ideas specific to the health issues in column one. Which activities are appropriate depends partly on the diagnosis and partly on the cognitive functioning of the individual.

# Therapeutic Intervention Grid

| Health Issue | Health Implications | Psychosocial Implications | Programming Ideas |
|---|---|---|---|
| **Dementia**<br>**Cognitive losses**<br>**Disorientation**<br>**Periods of confusion** | Short attention span<br>Anxiety<br>Wandering, restlessness<br>Catastrophic responses<br>Possible decrease in activity levels and physical fitness<br>Lost compensatory skills<br>Memory loss<br>Disorientation<br>Difficulty with directions (path finding)<br>Negative response to over-stimulation<br>Combativeness<br>Decrease in ability to learn new material | Depression based on realization of loss<br>No longer treated as an intelligent person due to loss of ability to communicate well in conversation<br>Increase in unstructured free time as the need for structure increases with confusion & disorientation<br>Decreased ability to interact appropriately in community settings<br>Helplessness/Hopelessness<br>Personal awareness of cognitive losses during more alert periods | Reality awareness<br>Validation therapy<br>Sensory stimulation<br>Music activities<br>Theme activities<br>Object identification, Sorting<br>Reading<br>Breathing<br>Remotivation, Reminiscing<br>Exercise/movement<br>Flash cards, Etch A Sketch<br>Velcro activities<br>Compensatory skills training<br>Promote outings and contact with family and the community<br>Decrease the stress and fear the individual may be experiencing by using structured & relaxing activities |
| **Sensory Deficits (vision, hearing, touch, taste, proprioception)** | Partial to total loss of one or more of the senses<br>Great potential for isolation<br>Potential limited hand strength<br>Potential pain<br>Stiff and swollen joints<br>Limited dexterity and coordination<br>Lack of color discrimination and/or blurriness | Perceived as mentally impaired or incapable of conversation and/or normal activity | Sensory stimulation<br>Weaving<br>Theme activities<br>Exercise/movement<br>Visual cues<br>Auditory cues<br>Activities to learn strategies to compensate for losses<br>Focus on senses still intact |
| **Language Barriers** | Inability to make needs known and to communicate in primary language | Perceived as mentally impaired or incapable of conversation and/or normal activity<br>Loss of familiar language, customs and music | Communication cards in primary language<br>Visual cues<br>Communication board<br>Tapes in primary language, music & foreign newspapers |

21

# Therapeutic Intervention Grid

| Health Issue | Health Implications | Psychosocial Implications | Programming Ideas |
|---|---|---|---|
| Comatose | Non-responsive<br>Limited or no vision<br>Communication deficit<br>Potential for skin integrity problems<br>Possible NG tube (feeding tube) | Isolation<br>Family and friends feel helpless or hopeless about visiting unless able to assist in the rehabilitative process | Music<br>Eye tracking experiences (mobiles, posters if eyes are open)<br>Soft range of motion exercises<br>Hand over hand activities<br>Tactile stimulation<br>Auditory stimulation<br>Reading out loud<br>Pet therapy<br>Pat mat |
| Head Injury | Need for compensatory skills<br>Impaired memory and judgment<br>Impulsivity<br>Weak problem solving<br>Catastrophic reaction to stress<br>Irritability due to limited cognitive, motor and language abilities<br>Slow processing of information and learning and remembering new information<br>Poor safety skills | If the injury is not visible, expectations are often greater than potential resulting in frustration for the resident and caregivers<br>Lack of initiative<br>Decreased ability to structure or manage time<br>Change in social relationships and behavior<br>Decreased ability in work, academic and leisure performance | Sequencing activities<br>Sensory integration<br>Sorting games<br>Word games<br>Body awareness and movement<br>Word search activities<br>Hangman<br>Crossword puzzles<br>Large sectional puzzles<br>Attention to task building activities<br>Pat mat<br>Theme activities<br>Links to community resources |
| Subacute<br>IV therapy<br>NG tube<br>Keosh feed line | Limited mobility<br>Low level of energy | Loss of control based on limited mobility<br>Feelings of vulnerability<br>Exhaustion due to condition and therapy | Music<br>Talking books<br>Oral history visits<br>Reinforcement of therapy goals<br>Environmental/relaxation tapes<br>Theme activities |

# Therapeutic Intervention Grid

| Health Issue | Health Implications | Psychosocial Implications | Programming Ideas |
|---|---|---|---|
| **CVA (stroke)**<br>**Left sided brain injury** | Right hemiparesis/hemiplegia<br>Language, reading/writing problems<br>Aphasia, word finding problems<br>Attention deficits<br>Decreased verbal learning<br>Difficulty distinguishing left and right<br>Visuospatial neglect<br>Memory deficits<br>Lability, mood swings<br>Low frustration tolerance<br>Sleep disturbances<br>Frustration with group experiences<br>Impaired verbal math skills<br>Lack of inhibition<br>Behavior is slow, cautious, anxious<br>Good attention span<br>Underestimates ability | Isolation depending on location of CVA and degree of impairment<br>Depression — both physiological and related to loss(es) or expectations beyond potential<br>Impatience, frustration with new functional status and lack of speedy recovery<br>Self-conscious about appearance and language difficulties | Involve in appropriate exercises as soon as possible after stroke<br>Activities which stimulate cognitive functioning<br>Body image activities<br>Retraining cognitive and perceptual abilities<br>Repetitive tasks and movements to achieve mastery and therefore transfer skills to other activities<br>Sensory integration activities<br>Sequencing activities<br>Communication group experiences<br>Working with significant others to identify leisure interests and opportunities<br>Exercise activities<br>Opportunities for community reintegration as part of rehabilitation<br>Life skills training<br>Focus on strengths vs. limitations |
| **CVA (stroke) —**<br>**Right sided brain injury** | Left hemiparesis/hemiplegia<br>Perceptual problems<br>Poor spatial orientation and concepts of direction<br>Gets lost easily<br>Decrease or increase in sensation<br>Change in vision<br>Seizures<br>Decreased eye-hand coordination<br>Impaired concrete thinking<br>Sleep disturbances<br>Left side neglect<br>Behavior is fast, impulsive, with lack of inhibition and verbal outbursts<br>Short attention span<br>Constant talking<br>Overestimates ability | | |

23

# Therapeutic Intervention Grid

| Health Issue | Health Implications | Psychosocial Implications | Programming Ideas |
|---|---|---|---|
| **Short term rehab**<br>**Pre-discharge/post therapy rehab residents (i.e. hip fracture etc.)** | Limited energy & easily fatigued<br>Primary focus on therapy goals<br>Disinterest in group activities<br>Self-consciousness | Relationships may be strained due to pain and due to the resident needing to adjust to new (usually lower) ability<br>Impatience with the current situation<br>Fantasies about home and about the ability to care for him/herself<br>Lack of information about home health care and unreasonable expectations can cause anxiety for resident and family | Reading<br>Relaxation tapes<br>Exercise/movement<br>Bird watching<br>Out of door social activities<br>Work/service oriented activities<br>Community integration<br>Reinforcing therapy goals<br>Resident council<br>Volunteering<br>Memory book |
| **Huntington's Chorea** | Severe mood swings<br>Involuntary movements<br>Twitching<br>Nervous behavior<br>Depression<br>Communication problems | Hopelessness, isolation and feelings of anger and abandonment<br>Guilt based on the genetic component of this disease<br>Inability to feel independent due to tremors | Exercise<br>Expressive opportunities<br>Weaving<br>Music for relaxation<br>Ceramics<br>Homemaking activities<br>Adaptive switches<br>Verbal word games<br>Communication groups<br>Theme activities |
| **Parkinson's Disease** | Resting tremors<br>Rigidity<br>Brady kinesia (slow movement)<br>Has difficulty with more than two movements at one time<br>Softness of voice<br>Depression<br>Need extra time to respond<br>Unsteady gait<br>Possible limb apraxia<br>Poor coordination<br>Possible dementia & hallucinations | Isolation as communication becomes more difficult<br>Perceived as having dementia when this is not necessarily true | Exercise<br>Expressive opportunities<br>Weaving<br>Music and relaxing<br>Ceramics<br>Homemaking activities<br>Adaptive switches<br>Verbal word games<br>Communication groups<br>Theme activities |

# Therapeutic Intervention Grid

| Health Issue | Health Implications | Psychosocial Implications | Programming Ideas |
|---|---|---|---|
| **Multiple Sclerosis** **Amyotrophic Lateral** **Sclerosis (ALS)** | Possible loss of fine and gross motor skills<br>Possible speech and language disorders<br>Possible vision impairments<br>Fluctuation both physically and emotionally<br>Possible fluid retention<br>Gastrointestinal problems<br>Depression<br>Possible limb apraxia — keep movements large and allow space | Total loss of control is possible<br>Anger<br>Attempts to manipulate the environment in order to have needs met<br>Fantasizing about home and the ability to care for oneself<br>Lack of participation in activities<br>Anxiety<br>Impatience and frustration over situation | Exercise<br>Movement<br>Need for energy conservation techniques<br>Relaxation<br>Creative outlets<br>Opportunities to socialize with peers in age-appropriate activities<br>Visualization<br>Empowerment activities<br>Adaptive switches<br>Communication activities with yes/no responses |
| **Cardiopulmonary Problems** **COPD** **Asthma** **Hypotension** **Hypertension** | Anxiety<br>Coughing<br>Light headed depending on body positioning<br>Inability to breathe deeply<br>Decreased endurance<br>Low tolerance to dust, odors and crowded spaces<br>Depression<br>Activities requiring raising the arms over the head are too taxing<br>Limited time up<br>Added stress on heart | Attempts to manipulate the environment and personnel secondary to feelings of anxiety and claustrophobia<br>Need to feel in control of personal environment as much as possible | Hand work<br>Breathing exercises<br>Relaxation<br>Energy conservation techniques<br>Need for balance of active and passive activities<br>Slow-paced activities<br>Activities which do not require lifting of heavy objects<br>Crossword puzzles<br>Puzzles<br>Reading<br>Creative writing<br>Theme activities |

25

# Therapeutic Intervention Grid

| Health Issue | Health Implications | Psychosocial Implications | Programming Ideas |
|---|---|---|---|
| **Critically Ill Terminally Ill Hospice** | Limited energy and time awake<br>Depression<br>Potential for pain | Changing moods depending on state of anger, depression and acceptance<br>Existential issues of life and death<br>May have unfinished business that needs to be done | Relaxation<br>Being read to<br>In room travel slides or environmental tapes<br>One-on-one volunteers<br>Memory book<br>Companionship<br>Visualization<br>Opportunity to talk<br>Light range of motion activities |
| **Ventilator Dependent** | Potential for sensory deprivation<br>Lack of mobility/freedom of movement<br>Potential for skin integrity issues<br>Communication problems<br>Lack of endurance<br>Potential for significant hours a day in bed<br>Pain related to injuries and condition<br>Cardiopulmonary issues<br>Partial to total loss of one or more senses<br>May be non-responsive<br>Potential for total care in ADLs<br>May have a tracheotomy<br>May be fed by tube | Inability to move around without equipment<br>Depression related to condition<br>Anxiety related to breathing<br>Need emotional outlets<br>Potential for social isolation<br>Short or long term need for ventilator<br>Potential for embarrassment in groups related to equipment and equipment sounds | Visualization & relaxation tapes<br>Mobiles<br>Music<br>Slide shows<br>Activities related to body awareness and directionality games<br>Opportunities to be outdoors<br>Range of motion activities<br>Pain management techniques<br>Reading and being read to<br>Intellectual activities<br>Pets<br>Theme related decorations<br>Volunteer visitors<br>Small fish bowl in room within visual range<br>Computer games<br>Dot to dot puzzles<br>Wrist bands with bell to enhance movement and auditory stimulation<br>Drinking straw with streamer attached to enhance breathing exercises |

# Therapeutic Intervention Grid

| Health Issue | Health Implications | Psychosocial Implications | Programming Ideas |
|---|---|---|---|
| **Spinal Cord Injury**[8] | Loss of mobility<br>Loss of motor strength<br>Loss of Sensory Awareness<br>Depression<br>Change in self-image<br>Change in physical fitness<br>Loss of bowel and bladder control<br>Susceptibility to pressure sores<br>Potential for long term pain | Change in vocational abilities<br>Change in independence<br>Change in self-image<br>Change in social relationships | Assess physical and psychological dysfunction<br>Increase functional abilities through the use of recreation/leisure oriented programs<br>Teach functional skills<br>Teach recreational skills and provide adaptive equipment<br>Provide opportunities for creative self-expression<br>Teach progressive relaxation techniques<br>Teach stress management skills<br>Build community resources and skills |

27

[8] Spinal Cord Injury information from the American Therapeutic Recreation Association, 1992, **Therapeutic Recreation Services**, ATRA, Hattiesburg, MS.

# Mobility Losses and Multiple Medical Issues[9]

Preventing loss of mobility is a primary goal of Physical Therapy and is greatly enhanced by exercises in a group setting or on a one-on-one basis provided by the Activity Professional. With the increasing constraints of insurance companies, many residents are no longer able to receive the extended therapy they need. This is resulting in greater numbers of residents who depend on the Activity Professional to continue this focus on therapy goals. The Activity Professional needs to have not only a basic knowledge of diagnoses but also the ability to blend this understanding with movements and exercises which will help to maintain and enhance functional skills.

Below is a list of the more common conditions encountered in a long term care setting with brief descriptions and suggestions about the best approach to exercise. Every disorder has a basic description but remember that every person you see will present himself or herself in a unique manner.

## Medical Groups

### Cardiac:
Residents with cardiac disorders may have sustained a myocardial infarction or have undergone open heart surgery for valve replacement, had a coronary artery bypass or even a heart transplant. Clinically, they may present varied appearances from no outward signs to shortness of breath with minimal activity.

Have the resident monitor his/her pulse before, during and after the sessions with caution not to exceed 20–30 beats above his/her resting heart rate. Some medications modify the resident's responsive heart rate so that this target heart rate will not be appropriate. If in doubt, ask the resident's physician or the nursing staff for assistance. Many areas also have a local cardiac rehab group which can provide the facility's staff with additional good information.

Suggestions for exercise:
- Limit upper extremity activity thus reducing stress on the heart. Do not use arm weights.
- Encourage activities which involve walking.
- Encourage stationary bicycles.
- Encourage dance activities.

### COPD:
Chronic Obstructive Pulmonary Disease. This medical condition results in the resident's decreased ability to breath normally. Many of your residents may need portable oxygen.

Suggestions for exercise:
- Sitting exercises.
- Decrease the number of upper extremity/arm exercises.
- Stop all exercises if the resident becomes winded.
- Pacing activities is the key to functional independence for the resident with COPD.

Note: The position where the resident will be most comfortable is with the head and shoulders forward. Continue to encourage activities to lengthen the trunk such as one armed overhead stretches.

---

[9] This section on Mobility Losses and Multiple Medical Issues was written by Mary Kathleen Lockett, RPT.

## Neurological Groups

**CVA:**
Cerebral Vascular Accident (CVA) is a neurological disorder also known as a stroke. Whether a resident has sustained a right CVA with resulting left-sided weakness or a left CVA with a right-sided weakness will determine the cognitive and physical deficits present. It is important to remember that residents can be affected very minimally with excellent recovery or have extensive damage with poor recovery.

**Left Hemiplegia (Right CVA):**
While language is mostly intact, beware of impulsive behavior and neglect of his/her left side. Encourage resident to keep his/her head centered in midline. Encourage left-sided activities and movements. Be aware that reasoning with a resident with a left hemiplegia is often difficult.

**Right Hemiplegia (Left CVA):**
Language is often affected resulting in aphasia, either receptive, expressive or global. Establish a communication task and expect the resident with a right hemiplegia to have fair reasoning skills.

Suggestions for exercise:
- The resident may go from having flaccid extremities to having spastic extremities.
- Be alert to painful shoulder syndromes seen with either condition.
- If the resident is in a wheelchair, make sure that his/her upper body is supported in midline.
- Be sure the affected arm is supported and have the resident use the non-affected leg to propel the chair.
- Lap boards are strongly encouraged by the therapists. Because they are considered to be physical restraints, interdisciplinary team approval in a long term care setting is required.
- If the resident is ambulatory, balance may still be affected so encourage sitting exercises. If standing, have the resident hold on to a secure surface.
- Expect frustration and occasionally inappropriate behavior especially with a resident who is aphasic. Ask his/her therapist for suggestions if you are having difficulty with a particular resident.

**MS:**
Multiple Sclerosis is a neurological disorder affecting more women than men. It can be very mild or very severe, there can be remissions for years or no remissions and can allow a person to remain ambulatory or cause them to be in need of a wheelchair for mobility. Common clinical presentations are tremors and sensory losses of the extremities, visual disturbances, unsteady gait and occasional personality disorders.

Suggestions for exercise:
- It is important for these residents to exercise with the goal of increasing strength and range of motion.
- Of equal importance is the need to avoid getting overly fatigued.
- Allow frequent rest periods.
- Encourage sitting exercises if balance is affected, otherwise allow standing exercises with support.

**Parkinson's:**
This chronic neurological disorder can present a range from mild rigidity with no cognitive deficits to severe rigidity with cognitive deficits.

Suggestions for exercise:
- Start the exercise session with head rotations to the right and left.
- Follow with reciprocal arm exercises and trunk rotation to the right and the left.
- Marching in place is an excellent activity both standing or sitting.
- Use a metronome for the resident to keep time to.
- It is felt that reciprocal and rotational activities help to decrease rigidity.
Note: Be very alert to these residents leaning or falling backwards and having trouble initiating movements.

**Head Injury:**
Many individuals who are in their teens, twenties and beyond are being admitted to long term care facilities with head injuries. It is highly recommended that these residents be screened for appropriateness by their therapist prior to entering your activities. This is due to their variable cognitive status and a decreased ability to tolerate certain levels of stimulation.

Suggestions for exercise:
- Limit auditory and visual stimulation to reduce the possibility of over-stimulation.
- Try and work on a one-on-one basis and gradually incorporate them into a group setting (small first).
- A calm and firm voice works best. Avoid yelling or speaking too loudly.
- Be patient but do not tolerate any aggressive behavior.
- Again, ask the therapist for appropriate interventions.

## Orthopedic Groups

Many residents with THR (total hip replacements) and with TKR (total knee replacements) come for short term rehab and are not always interested in participating in social activities. But many residents also have to undergo procedures and are quite willing to participate in activities.

**Total Hip Replacement:**
If your resident is between one and eight weeks following a total hip replacement, s/he has some very important precautions.
- S/he cannot bend at the hip greater than 90 degrees. Therefore, s/he must be in a semi-reclining position with a firm seat. (No low seated chairs)
- Keep the knees up in a V-position, with pillows below both knees.
- Do not let operated foot turn inward.
- S/he will ambulate either with crutches or walker. No canes at this point. S/he may not be able to bear full weight on the affected leg, so no standing exercises or leaning forward.

Note: After his/her hip has healed (six to eight weeks post op) s/he may return to full weight bearing ambulation and with no bending restrictions.

**Total Knee Replacement:**
A resident with total knee replacement may have restrictions as to his/her weight bearing ability, but many are full weight bearing. S/he will use either a walker or crutches and, depending on his/her physician's request, may or may not be wearing a leg brace. Compared to a the resident with a total hip replacement, there are fewer restriction but s/he may have a bit more pain.

Suggestions for exercise:
- Encourage sitting exercises with the brace removed.
- There is no limit to upper extremity exercises.

**Weight Bearing Status**
For your information, the following abbreviations are frequently used:
FWB     Full Weight Bearing
NWB     Non Weight Bearing
PWB     Partial Weight Bearing (refers to 25% to 75% of weight on leg)
TTWB    Toe Touch Weight Bearing (allows resident to rest leg on floor, but *no* weight may be put on it.)

As previously recommended, stay in close communication with the therapists working in your facility. Your role as an Activity Professional — and a team member — is a very important one.

# Cognitive Impairments

Many of the residents in long term care facilities have some form of cognitive impairment. We need to understand the impairment to understand the possibilities for the resident. There are two ways to divide the impairments:

1. whether the impairment is dementia-like or due to a psychiatric diagnosis
2. whether the impairment is acute or chronic.

Dementia is caused by a physical (usually known) impairment in the brain such as Alzheimer's, vascular disease and other causes. Psychiatric impairments are disturbances related to personality and life experiences which do not have an obvious organic cause. Examples include phobias and psychoses.

Acute cognitive impairments include any situation which changes quickly (within hours or days) and has a reasonable chance of returning to normal. Alcohol intoxication and overdoses of medication are acute impairments. Chronic impairments change slowly and usually do not allow the resident to return to normal functioning. Dementia and other damage to the brain such as that resulting from long-term alcohol abuse are chronic.

There are a few diagnoses which cover most of the impairments that we see. Before we look at the list, there is an important point to be made about some of these diagnoses — they don't always give us a clear enough picture. For example, dementia is the most common cognitive impairment seen in residents of long term care facilities. Of the 1.3 million residents, approximately 60 per cent are estimated to have some form of dementia. (Dementia means that the resident has "multiple cognitive deficits that include memory impairment and at least one of the following cognitive disturbances: aphasia, apraxia, agnosia or a disturbance in executive functioning"[10])

If you are working with a resident who has "dementia," you need to know more. You need to know why the resident has been diagnosed as having dementia:

- Is it because s/he drank a fifth of whiskey every day and destroyed too many of his/her brain cells? (Provide appropriate sensory stimulation activities. Don't expect to see significant improvement.)
- Is it because the doctor prescribing the pain medication didn't realize that the dentist prescribed pain medication and the resident is overdosing on medications? (Speak up at team meetings about your medication concerns. Expect the dementia to improve if the medication dosages are more appropriate.)
- Is the resident simply not hearing what is said so s/he can't respond appropriately? (Work on alternate means of communication and expect an improvement.)

There are many more examples, of course, but the idea is to understand that a diagnosis is not always the final answer when you are working with a particular resident.

There are eight types of cognitive impairments which are typically seen in long term care facilities:

1. **Dementia** is not a disease but rather a cluster of symptoms. These symptoms significantly limit a person's ability to perform normal, complex tasks associated with taking care of him/herself. Dementia means a loss of memory (newly learned information and, later, previously learned information) and at least one of the following:

---

[10] American Psychiatric Association, 1994, **Diagnostic and Statistical Manual of Mental Disorders IV**.

a.   deterioration of the ability to communicate. This includes: Aphasia, the ability to recognize an object or a person but the inability to find the right word to describe the object or person resulting in the excessive use of words such as "thing" or "it." Apraxia, the inability to remember how to move your mouth and tongue to correctly pronounce words. Agnosia, the inability to recognize what an object is or who a person is.

b.   deterioration of executive function. This is a significant impairment in the ability to think through problems, to initiate purposeful activity, to decide in what order actions should be done (as in dressing), to appreciate the significance of one's actions (picking up the unit's cat by the tail may make the cat angry) and to be able to stop what one is doing (to stop pouring milk when the glass is full).

Approximate 50-60 per cent of dementias are irreversible. This means that anywhere from 650,000 to nearly one million people with dementia are being cared for with no hope of significant improvement. Dementia may be chronic or acute. It is organic.

The types of dementia are
- Dementia of the Alzheimer's type
- Vascular dementia
- Dementia due to HIV disease
- Dementia due to a head trauma
- Dementia due to Pick's disease
- Dementia due to Huntington's disease
- Dementia due to Parkinson's disease
- Dementia due to Creutzfeldt-Jakob disease
- Dementia due to other general medical conditions
- Substance-induced persisting dementia
- Dementia due to multiple etiologies (causes)

Dementia of the Alzheimer's type is the most common type of dementia. It is an incurable neurological disease in which changes in the nerve cells of the outer layer of the brain result in the death of a large number of cells. This disease is organic, chronic and irreversible.

2. **Pseudodementia** refers to a condition which resembles dementia but is not the result of an organic factor. Typically depression is the culprit, producing dementia-like symptoms which include memory problems, confusion and attentional disturbances or deficits. Apathy, withdrawal and inability to care for oneself are a part of the picture. Whether the pseudodementia is acute or chronic depends on the underlying cause. (Pseudodementia is not an official **DSM-IV** diagnosis.)

3. **Delirium** involves disorganized thinking and an inability to attend to external stimuli and appropriately shift to new external stimuli. It typically occurs suddenly and lasts a short time. (It's acute.) The causes are organic and include infection, fever, post-op condition, drug-induced states, etc.

4. **Stroke** refers to any damage to the brain resulting from lack of blood supply to the affected part. It usually results in the loss of particular functions which vary greatly depending on the part of the brain that is affected. It is organic and has both an acute phase and a chronic phase. Some recovery is usually seen.

5. **Traumatic Brain Injury** describes damage to the brain caused by physical injury to the brain including car accidents and gunshot wounds. The impairment is organic and has both an acute and chronic phase. Recovery may go on for ten or more years after the accident.

6. **Depression** is characterized by "being down in the dumps" or sad for most of the day for many weeks. Over a period of time, this sadness is present more days than not. A resident who is depressed may also experience a change in eating patterns (poor appetite or overeating), a change in sleeping patterns (insomnia or hypersomnia), a drop in energy (fatigue), a drop in self-esteem, a drop in the ability to concentrate long enough to make decisions or to respond to situations and a decrease in the ability to be hopeful. Between 20% – 25% of residents with major medical problems (e.g., stroke, heart disorders, cancer, diabetes) will experience a major depression disorder. Depression may be chronic or acute.

7. **Anxiety** is the most common psychiatric disorder experienced by the general population. There are twelve major psychiatric disorders grouped under the heading of Anxiety Disorders including: Panic Disorder, Agoraphobia and Post Traumatic Stress Disorder. Anxiety impairs the resident's ability to respond to events and people in normally expected manners. Anxiety may be due to a variety of organic and nonorganic causes and may be either acute or chronic.

8. **Psychotic Disorders** are psychiatric disorders where the resident may experience hallucinations; have disorganized actions or speech or, as an extreme, catatonic behavior; and/or delusional ways of looking at the world (severe lack of normal insight). Psychotic disorders include schizophrenia, delusional disorders and other conditions.

# Classification of Cognitive Impairments

| | Organic Impairments (related to impairments in brain and brain tissue) (reversibility depends on cause) | Psychiatric Impairments (Related to personality and life experience, may be organic in nature) (frequently treatable) |
|---|---|---|
| **Acute** | **caused by trauma, infection, diabetes, chronic heart failure, drugs and alcohol, reversible to some degree**<br>Delirium<br>Medication Overdose<br>Alcohol Intoxication<br>Stroke (acute phase)<br>Traumatic Brain Injury (acute phase) | **caused by events in the resident's life, his/her perceptions of life and may be organic in origin, can be treated with psychological intervention, reversible although there may be recurrences**<br>Depression<br>Anxiety<br>Panic Attacks<br>Phobias |
| **Chronic** | **caused by physiological degeneration or damage to the brain, generally irreversible, some variation in skill level is seen day to day**<br>Dementia (due to Parkinson's Disease, Pick's Disease, HIV Disease, Creutzfeldt-Jakob Disease, etc.)<br>Alzheimer's Disease<br>Substance Induced Persisting Dementia<br>Stroke (chronic phase, psychosis is a possible result)<br>Traumatic Brain Injury (chronic phase) | **caused by events in the resident's life, has not been helped by psychological intervention, probably irreversible**<br>Pseudodementia<br>Depression<br>Psychosis |

# Sensory Loss

Everyone who has ever read the literature about Helen Keller has marveled at her ability to adapt to her sensory losses. Her compensatory skills were incredible; her will and her talent, monumental; her support system, constant. But what happens to everyday people like our residents when they suffer sensory losses? Do they have the skills and the talent to compensate adequately for their losses? How does loss influence one's adjustment and involvement in the long term care facility?

Sadly, by the time most older people come into long term care, they have already experienced diminished visual or auditory capacity — or both. Vision and hearing can be a factor in the smooth and complete integration into facility life. Loss of one or the other can create a barrier to adjustment and, frequently, to the ability to socialize. As sensitive health care providers, we must be acutely aware of the potential for isolation inherent in this and make every effort to increase the opportunities for interaction.

Imagine how we become comfortable in new surroundings, such as a hotel. We use our vision to orient ourselves to the placement of doors and windows. We find the bathroom. We learn to identify, by sight if not by name, those who might be useful in assisting us with information or problem solving. If we can't see, we depend on our auditory sense to sharpen our awareness of traffic patterns, new or identifiable noises around us and the daily rhythm of activities.

As we age, it is possible that, even if we do not lose total capacity, our senses may diminish enough to make most situations (especially new ones) awkward. In defense, compensatory skills are developed to mask the deprivation and to allow at least the illusion of normalcy. For example, some one with a hearing loss may smile at everything they think they hear in every interaction or s/he may answer yes to all questions. Frequently people are embarrassed to ask us to repeat ourselves; sometimes repeating is to no avail anyway if the hearing loss is significant.

So what is the issue here? That this person may be labeled confused or senile and left to his/her own memories. With the additional loss of social stimulation, memory loss may become an actual problem and we still haven't solved the original problems: a lack of social interaction and the possibility of an incorrect interpretation of the resident's condition.

So what do we do? Look for the problem. If it's there, make sure that others know the problem is with hearing and not cognition, speak clearly, face the resident directly, repeat as necessary, use gestures, communication boards, if possible, and in a surprisingly small number of cases, a hearing aid.

As for visual loss, with a resident who is alert, although sight is denied him/her, a vivid word picture can create a colorful image. Of course the individual with a visual impairment is more likely to need assistance to move around the facility and cueing at meals, but coupling this resident with a resident volunteer can avoid a potential problem.

The really unfortunate thing is that sometimes nothing works well. As a result, we find that residents engage in parallel existences. How often family members will say, "My mother has such a nice roommate; I wish they would talk to each other." In actuality, we have attempted on numerous occasions to introduce new roommates to each other only to be thwarted in our efforts by each one's inability to hear the other's voice. What happens? They only coexist, their lives never really touching in a meaningful way; two oriented, interesting and social people unable to fully enjoy the company of the person they live with. This same problem will preclude involvement in many activities. But, all is not bleak as the truly interested individual will (if able) develop a level of involvement s/he is comfortable with and many times this means establishing a relationship with one or more staff members.

It is not uncommon for residents to choose staff as kindred spirits. Part of this may be desire; part a refusal to identify with the other residents; but a large part of this may be because the residents can hear the staff when they are educated to be patient, to repeat as necessary and to speak loudly. Staff also have the ability to be heard by projecting their voices whereas another resident may not have this ability.

Sensory losses pose terrible dilemmas and in many cases frustrate the resident, the family and even the staff. Staff should employ a great variety of creative skills and sensory tools to alleviate isolation and communication barriers. If all else proves to be unsuccessful, remember that the sense of touch is likely to remain intact until near death. A kind and gentle touch will almost always be received.

# 3. Work Descriptions

This chapter describes the work done by Activity and Social Service Professionals. For each of these positions we have included a description of the work that they do, an example of a typical day and a formal position description.

These are rewarding professions, but they can be difficult at times. Significant complications will arise if you are disorganized. We have included some ideas for controlling the chaos of a health care setting so that the human needs and the bureaucratic needs can both be met without total loss of sanity. (Some loss of your sanity, some of the time, and the ability to gain it again are part of the informal work description for both of these professions.)

## Activity Professional

The Activity Professional plays many diverse roles within the care facility, but they are all directed at satisfying the goal of creating a homelike environment where the residents have control of their lives. There are administrative responsibilities and resident care duties and plenty of other tasks that keep the work interesting.

The administrative role is as the director of the Department of Activity Services. In that role the Activity Professional is responsible for creating policies and procedures that lead to programs which meet the needs of the residents and comply with all appropriate government regulations. S/he is the supervisor for all of the activity staff and all activity volunteers within the facility.

The resident care role requires the Activity Professional to act as a member of the interdisciplinary team in assessing residents, writing and carrying out care plans and updating the plans at appropriate intervals. S/he needs to work with the residents to find out what their capabilities are and to plan activities which maintain and/or enhance those capabilities.

Other tasks like facilitating the Resident Council, publishing a newsletter, coordinating a casino night, helping public relations, conducting community outings and all the rest are part of the work of providing the best possible environment for the residents of the long term care facility.

Some of the specific tasks for Activity Professionals require them to:

- Assess each resident for individual needs and interests
- Complete an initial activity assessment for each resident
- Complete the Minimum Data Set (MDS) comprehensive assessment form — Section I (United States)
- Identify a priority care plan need or problem for each resident if indicated by the assessment
- Develop a monthly calendar of activities which meets the assessed needs of all residents in the facility
- Organize, plan and coordinate the activity program
- Schedule and lead activity groups
- Supervise adult education instructors while on site
- Arrange special events and outside entertainers
- Train staff and volunteers
- Establish and develop community contacts and resources
- Manage and supervise the volunteer program
- Be a member of the weekly Resident Care Conference meetings
- Keep daily record of each resident's leisure involvement
- Keep a bedside log of date, length of visit, type of visit and response to visit for all residents in need of one-on-one visits
- Document the treatment plan in the progress notes at least once a quarter
- Document and address changes in condition
- Assure compliance with federal and state regulations and corporate policies and procedures
- Keep current through national, state and local professional affiliations to update skills and secure continuing education
- Edit the monthly newsletter
- Prepare and keep the budget for the department
- Evaluate programs to assure appropriateness for the current census of residents

# The Life of an Activity Professional

A typical day at work may look like this:

| | |
|---|---|
| 9:00 – 9:30 | Check on census, resident status, new admits<br>Change Reality Orientation board<br>Change arrow on calendar<br>Check with nursing regarding any changes of condition, discharges, etc. |
| 9:30 – 10:00 | Announce activities<br>Set up room<br>Assist with transporting residents |
| 10:00 – 12:00 | Lead activity groups or supervise other leaders<br>Attend resident care plan meetings<br>Attend department head meetings<br>Attend MDS meetings<br>Take attendance for groups<br>Visit one on one |
| 12:00 – 1:00 | Lunch |
| 1:00 – 1:45 | Documentation (new admits, care plans, quarterly notes)<br>Interview new residents<br>Coordinate departmental responsibilities<br>Return phone calls<br>Volunteer recruitment, interviewing and orienting |
| 1:45 – 2:00 | Announce activities<br>Set up for activities<br>Assist with transporting residents |
| 2:00 – 4:00 | Lead activities or supervise leaders<br>Visit one on one<br>Take attendance for groups<br>Documentation (assessments, care plans, etc.)<br>Special event coordination<br>Lead a special needs group |
| 4:00 – 5:00 | Organize files and office for next day<br>Write a to do list for tomorrow<br>Make end of the day farewell visits |

On a monthly basis the Activity Professional is responsible for planning and leading a set of activities designed to meet the needs of the residents of the facility. The following page shows a schedule prepared by Sherry Cardenas, AC of The Meadows of the Napa.

OBRA requirements normally mean that there must be some leisure activity in the morning, afternoon and evening seven days a week for all residents. This includes activities for residents who are unable to participate in the group activities. The activity department needs to help facilitate evening and weekend activities whether the staff person is there or not.

# May 1996

## THE MEADOWS OF THE NAPA 1900 ATRIUM PARKWAY NAPA CA

| Sunday | Monday | Tuesday | Wednesday | Thursday | Friday | Saturday |
|---|---|---|---|---|---|---|
| | | | **1**<br>9:00 AM RISE AND SHINE EXE.<br>9:00 AM SENSORY EXERCISE<br>9:30 AM NEWS AND R/O<br>10:00 AM SENSORY COOKING<br>10:30 AM TREASURED POEMS<br>2:30 PM WILD LIFE ADVENTURES<br>4:00 PM BINGO BUDDIES<br>4:00 PM TRIVIA CHALLENGE<br>ROOM VISITS | **2**<br>9:00 AM RISE AND SHINE EXE.<br>9:30 AM NEWS AND R/O<br>10:30 AM LIVING HISTORY<br>11:00 AM BIBLE STUDY<br>11:00 AM CINE DOME THEATRE OUTING<br>2:30 PM 100 BLOCK TALK<br>4:00 PM SENIOR OLYMPICS | **3**<br>9:00 AM RISE AND SHINE EXE.<br>9:00 AM SENSORY EXERCISE<br>9:30 AM NEWS AND R/O<br>10:30 AM HOBBIES UNLIMITED<br>11:00 AM SENSORY NATURE<br>2:30 PM MUSIC AND MORE<br>3:00 PM RYTHM BAND<br>4:00 PM CINCO-DE-MAYO PARTY | **4**<br>10:00 AM MUSICAL STRETCH<br>10:30 AM BINGO SOCIAL<br>11:00 AM SENSORY CIRCLE<br>2:00 PM NATURE WALKS<br>2:30 PM PAINTING CIRCLE<br>3:00 PM HANDS OF FRIENDSHIP<br>3:30 PM KNITTING CIRCLE |
| **5**<br>10:00 AM MUSICAL STRETCH<br>10:30 AM SUNDAY NEWS<br>11:00 AM BOOK CHAT<br>2:00 PM BAPTIST FELLOWSHIP<br>3:00 PM TRAVEL ADVENTURES<br>HAPPY CINCO-DE-MAYO DAY<br>ROOMVISITS | **6**<br>9:00 AM RISE AND SHINE EXE<br>9:00 AM SENSORY EXERCISE<br>9:30 AM NEWS AND R/O<br>10:30 AM HISTORY CHALLENGE<br>11:00 AM SENSORY FUN<br>2:30 PM MUSICAL TUNES<br>4:00 PM GARDEN SOCIAL | **7**<br>9:00 AM RISE AND SHINE EXE.<br>9:30 AM NEWS AND R/O<br>10:00 AM MUSICAL TRIVIA<br>10:30 AM MUSICAL SLIDES<br>1:00 PM BINGO FOR $<br>2:30 PM DOMINOES<br>3:00 PM CATHOLIC COMMUNION<br>4:00 PM OUR HISTORY | **8**<br>9:00 AM RISE AND SHINE EXE.<br>9:00 AM SENSORY EXERCISE<br>9:30 AM NEWS AND R/O<br>10:00 AM SENSORY COOKING<br>10:30 AM TREASURED POEMS<br>2:30 PM WILD LIFE ADVENTURES<br>4:00 PM BINGO BUDDIES<br>ROOM VISITS | **9**<br>9:00 AM RISE AND SHINE EXE<br>9:30 AM NEWS AND R/O<br>10:30 AM LIVING HISTORY<br>11:00 AM OLIVE GARDEN<br>1:00 AM RESIDENT COUNCIL<br>2:30 PM 200 BLOCK TALK<br>4:00 PM SENIOR OLYMPICS | **10**<br>9:00 AM RISE AND SHINE EXE.<br>9:00 AM SENSORY EXERCISE<br>9:30 AM NEWS AND R/O<br>10:30 AM HOBBIES UNLIMITED<br>11:00 AM SENSORY NATURE<br>2:30 PM MUSIC AND MORE<br>3:00 PM RYTHM BAND<br>4:00 PM MOTHERS DAY TEA | **11**<br>10:00 AM MUSICAL STRETCH<br>10:30 AM BINGO FUN<br>11:00 AM NATURE WALKS<br>2:00 PM PAINTING CIRCLE<br>2:30 PM PAINTING CIRCLE<br>3:00 PM HANDS OF FRIENDSHIP<br>3:30 PM KNITTING CIRCLE |
| **12**<br>10:00 AM MUSICAL STRETCH<br>10:30 AM SUNDAY NEWS<br>11:00 AM BOOK CHAT<br>2:30 PM BAPTIST FELLOWSHIP<br>3:00 PM TRAVEL ADVENTURES<br>7:00 PM FAMILY VIDEO<br>HAPPY MOTHERS DAY<br>ROOMVISITS | **13**<br>9:00 AM RISE AND SHINE EXE.<br>9:00 AM SENSORY EXERCISE<br>9:30 AM NEWS AND R/O<br>10:30 AM MATH CHALLENGE<br>11:00 AM SENSORY FUN<br>2:30 PM MUSICAL TUNES<br>4:00 PM POKER AND MORE | **14**<br>9:00 AM RISE AND SHINE EXE.<br>9:30 AM NEWS AND R/O<br>10:00 AM NEWS SLIDES<br>10:30 AM MUSICAL TRIVIA<br>1:00 PM BINGO FOR $<br>2:30 PM CHECKERS<br>3:00 PM CATHOLIC COMMUNION<br>4:00 PM LEATHER WORKS | **15**<br>9:00 AM RISE AND SHINE EXE.<br>9:00 AM SENSORY EXERCISE<br>9:30 AM MYSTERY DRIVE<br>9:30 AM NEWS AND R/O<br>10:00 AM SENSORY COOKING<br>10:30 AM TREASURED POEMS<br>2:30 PM WILD LIFE ADVENTURES<br>4:00 PM BINGO BUDDIES<br>ROOM VISITS | **16**<br>9:00 AM RISE AND SHINE EXE.<br>9:30 AM NEWS AND R/O<br>10:30 AM LIVING HISTORY<br>11:00 AM "THE SPOT" OUTING<br>2:00 PM 300 BLOCK TALK<br>2:30 PM BIBLE STUDY<br>4:00 PM SENIOR OLYMPICS | **17**<br>9:00 AM RISE AND SHINE EXE.<br>9:00 AM SENSORY EXERCISE<br>9:30 AM NEWS AND R/O<br>10:30 AM HOBBIES UNLIMITED<br>11:00 AM SENSORY NATURE<br>12:00 PM NATIONAL NURSING WEEK BBQ<br>2:30 PM MUSIC AND MORE<br>3:00 PM RYTHM BAND | **18**<br>10:00 AM MUSICAL STRETCH<br>10:30 AM BINGO SOCIAL<br>11:00 AM NATURE WALKS<br>2:00 PM PAINTING CIRCLE<br>2:30 PM PAINTING CIRCLE<br>3:00 PM HANDS OF FRIENDSHIP<br>3:30 PM KNITTING CIRCLE |
| **19**<br>10:00 AM MUSICAL STRETCH<br>10:30 AM SUNDAY NEWS<br>11:00 AM BOOK CHAT<br>2:00 PM BAPTIST FELLOWSHIP<br>3:00 PM TRAVEL ADVENTURES<br>7:00 PM FAMILY VIDEO<br>ROOMVISITS | **20**<br>9:00 AM RISE AND SHINE EXE.<br>9:00 AM SENSORY EXERCISE<br>9:30 AM NEWS AND R/O<br>10:30 AM SCIENCE CHALLENGE<br>11:00 AM SENSORY FUN<br>2:30 PM MUSICAL TUNES<br>4:00 PM GARDEN SOCIAL | **21**<br>9:00 AM RISE AND SHINE EXE.<br>9:30 AM NEWS AND R/O<br>10:00 AM MUSICAL TRIVIA<br>10:30 AM MUSICAL SLIDES<br>1:00 PM BINGO FOR $<br>2:30 PM CARDS AND MORE<br>3:00 PM CATHOLIC COMMUNION<br>4:00 PM OUR HISTORY | **22**<br>9:00 AM RISE AND SHINE EXE.<br>9:00 AM SENSORY EXERCISE<br>9:30 AM MYSTERY DRIVE<br>9:30 AM NEWS AND R/O<br>10:00 AM SENSORY COOKING<br>10:30 AM TREASURED POEMS<br>2:30 PM WILD LIFE ADVENTURES<br>4:00 PM BINGO BUDDIES<br>ROOM VISITS | **23**<br>9:00 AM RISE AND SHINE EXE.<br>9:30 AM NEWS AND R/O<br>10:30 AM LIVING HISTORY<br>11:00 AM SURPRIZE TRIP<br>2:00 PM 400 BLOCK TALK<br>2:30 PM BIBLE STUDY<br>4:00 PM SENIOR OLYMPICS | **24**<br>9:00 AM RISE AND SHINE EXE.<br>9:00 AM SENSORY EXERCISE<br>9:30 AM NEWS AND R/O<br>10:30 AM HOBBIES UNLIMITED<br>11:00 AM SENSORY NATURE<br>2:30 PM MUSIC AND MORE<br>3:00 PM RYTHM BAND<br>4:00 PM HAPPY HOUR | **25**<br>10:00 AM MUSICAL STRETCH<br>11:00 AM SENSORY CIRCLE<br>2:00 PM NATURE WALKS<br>2:30 PM PAINTING CIRCLE<br>3:00 PM HANDS OF FRIENDSHIP<br>3:30 PM MENS WORKSHOP |
| **26**<br>10:00 AM MUSICAL STRETCH<br>10:30 AM SUNDAY NEWS<br>11:00 AM BOOK CHATS<br>2:30 PM BAPTIST FELLOWSHIP<br>3:00 PM TRAVEL ADVENTURES<br>7:00 PM FAMILY VIDEO<br>ROOMVISITS | **27**<br>9:00 AM RISE AND SHINE EXE<br>9:00 AM SENSORY EXERCISE<br>9:30 AM NEWS AND R/O<br>10:30 AM GEOGRAPHY CHALLENGE<br>11:00 AM SENSORY FUN<br>2:30 PM MUSICAL TUNES<br>4:00 PM POKER AND MORE | **28**<br>9:00 AM RISE AND SHINE EXE.<br>9:30 AM NEWS AND R/O<br>10:00 AM NEWS SLIDES<br>10:30 AM MUSICAL TRIVIA<br>1:00 PM BINGO FOR $<br>2:30 PM POKER HOUR<br>3:00 PM CATHOLIC COMMUNION<br>4:00 PM WOOD SHOP | **29**<br>9:00 AM RISE AND SHINE EXE.<br>9:00 AM SENSORY EXERCISE<br>9:30 AM MYSTERY DRIVE<br>9:30 AM NEWS AND R/O<br>10:00 AM SENSORY COOKING<br>10:30 AM TREASURED POEMS<br>2:30 PM WILD LIFE ADVENTURES<br>4:00 PM BINGO BUDDIES<br>ROOM VISITS | **30**<br>9:00 AM RISE AND SHINE EXE.<br>9:30 AM NEWS AND R/O<br>10:30 AM RED LOBSTER OUTING<br>2:00 PM 500 BLOCK TALK<br>2:30 PM BIBLE STUDY<br>4:00 PM BEACH PARTY | **31**<br>9:00 AM RISE AND SHINE EXE.<br>9:00 AM SENSORY EXERCISE<br>9:30 AM NEWS AND R/O<br>10:30 AM HOBBIES UNLIMITED<br>11:00 AM SENSORY NATURE<br>2:30 PM MUSIC AND MORE<br>3:00 PM RYTHM BAND<br>4:00 PM BIRTHDAY PARTY | |

## ACTIVITIES CALENDAR : BY SHERRY CARDENAS A.C.

# Position Description

**Title**                      Activity Professional

## Purpose of the Position

Under the direction of the Administrator, the Activity Professionals, lead by the Activity Director, are responsible for the planning, coordination and implementation of the activity programs. Activities shall be done on a daily basis and shall make every effort to meet the residents' needs and interests.

## Qualifications

A qualified professional who: "*Is a qualified therapeutic recreation specialist or an activities professional who is licensed or registered, if applicable, by the State in which practicing; and is eligible for certification as a therapeutic recreation specialist or as an activities professional by a recognized accrediting body on or after October 1, 1990; or has 2 years of experience in a social or recreational program within the last 5 years, 1 of which was full-time in a patient activities program in a health care setting; or is a qualified occupational therapist or occupational therapy assistant; or has completed a training course approved by the State.*"[11]

## Duties and Responsibilities

Activity programs are developed within the framework of the facility organizational structure in accordance with federal regulations and the approval of each resident's attending physician. The programs are coordinated in a team effort with related facility services and staff. Programs are to include activities for residents who are ambulatory, non-ambulatory and on bedrest and the activities are to be planned for both group and individual participation.

With understanding of the adverse effects of institutionalization which can promote isolation, sensory deprivation and dependence, the Activity Professional shall build into the program a variety of means to counteract these effects. S/he shall:

1.  Evaluate each resident according to his/her background, interest, leisure, previous lifestyle, abilities, physical and cognitive limitations and needs. This shall serve as the base from which the individual activity program shall be developed.

2.  Document the individual activity program using the appropriate assessment forms to be found in the medical record, completing the activity plan within the required time after admission (14 days for federal regulations, 7 days for some states).

3.  Attend Resident Care Conferences and record in the resident care plan on a quarterly basis (or sooner, as needed).

4.  Maintain timely progress notes specific to the residents' activity plans, recording at least quarterly in the medical record and more frequently when appropriate.

5.  Develop appropriate records which indicate resident attendance and participation in the program with reference to resident's response to the program. It is important to note active participation as compared to perimeter participation. These records should also include a bedside log for special programming.

---

[11] OBRA, Tags F248 and F249.

6.  Develop, implement, lead and monitor individual and group activities and meet specific needs of the residents.

7.  Develop activities providing the opportunity for residents to experience sensory input (touch, smell, taste, etc.), group interaction and personal achievement.

8.  Include activities which encourage residents to make decisions, participate in planning and assume a degree of responsibility and independence.

9.  Develop a method to implement programs within a designated budget allocated by the Facility Administrator. Keep a ledger and inventory of supplies.

10. Establish an active volunteer program which includes the screening, orientation, training, supervision and evaluation of volunteers.

11. Develop methods for effective utilization of community resources.

12. Serve as a facility liaison to promote positive community support.

13. Interpret to residents, other staff members and the outside community the purpose and achievements of the activity program through at least yearly in-service training and presentations.

14. Attend and participate in staff meetings, department head meetings, designated committee meetings and resident care conferences.

15. Develop a method for obtaining current knowledge of federal and state regulations pertaining to activity programs.

16. Other responsibilities as defined by the administrator.

# Social Service Professional

The Social Service Professional's main responsibilities as part of the resident care team can be summarized as follows:
- Assess resident needs
- Update resident status
- Interpret observed behaviors
- Counsel residents and families
- Field grievances from residents and families
- Ensure resolution of grievances
- In-service other staff and members of the community
- Role model professional attributes

**Assess resident needs**

Some of the talents which help in this aspect of a Social Service Professional's work are being naturally curious, genuinely interested, consistently diplomatic and, sometimes, persuasive. During the initial assessment, the resident moves from the one-dimensional, merely charted person to the three-dimensional person with a past, present and future. Background information such as birthplace, siblings, education, marriage, children, occupation, life style, religion, retirement and hobbies emerge to paint a picture of a person in society — his/her past. Next, we find what the circumstances were which brought him/her to the long term care facility; what series of illnesses, failures in the living situation or changes in health status necessitated placement — his/her present.

By combining past and present, the Social Service Professional should be able to develop an idea of the resident's reaction to illness: how s/he will live with it, be controlled by it or develop the use of a sick role.

In the course of the assessment, it is important to look for and define orientation. Is the resident alert and aware of time, place and events (also referred to as oriented x3) or alert and able to answer simple questions that do not test the memory? Do sensory impairments (especially deafness) impact orientation? Who visits? Who tends to concrete needs? Is the relationship loving or dutiful? What are the special identifying traits? Does the resident always wear hats? Like to wear certain colors? Grab at all passersby?

There are several factors that work in your favor as you approach an assessment interview:
1. Most people like to talk about themselves.
2. Families of residents also enjoy reminiscing about the past and equate your gentle inquiries with caring about the well-being of the resident and about themselves as well.
3. This is an opportunity to acknowledge the pain of separation (either family from resident or resident from what had been his/her world) and to divide the past from the reality of the "now" and the uncertainty of the future.

A positive experience at this juncture can disarm the resident's anger, as well as the family's depression created by the unnecessary guilt of placing someone in a long term care facility. The assessment can set the tone for all future interactions.

Why should assessment — developing the case history — be so important? Do the "who, what, where, when and why" of a person's past make a difference?

Assessment is important because unless we develop an image of the resident as a complete person, we will always be taking care of faceless "sick folks." We will not ever learn to take care of people. The sadness for Social Service Professionals is that we will never know the residents in the context of their previous lifestyle; we will never see them "well." We can, however, glimpse a person's totality if we ask questions appropriately and use that information to help plan the resident's future.

Once the initial assessment interview has been completed with the help of the resident, family and medical data base, it is necessary to complete the Minimum Data Set (MDS). (The MDS is the comprehensive, interdisciplinary assessment which is required for every resident in long term care throughout the United States.) Combing through the information you have gathered should provide the information for the MDS. Essentially the MDS distills what you have learned. But, because it is only a summary of all the facts you have at your finger tips, it would be wise to record the salient data that has not been used on an assessment form or as a narrative statement so that nuances of personality and behavior do not become lost to you.

Depending on the information recorded on the MDS and aided by your fact-gathering, you will make an entry on the resident care plan. We have sometimes gone into an interview thinking that we know what a person's care entry will be and have been very wrong. One must never assume.

Generally, just rewriting what you have learned will crystallize the problem/need/concern without any need for preconceptions. At the end of this assessment/MDS process, the Social Service Professional will know what follow-up each person requires. For example, is discharge back home or to a lesser level of care of primary concern? Is the resident in the long term care facility for terminal care (i.e. related to illness) as opposed to custodial care? Is the resident having problems adjusting to the change from home to a long term care environment? Or is the resident unable to give you any clues (because of inclination or disease state) and will the Social Service Professional have to use his/her skills to repeatedly assess needs? In any case, there is a job to do.

## Update Resident Status

Things change! A resident might suffer a health crisis which impairs orientation. A husband or a child might die. Teeth might get lost. Financial circumstances might be altered. The resident might return to the previous level of function (presumably higher).

A change of condition or social status must be noted so that this information is available to all members of the care team. Never forget that people who are ill in a long term care facility live in a well-controlled balance. Many of their outside influences have been removed from their lives or have been altered or diminished by attrition or choice. As a result, changes which are more easily absorbed by a well person can greatly influence the physical and emotional personality of a resident. Obviously, illness will make a difference, but even something as subtle as a change in the visiting pattern of a family member, an argument or the switch from private payment to Medicaid can result in behavior change. Whatever it is, a social service note is important. This will lead to a more accurate interpretation about the resident, as described below.

## Interpret Observed Behaviors

We help interpret the psychosocial needs of the resident for other members of the care team. These needs are based on a resident's personality, his/her reaction to illness and his/her reaction to outside influences. Anger, aggression, passivity, anxiety: these are responses. As a Social Service Professional, you have the information gathered from the data base to assist the resident care team with interpretation and determination of why the resident is giving this response to his/her environment. The key to the puzzle is not the response; it is why this response is being used. Use every opportunity (resident care conferences, rehab meetings) to share what you know, especially if it will have a positive effect on resident care.

## Counsel Residents and Families

We are in the facility, first and foremost, to tend to the resident. However, most residents come to us with a family and, in many cases, the family also needs our care. The Social Service Professional forms a bridge between community and facility. S/he provides important resource information but, even more importantly, emotional information. If we are successful at interpreting behavior, facility policies and the bureaucracies, the resident and the family will find it easier to accept the placement. If their concerns are not dealt with, they will resist and may never deal with feelings of abandonment, guilt, loss and defeat. This is true for both the resident and the family. Every facility has rules and regulations. We think it is best to give this information to the resident (if well enough) or to the responsible party at the time of admission.

The problem is that so much emotional baggage is being brought into the facility during admission that most of the information cannot be comprehended, no matter how lucidly conveyed or how sincerely received. Therefore, advise family members that they are not expected to know and understand everything. Advise them to observe, make lists and ask questions. There is usually a very good explanation for everything, but one must be in a state of mind which is receptive to understand it. The time of explanations is an excellent opportunity for family/resident/Social Service Professional to become connected initially. From then on, you will often be sought out because you are constant in an ever-changing environment.

Follow-up on all reasonable requests. One of OBRA's premises is that the residents (and families) have the *right* to make reasonable requests for change and the facility has the *responsibility* to act on the request in a reasonable manner. Get answers for things you don't know. Always be willing to listen to a frustration or a sorrow. You will find that it takes very little to ease a troubled mind — interest and information will do.

### Field Grievances from Residents and Families

Never forget that the long term care facility is a new bureaucracy to most people. It is an emotional experience which may create barriers to understanding as well as feelings of impotence. The Social Service Professional has a major role in interpretation: complaints/grievances often are not what they seem to be. Frequently they are a form of communication, a way of entering into conversation and eliciting assistance in a foreign and not always welcoming milieu.

Listen with compassion, not judgment; seek to sort out the real complaint and refer it to the appropriate department unless you are able to deal with it yourself. Listen, write down key words, dates and times, make a list of concerns and tackle them one at a time. Then, return with your follow up information.

You should expect to hear more complaints at the beginning of a placement. This has a great deal to do with personal pain (resident and family) and with misunderstanding or miscommunication. Are clothes being lost in the laundry? Has the family been informed about the facility policy for marking them?

Do not ever assume that someone is simply a chronic complainer. Listen, try not to be defensive and remember that any attempt at a solution goes a long way toward establishing good relationships.

Sometimes, in order to diffuse a volatile situation, we will listen, try to relate to all concerns and ask, near the end of the interview, if the family feels the resident is cared for, liked and responded to. We feel that putting things at this very basic level will sometimes produce a more satisfying outcome — especially if the response is yes. We don't forget about the lost slippers, but their importance will assume the appropriate place in the hierarchy of "what comes first."

Occasionally when we ask a resident if all is going well, s/he won't want to say that it is not for fear of getting someone in trouble. The same is true of families. Both resident and family may feel very vulnerable in these instances and are afraid of reprisal: physical or emotional abuse heaped onto the resident by a vengeful employee. It is important to describe the grievance procedure early in the new resident/family relationship and to impress upon them the importance of the correct process.

To summarize the grievance procedure:
1. establish this avenue of communication with residents and families early in the relationship,
2. reassure the timid that you will take action and there will be no reprisal and
3. follow-up on all concerns.

**Ensure Resolution of Grievances**

Most facilities post the grievance procedure. In cases when the consumer is not satisfied with your response, s/he should be instructed and encouraged to see your administrator. If this is still not satisfactory, the state ombudsman should become involved. The ombudsman's role is often misunderstood, but with their increasing involvement in the survey process, it behooves us to educate ourselves about who they are and what they can do to help us.

There are very few of us who have not at one time or another been afraid of the ombudsman's presence in the facility. Unfortunately, they have usually been viewed as enforcers. This is not their intended role. In fact, they are meant to be neutral and available to assist both residents/families and the facilities.

If you have not already established a relationship with your area's or state's ombudsman office and your facility ombudsman do it now. You will find that familiarity will break down barriers of mistrust and fear of the ombudsman.

**Inservice Other Staff and Members of the Community**

Although there is no actual mandate which says what or how many inservices Social Service Professionals are responsible for, it makes sense that we focus on those topics that we know best. The reason that Social Service Professionals are reluctant to give inservices is that often we don't have confidence in what we know. Yet, our perspective is unique in the facility and we have a special feeling about residents and their feelings.

An inservice about your role in the facility is a good start! Or, there may be a particular topic you have learned a great deal about and feel comfortable sharing. (Alzheimer's Disease and its impact on resident and family interests us a great deal.) Talk about Resident's Rights and our responsibilities toward meeting them. Discuss the psychosocial needs of the elderly; demystify the needs of the dying resident; speak of resident dignity and privacy and the right of confidentiality. If you still feel stumped for a topic of interest, examine the elements of communication and what a difference it can make to communicate efficiently.

Prepare three to four topics for discussion so that when you are asked to present, you will be ready and confident. It will be invigorating to share your knowledge and elicit responses from the group, especially if you are speaking about something you are very comfortable with.

**Role Model Professional Attributes**

This is the Social Service Professional's most subtle activity in the facility. If you are doing it well, some things you normally do will get done even when you are not there.

Nothing that a Social Service Professional does is either secret or magic — it only seems that way. By being open and friendly with other staff members at all levels (from the Administrator to the Certified Nursing Assistants to the housekeeping staff) you are modeling, teaching, being an example of how to do your work so that your absence does not create a void — as it shouldn't.

Always answer questions honestly; discuss such things as how to talk with residents who are dying or how to respond to bereaved family members. Your example may give courage to others to offer solace and support.

Be proud of your professional approach to your work and you will be role modeling and influencing behavior. And even though you will not always be in the facility, your social service skills, your being-there-for-people skills should pervade the entire facility and create a positive atmosphere.

You will know you have succeeded when a staff member comes up to you and says, "When you weren't here the other day, I remembered that you always take Lucy to a quiet spot and speak calmly to her when she is upset. I tried it and it worked for me, too."

# Teamwork

The moment you walk into a facility, you have joined a team. It is not just you, the residents and the families; the team also includes all of the other workers in your long term care facility:

- nursing (including aides)
- activity staff
- social service staff
- therapists
- dietary workers
- administration
- business office staff
- physicians
- housekeeping staff

While most of the components of the health care team use concrete information (such as a health history) from which to draw their information about a resident, social services is a bit different. We deal with communication and emotion, helping the residents and guardians to express their feelings about what is happening and what is being planned. It makes our perspective different from the others. Social Service is a soft science, therefore a bit unpredictable, as is human behavior.

Using the data presented to the health care team by each member of the team and input from the resident and his/her family, we develop a resident profile. We are working together to figure out what is best for the resident. Mutual goal setting is a powerful tool for finding the best care plan. It involves give and take of ideas and is stimulating for everyone. With the resident's good in mind and with the resident and/or responsible party being involved to the maximum extent possible, we find that the plans we make usually work well when we implement them.

Sometimes there is a tendency to be elitist in health care settings. It is a mistake. We find the certified nursing assistants (CNAs) to be invaluable sources of information. They are with the residents in a much more intimate way than we are (except perhaps at death) and are sometimes in a far better position to recognize and describe mood changes. CNAs see a lot of visitors, view interactions, share confidences. They know when a resident needs new clothing, is upset by a roommate or just doesn't seem the same. All disciplines can profit from information the CNAs have. Make sure you solicit information, pay attention and then follow up. Make the CNAs your allies. Respect and respond to their inquiries and their requests.

With the new emphasis of the survey process of OBRA's Final Rule, it is more important than ever that we use all available sources to assess the residents' needs. It is essential that we either know or can anticipate what a resident is capable of and of his/her frailties and needs. Using this information, we must have a plan that everyone knows and, to an extent, participates in.

# The Life of a Social Service Professional

We'd like to think when we go to work in the morning that our day will end up the way we had imagined it would. This almost never happens. Chores we had expected to tackle first may remain undone, sometimes until tomorrow or the next day. People we needed to phone may have been unavailable, so our task is incomplete. Paperwork finished — well, that rarely happens.

By its very nature, the work of a Social Service Professional is full of distractions and unanticipated emergencies. It is rare to go from Resident A to Resident B in a straight line! Some days it will feel that your feet don't even touch the floor and that nothing has really been accomplished. This actually means that you abandoned your game plan sometime in the first hour of the day and never returned to it. Remember, though, that unanticipated work is still work!

It is best to begin with a plan of action. This can actually be broken down into segments. Having the full picture, specifying a month's worth of responsibilities, will bring focus to each day.

## Daily

Upon arrival in the morning, check in with the Director of Nursing or the Nursing Supervisor. Ask about:
- Anticipated admissions
- Room changes
- Emergency discharges
- Deaths

Check with the staff nurses and aides about:
- Behavior changes
- Change of condition
- Resident needs
- Lost dentures or glasses

Make a list and decide how you will follow up.

## Weekly

- Do new resident assessments
- Write quarterly and annual updates for the week
- Chart on new residents, checking for adjustment or progress toward discharge
- Attend weekly resident care plan meetings
- Attend weekly rehabilitation meetings

## Monthly (if applicable)

Send out notices for next month's resident care conferences to family members, guardians and other appropriate individuals.

## Ongoing

Family and resident contact: the real reason we go to work every day.

Every day is a new day. Remain hopeful that you will "finish," but accept the challenge of a changing environment, while trying not to become too frustrated.

# Position Description

**Title**          Social Service Professional

## Purpose of the Position

Under the direction of the Administrator, the Social Service Professionals, lead by the Social Service Director, are responsible for assuring that quality social services are provided to residents and their families, assisting them with the social and emotional aspects of illness and disability; also, to promote a therapeutic community including residents, families and the entire staff so that supportive relationships will be developed, thus enhancing the care given.

## Qualifications

A qualified Social Service Professional (required by OBRA law in a facility with more than 120 beds) is an individual with *"a bachelor's degree in social work or a bachelor's degree in a human service field including but not limited to sociology, special education, rehabilitation counseling and psychology; and one year of supervised social work experience in a health care setting working directly with individuals.*"[12]

## Duties and Responsibilities

Provide social services to attain or maintain the highest practicable physical, mental and psychosocial well-being of the resident as discussed below:

1. Complete a psychosocial assessment and a social history within the required time after admission (14 days for federal regulations, 7 days for some states). This is to include the MDS and appropriate follow-up to that documentation.

2. Process all social service paperwork required by managed care systems in a timely manner.

3. Begin a discharge plan.

4. Enter on the resident care plan if there is an identified social service problem.

5. Always chart when a social service intervention has been indicated.

6. Complete a quarterly social service progress note.

7. Update the discharge plan annually for long term care residents and at least quarterly for residents who display a potential for discharge to a lesser level of care.

8. Reassess the social service entry on the resident care plan at least quarterly, updating problems, goals and approaches as appropriate.

9. Interpret psychosocial needs, goals and plans to appropriate staff.

10. Counsel residents and families during orientation and adjustment to the facility and during other times of crisis or trauma.

---

[12] OBRA Tag F251.

11. Participate with the interdisciplinary team in resident care conferences, presenting the psychosocial components of the resident's needs and formulating a coordinated plan.

12. Identify changes in responses, behavior or personality, such as depression, anxiety, withdrawal or aggressiveness and discuss this with the interdisciplinary team; chart to this.

13. Maintain a file of community resources including community social and mental health agencies; appropriate referrals are made when necessary.

14. Maintain a knowledge of current facility, state and federal regulations, policies and procedures as they apply to social services.

15. Facilitate and convene a Family Council as indicated by facility need.

16. Attend and participate in staff meetings, department head meetings, designated committee meetings and resident care conferences.

17. Participate in the facility inservice education program, especially as it applies to the psychosocial needs of the resident; this is coordinated with the Staff Developer.

18. Other responsibilities as defined by the administrator.

# Professionalism

Professionalism is a term that we hear used everyday. What does it actually mean to you as an Activity or Social Service Professional? Perhaps the easiest way to define professionalism is to identify an individual whom you regard as a professional. What is it about them that creates that feeling of respect and recognition? Is it something concrete about what they do or just a feeling associated with who they are as a person?

You will most likely answer "something concrete" along with a feeling of confidence that the individual carries with him/her in his/her work. The concrete substance that creates a professional is a combination of purpose, vision, goals, skills, hard work, solid ethics and constant upgrading of education and skills. Each professional field has its own purpose, vision, goals, ethics and skills learned through schooling and apprenticeships. While each professional group is unique in many ways, working as a team means that they also need to have much in common.

Activity and Social Service Professionals share a common goal. That goal is to enhance the quality of life of residents living in a long term care facility. This creates the vision of how life and programming could be in these settings. It creates a vision of residents coming first and policies being created with considerations of the residents coming before concerns about the staff. This sensitivity helps create programs which have a purpose and a goal specific to the quality of life issues we address for all residents regardless of limitations and special needs. We make the positive happen through the use of our skills.

The reality is that this is quite a challenge for the team to meet. OBRA mandates that a qualified professional direct these services. This individual needs to be prepared to work hard at educating people about the impact their work and programs have and, at the same time, continue to build onto his/her own skills and knowledge.

The position of Activity or Social Service Director is a department head position. This means that not only is this individual responsible for all the duties and services provided by the Activity and Social Service Professionals in his/her department, but s/he is also responsible to every other staff member because of the team emphasis.

In other words, an area of information forgotten, a resident incompletely assessed, documentation past due or a lack of appropriate programs reflects on everyone else on the team. Being a professional means taking responsibility. If there is a diagnosis that you do not understand or a resident that you don't know how to care for, you must bring this up and work with other disciplines to seek a solution. This obviously goes both ways in that other departments need to work with you in meeting common goals and understanding your goals and priorities.

One sure way of not only being a professional but feeling that sense of confidence associated with professionalism is to network and be a member of local, state and national activity and social service organizations. Not only will you share common issues and concerns, you will also gain important continuing education in the educational meetings, workshops and conventions as well as a tremendous amount of support. So much of this type of work is done individually and it is easy to feel "out of the mainstream" as pressures at work mount. Keep yourself balanced by taking care of yourself, your own leisure needs and interests and professional development. The residents benefit from a well balanced professional and a happy team.

# A Personal Note

After all of the somewhat dry descriptions of the job, Mary Anne Weeks contributed a more personal note on what the job feels like to her.

## Is This What a Profession Is?

*Monday seems to roll around far too frequently for my taste, so when it does, it is best that I am going somewhere that I want to be!! You know that feeling — that examination of motivation when you realize that you face another week of work.*

*We've all had to go places and be places that simply have not suited us; in fact, we will probably always have obligations that take us into situations we would rather avoid. Hopefully, though, where one spends 8 hours a day is not such a place. I mean, of course, the WORK PLACE.*

*It is interesting for me to reflect and to see how I happened into my profession (please note, I did not say JOB!). It helped that I was in the right place at the right time, but events in my life had always been leading me in the direction of working in the field of geriatrics. Somehow, no matter what interest I was pursuing, work with older adults was always there. Perhaps I made it happen because my comfort level was so pronounced at such times; maybe I was just lucky. In any case, without setting a goal that thrust me in the direction of geriatric social work, this innocent stumbled happily upon what I like to think of as my vocation.*

*Jobs come and go; some people fall in and out of jobs as easily as they change shirts. It is when you find your profession, however, that you realize that you have the potential within you to make a difference, if only (and I am not saying this to negate its power) in your own life.*

*On Mondays when I awaken and do a mental forecast of the week ahead I find that, even after more than a decade, I am still interested in what is ahead, curious about what the week will bring and grateful that I can go somewhere that I want to be.*

## Being There

*I would be untruthful if I said that every minute of every day that I am in my facility stands out as memorable, worthwhile, fun or even interesting. But ... just when I am the lowest or the most uninspired, someone will come along and, once again, I will be revitalized. Note that I wrote someone, as my warmest experiences are almost always related to a person and his/her actions.*

*I can still elicit the feeling I had one cold and dreary winter morning just as I was beginning my day. It seemed as though I was facing 8 hours of charts and computer input and grievances; I felt that I wasn't ready to begin. Then the daughter of a resident came in to take her mother out to the eye doctor; she had a positive attitude, kind words and a friendly smile for everyone and I can still remember thinking how very lucky I was to be somewhere that I had ready access to truly nice people — every day of the week. In a nut shell, that kind of experience keeps me going.*

*Casual visitors entering a long term care facility are usually:*
*1. intimidated,*
*2. horrified,*
*3. depressed,*
*4. stunned and/or*
*5. overwhelmed by the experience.*

*Becoming truly non-threatened and comfortable in our environment is a matter of time and experience. How often have you heard: How can you stand it here; don't you get depressed? "Imagine," I might ask in return, "going somewhere every day only to be depressed and unhappy!!" Instead, my usual response is that I so enjoy the residents, the families and the friends. I learn from them, they learn from me and — best of all — we share a lot of laughter.*

*I believe that by working in long term care, I have been given the tools I need to live a full life. In the course of interviewing residents, the most common thread is of lives well-spent, lives of satisfaction and accomplishment with little room left for regret. This has helped me frame a positive philosophy of life: fill life with experiences worth appreciating rather than living a life of "wishing it had been." The sadness that comes across to me, usually as a spouse fails, is the grief for life as it had been — not life misspent. How true it is that happy memories create the deepest pain in the early stages of separation and grief.*

*I was told many years ago by a very wise man that when we are old, sometimes all we have left to us are our memories; it is our responsibility to make them good ones. I like to think that we can all live our lives that way so that should we be in a wheelchair one day in a long term care facility, we will have plenty to think about!!!*

*If I were to summarize why I do what I do, I would have to say that I have found a place where give and take happens every day; a place where people are vulnerable yet open-hearted, sometimes lost and searching, yet open-minded for change. Listening well to everyone's unique position provides me with the words/ideas/information I need to provide service.*

# 4. Environment

This chapter will look at two aspects of the environment in a long term care facility: the environment as it is perceived by the resident and the environment you will be working in as an Activity or Social Service Professional.

## Resident's Environment

If an Activity or Social Service Professional is not aware of the profound importance and significance of a person's personal environment, s/he needs only look around his or her own home or room. Objects and mementos that could be easily overlooked by the rest of the world have special meaning. They give comfort and joy. They help create a place where a person enjoys spending time. Friendships and feeling like part of the community are important aspects of our lives. Our friends and our culture help us know who we are. Our ability to express our spiritual feelings is vital for understanding the purpose of our lives. This chapter talks about designing an environment in a long term care setting so that each resident will have the best possible opportunity for a high quality of life.

### Physical Environment

The physical plants of most facilities were originally designed in the early 1960's when the philosophy for long term care facilities was focused on the bedroom and not the living space or environment. It was believed that, since most long term care residents would be spending most of the day in bed in frail health and eventually die, they did not need a living space or larger environment.

This was a damaging myth. Unfortunately for those resilient individuals who helped prove this myth false, there were no areas designated for resident activities and the places in which residents did congregate had to be shared with at least two other services in the long term care facility. With many adaptations and remodeling over the years, the industry has tried to work within the original structure of the long term care facility while being sensitive to personal needs for space. The goal is not to remodel the long term care facility, but rather to affect change within the existing structure.

How do we create an environment around a resident to stimulate him/her?

Begin with all of the orientation tools available. Ideally each room should have a clock, a calendar and large-print room numbers. The room itself should have aesthetically pleasing pictures or mobiles. For an individual who enjoys pets, provide opportunities to see and read or look at books and posters about animals.

For someone who is restricted to bed, have the bulletin board within visual range. If they can only focus up towards the ceiling, place an easy to see poster on the ceiling. Mobiles are also effective for residents who are restricted to bed. (Before placing any object on the ceiling, be sure that it is allowed by local fire codes.)

When there is a special event occurring in the facility, bring theme props to the room so that the resident has the opportunity to feel a part of the community.

Remember that as people age, they require more light to see clearly. Be sure that there is enough light for the resident to see all of the things in his/her room.

Give the residents the opportunity to request and be involved in changes which will enhance further independence and involvement (bookshelves for reading, opening doors or windows, reading lights, calendars, clocks) in accordance with OBRA standards. (OBRA Tag F246, Accommodation of Needs: "A resident has the right to reside and receive services in the facility with reasonable accommodations of individual needs and preferences, except when the health or safety of the individual or other residents would be endangered ...")

In the United States there are laws which outline minimum measurements for objects and structures in the resident's environment (The **Americans with Disabilities Act** or **ADA**). The next four pages provide you with a sample of the requirements. The first two pages are a checklist for permanent signage — those signs that would stay up year after year. The sign for the activity room, residents' lounge and potentially the sign for the bulletin board used for the monthly calendar would all fall into this category.

The other two pages show diagrams for minimum clearance for rooms and hallways. Remember, any object placed in the hallway reduces the space available. Minimum clearances do not mean from wall to wall but the actual space available. Fish tanks and wheelchairs "parked" along the wall make it harder for residents to get around. Chairs and couches, while homelike, may place the facility in violation of the **ADA.**

Remember that the **ADA** is a civil rights law. Any violation of this law is a violation of someone's civil rights and civil rights laws are considered more important and more significant than Medicare or Medicaid laws.

# Survey Form 19: Signage

**Facility Name:** _____ **Facility Location:** _____

**From:** _____ **To:** _____

| Section | Item | Technical Requirements | Comments | Yes | No |
|---|---|---|---|---|---|
| **4.1.2(7)** **4.1.3(16)** **4.30.1** | **Directional and Information Signs** | Do signs which provide direction to or information about, functional spaces of the building comply with 4.30.2, 4.30.3 and 4.30.5 (See below)? **EXCEPTION: Building directories, menus and all other signs which are temporary are not required to comply.** | | | |
| 4.30.2 | Character Proportion | Do the letters and numbers on such signs have a width to height ratio between 3:5 and 1:1; and a stroke width-to-height ratio between 1:5 and 1:10? | | | |
| 4.30.3 | Character Size | Are the characters on such signs sized according to viewing distance with characters on overhead signs at least 3 inches high? | | | |
| 4.30.5 | Finish | Do the characters and backgrounds on such signs have a non-glare finish? | | | |
| | Contrast | Do the characters contrast with their background (light-on-dark or dark-on-light)? | | | |
| **4.1.2(7)** **4.1.3(16)** **4.30.1** | **Room and Space Identification Signs** | Do signs which designate permanent rooms and spaces comply with 4.30.4, 4.30.5 and 4.30.6 (See below)? | | | |
| 4.30.4 | Raised and Braille Characters | Are the characters on such signs raised and accompanied by Grade II Braille? | | | |

Survey Form

19 – 1

| Section | Item | Technical Requirements | Comments | Yes | No |
|---|---|---|---|---|---|
| | Pictograms | If a pictorial symbol (pictogram) is used to designate permanent rooms and spaces, is the pictogram accompanied by the equivalent verbal description placed directly below the pictogram? (The verbal description must be in raised letters and accompanied by Grade II Braille.) (If the International Symbol of Accessibility or other information in addition to room and space designation is included on the sign, it does not have to be raised and accompanied by Grade II Braille.) | | | |
| | | Is the border dimension of the pictogram at least 6 inches high? | | | |
| | Character Size | Are the raised characters on such signs between 5/8 inch and 2 inches high and raised at least 1/32 inch? | | | |
| | Upper Case | Are the raised characters on such signs upper case and sans serif or simple serif? | | | |
| 4.30.5 | Finish | Do the characters and background on such signs have a non-glare finish? | | | |
| | Contrast | Do the characters on such signs contrast with their background (light-on-dark or dark-on-light)? | | | |
| 4.30.6 | Mounting Location | Are such signs mounted on the wall adjacent to the latch side of the door? (At double leaf doors, are the signs placed on the nearest adjacent wall?) | | | |
| | Mounting Height | Are such signs mounted with their centerline 60 inches above the ground surface? | | | |
| | Approach | Can a person approach to within 3 inches of such signs without encountering protruding objects or standing within the swing of the door? | | | |

Survey Form

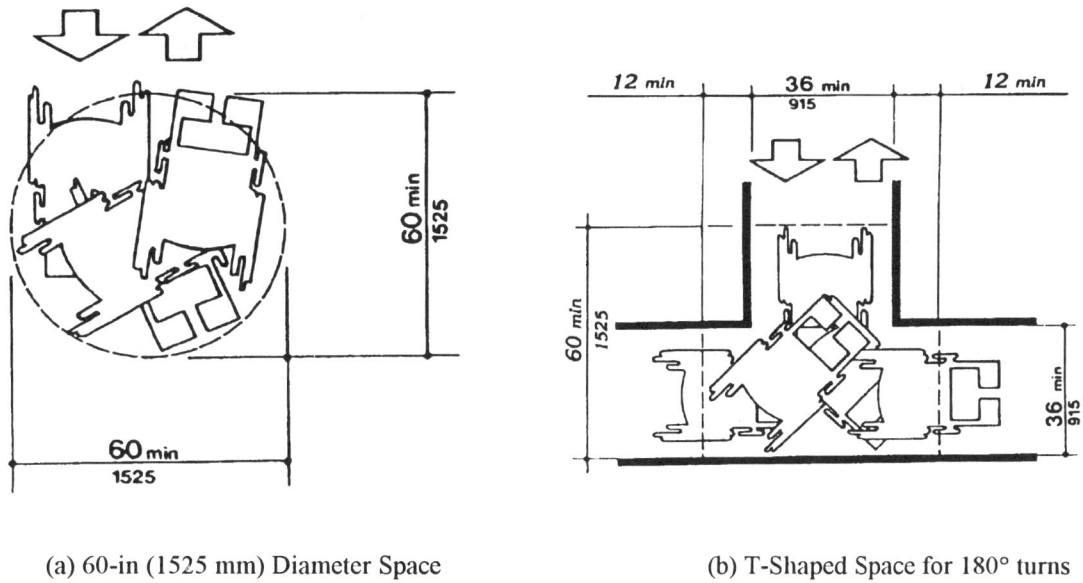

(a) 60-in (1525 mm) Diameter Space        (b) T-Shaped Space for 180° turns

**Figure 3: Wheelchair Turning Space**

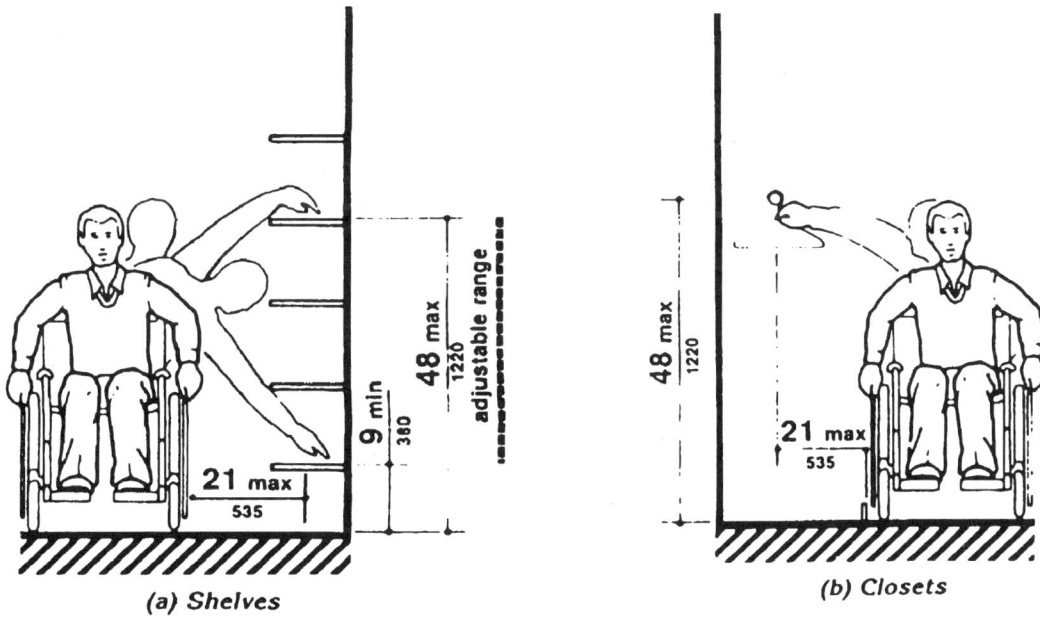

(a) Shelves        (b) Closets

**Figure 38: Storage Shelves and Closets**

accessible path of travel

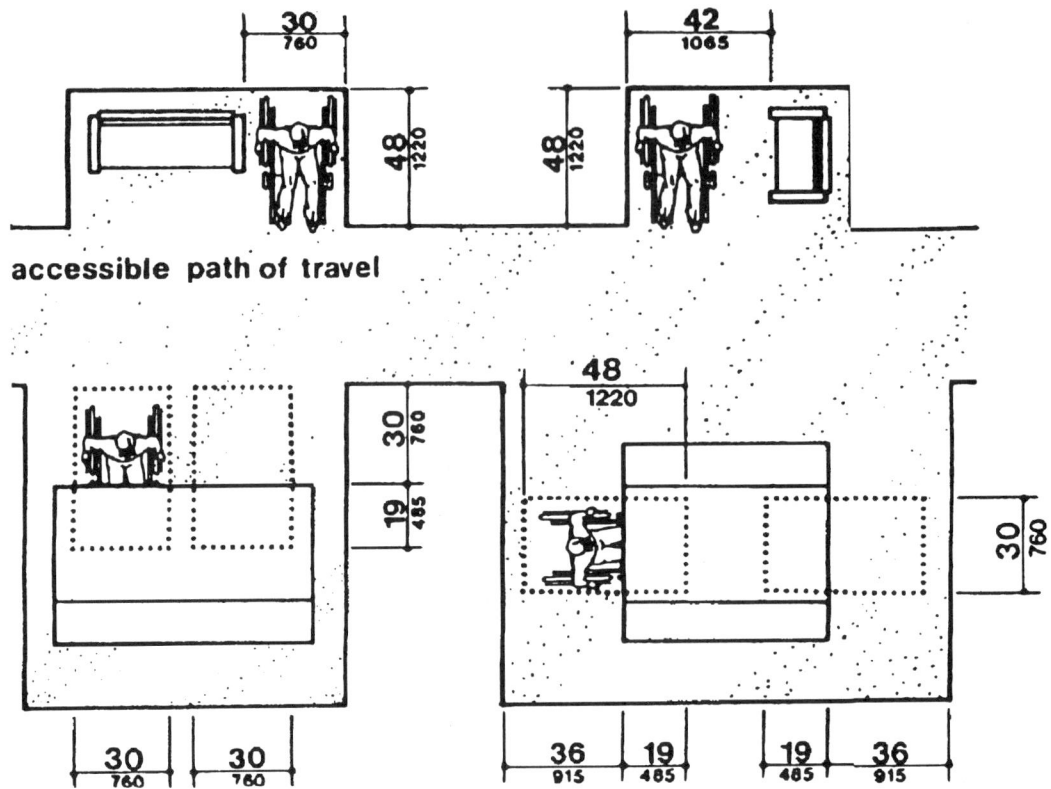

Fig. 45
Minimum Clearances for Seating and Tables

# Personal Environment

One of the most important elements of our personal environment is the space around us. Residents in long term care facilities do not have much space, certainly not as much as they had in their own homes. This space is territory and must be respected with vigor so as to give dignity to each and every resident.

The lack of space makes a resident's close personal space all the more important. We need to respect the resident's concerns about that space.

For example, you are sitting at the nurses' station doing your charting and suddenly you hear a resident yelling out, terrified. You look up and see nothing unusual. The yelling resident remains in her wheelchair, holding her book. She is surrounded by others in their wheelchairs and all of them seem to be oblivious to her. However, if you know her well; you have learned to identify, through ongoing assessment, what triggers her yelling. In this case, someone in one of those wheelchairs is just a little too close to her!

How will you know that this is true? By asking her and using her verbalization (which you have already heard) and her nonverbal cues (panic in her face) to verify what she is telling you. She needs more personal space. It is your responsibility to see that she gets it.

All residents establish their own definition of personal space. The more disabled they are, the more vulnerable they may feel and the wider the personal space they are likely to need. Our residents have little enough left that is personal; losses abound. But our person, our body, always belongs to us despite the physical and emotional insults it has incurred. We always need to control our physical space.

Culturally, we define this space, these invisible boundary lines. Intrusion into them is a violation of us personally. In the United States, we have a relatively wide personal space and even allowing others in to touch or hug can cause emotional flinching.

Personal space must be respected wherever it exists. Meeting the personal space needs of each resident is a requirement for a good personal environment.

The personal environment also includes the things we put in the space around us and in our rooms. Within the interpretive guidelines for environment is the mention of **Individuality and Autonomy** (OBRA Tags F240 to F245). We can improve a resident's personal environment by seeking out ways to celebrate the resident, his/her life, family accomplishments and interests. Any touch from home that adds a personal touch to the environment is important. Self-expression enhances quality of life. This expression can change one's residence from an institutional setting to a warm environment.

Being surrounded by familiar possessions serves another function — the stirring of memories. For those who have very limited access to the physical environment, memories provide a safe and comfortable dwelling place. Even a resident with dementia may be refreshed and reminded of family and events if given photos or memorabilia which provide entrance into a long-ago past.

Autonomy is defined as "a cluster of notions including self-determination, freedom, independence, liberty of choice and action."[13] To have physical autonomy over your environment, you need to feel that there is freedom to go where you choose in the least restrictive manner.

The psychological aspect of autonomy in a long term care setting is the ability to be a part of the plan of care and daily life of the facility. It is of utmost importance that the resident feels that there are options and that the staff is not trying to inhibit his/her active involvement for the purpose of management.

## Spiritual Environment

The spiritual aspects of the environment involve the questions of purpose and meaning in one's life. This involves personal values and belief systems. For many, it also involves a special routine and religious social contacts. For some residents the day of worship was different from the other six days of the week. The pace was different and frequently offered extra time for family and friends.

Another aspect of spiritual environment has to do with a feeling of reverence toward God. Staff or other residents who make fun of another person's beliefs or who use swear words decrease the quality of a resident's spiritual environment. Empowerment of, and respect for, the resident increases it. Making a better spiritual environment for each resident is one of the responsibilities of the Activity and Social Service Professionals.

> People say that what we're all seeking is a meaning for life. I don't think that is what we're really seeking. I think that what we are seeking is an experience of being alive, so that our life experiences on the purely physical plane will have resonances within our own innermost being and reality, so that we actually feel the rapture of being alive.
>
> — Joseph Campbell[14]

# Cultural Environment

Culture in the long term care facility is a concept that may be new to Activity or Social Service Professionals. It refers to a sense of belonging to a group or community which holds significance and value for its members. In order to provide a sense of belonging and meaningful life within a long term care facility, it is imperative to create and enhance a sense of culture. Culture, in this context, can go a long ways toward giving purpose to employees, volunteers and residents within a specific setting. The feeling of being part of a larger whole can be empowering, particularly for individuals who may feel wrenched from familiar settings, values or capabilities.

Culture contributes to the sensation of life in the environment. It can create:
- A sense of belonging
- A feeling of security and safety
- An affirmation of individuality, autonomy and personal accomplishments
- Respect for diversity
- A sense of purpose and involvement
- Enhanced independence as opposed to learned helplessness
- Opportunities for new and pleasantly surprising experiences
- Growth

---

[13] American Society on Aging, **Generations** Vol. XIV, 1990.
[14] Campbell, Joseph with Moyer, Bill, 1988, **The Power of Myth**, p. 3, Doubleday, New York, NY.

- Enjoyment
- A nurturing community

The Activity or Social Service Professional can nurture the creation of this new culture by:

- Encouraging all members, residents, employees and volunteers — professional and non-professional to think about and evaluate ideas about lifestyle, leisure and potential
- Encouraging innovation
- Adding the element of appropriate risk-taking for both staff and residents
- Looking for the uniqueness of each person and promoting that quality
- Encouraging leadership
- Becoming a facilitator in as many situations as possible
- Finding the child within ourselves and recognizing that playfulness is a necessary component of growth
- Listening well and communicating clearly
- Lending support in as many ways as possible
- Sharing the control
- Giving everyone responsibility for a positive environment

# Working Environment

The working environment involves at least four different groups of people who are concerned about a resident's health and well-being. If we could view these interactions from above, this is what we might see:

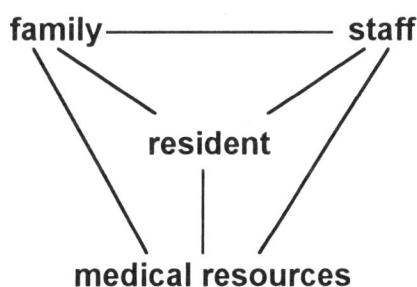

These interactions are complicated and complex and if all parties involved are not scrupulously careful, they will shortly resemble a game of gossip, with a "he said/she said" mode of communication leading to misinterpretation of facts and volatile situations. No one wants to lose control and no one — from resident to family to long term care facility staff to medical staff — wants to be the last to know! We cannot state clearly enough that communication between all of the interested parties is the most important component in resident care.

Activity and Social Service Professionals have varied responsibilities which require direct time with residents, staff and families, but they also have responsibilities for planning, coordinating, documenting and attending meetings. Department heads also need to supervise and keep an overview of the departmental services and responsibilities. Gone are the days when the Activity Professional was given a desk in the day room with the expectation of spending the day supervising the residents who came into the day room. Department heads now spend only 20% or 30% of their time directly with residents. Understanding the current requirements of your job is an important aspect of your working environment.

# Environmental Assessment Form

The **Environmental Assessment Form** is designed to encourage the Activity Professional, Social Service Professional and others to not only assess the environment of their facility, but to then act to remedy situations that need improvement.

Part 1 — "Psychosocial/Supportive" presents specific beneficial characteristics of a positive environment. Commonly found obstacles are included to help sharpen the focus on problems and point to interventions.

Part II — "Physical Factors" presents physical characteristics of the facility and obstacles in the same format as Part 1.

Part III — "Department Environment" looks at some of the requirements of the work environment for Activity and Social Service Professionals.

This form represents a generic version of an instrument that, hopefully, will become individualized and specific to the setting in which it's used. Use of this form on a regular basis can serve as an on-going progress report on the environmental state of the facility and the level of cooperation among staff members and residents for the benefit of all.

**How to use the form:**

**Step One:**       Read first characteristic in column one.

**Step Two:**       Read "obstacles" in column to the right. Do these obstacles exist? Are there others?

**Step Three:**    Use this blank column to identify solutions which work for both residents and staff. Think about human and physical resources needed. Think about what is on hand and how it can be used. Be creative.

**Step Four:**      Repeat steps one through three until all items have been covered.

**Step Five:**       Add concerns not noted on the form and continue the process until all items have been addressed.

# Environmental Assessment Form

## Psychosocial/Supportive

| STIMULATING ENVIRONMENT | OBSTACLES | INTERVENTIONS |
|---|---|---|
| Reality Awareness Objects | No clocks.<br>No calendars. | |
| Sense of Surprise/Newness | No change in schedule or activities offered — every day is the same. | |
| Variety/Diversity | Lacking programs that meet individual needs. | |
| Promotes Independence | No opportunity to engage in individual leisure interests.<br>No opportunity for decision making. | |
| Curiosity | No build-up to an event.<br>No one seems to care. | |
| Communication | No feeling of inclusion.<br>Confusion as to undiscussed changes. | |
| Meaningfulness | Feeling of being disenfranchised.<br>No individualization.<br>No feeling of being needed or of a sense of purpose. | |
| Normal Schedule | Schedule changes with little notice.<br>Canceled activities. | |
| Motivation | No desire to try something new.<br>Lack of stimulating curiosity.<br>Preferred activities not offered. | |
| Education | Too advanced/intimidating.<br>Too basic. | |
| Welcoming | Lack of social interaction between staff and residents or residents and other residents. | |
| Attitudes | Staff fail to see the individual and his/her potential.<br>Unrealistic expectations. | |
| Community | Sense of isolation. | |
| Involvement | Lack of intergenerational programs.<br>Lack of opportunities to help. | |
| Normal Life Setting | Lack of plants/animals.<br>Lack of normal structure of the daily routine. | |
| Cohort Factors | No provision of design appropriate to the familiar themes of past lives. | |
| Multi-Cultural | No diversity in cultural beliefs, customs and environment. | |

# Environmental Assessment Form

## Physical Factors

| FACTORS | OBSTACLES | INTERVENTION |
|---|---|---|
| Light | Privacy curtains pulled near window — no light. Dining room too bright. Bedroom too dark — want to read at night. | |
| Sound | Roommate's TV too loud. Radio on all day — wrong station. | |
| Available Space | Can't maneuver with chair in room. Too much furniture in living room or dining room. | |
| Accessibility | Controls out of reach. Bulletin boards behind bed. Can't get to clothes in cupboard. | |
| Decor | Beautifully decorated, BUT not functional for daily use. Lack of contrast in colors and design. Resident has no personal belongings in the room. | |
| Quiet Spaces | No place to go for privacy. | |
| Orientation Objects | Disorientation due to lack of clocks and calendars for individual use. Poor signage — not appropriate size or placement. Facility name not available. | |
| Color | Light shades of color hard to discern if visually impaired. Too bright — hard to relax. | |
| Visibility | Calendar too small. Room numbers unavailable. | |
| Adaptability | Need board lower on wall. Light above bed hard to reach. Light switch too small. | |
| Odors | Always smells. Soiled linen containers. | |
| Activity Space | Lack of small areas for residents to sit and watch activities with opportunity for physical distancing from others to avoid over-stimulation. | |
| Technology | Inappropriate level of technology. Too high tech or too antiquated for age group of resident. | |

# Environmental Assessment Form

## Department Environment

| FACTORS | OBSTACLES | INTERVENTION |
|---|---|---|
| Supply Space | No space for supplies and materials needed to run programs. | |
| Meeting Space | Inadequate private space to meet with residents for assessments and/or discussions. | |
| Meeting Space | Inadequate space for meetings with volunteers. Lack of space for other community integration activities. | |
| Meeting Space | Inadequate space or privacy for meetings with families. | |
| Work Areas | Private areas for each staff member to keep his/her work materials. | |
| Work Areas | Quiet areas for making phone calls, doing planning and conducting interviews. | |
| Quality of Life Services | Department doesn't reflect the facility philosophy for quality of life. | |

**Plan of action to improve environment:**

# 5. Programs for Your Facility

This chapter looks at the specifics of matching the assessed needs of the resident with activities and other care program ideas so that you can provide the most appropriate care to each resident. Assessment is the process of discovering who the individual is and what their physical and psychosocial needs are in terms of optimum care and functional status. After the assessment, care plans are created for each resident which outline the path the staff will take to meet the resident's needs. Every goal listed on the resident's care plan should be able to be traced back to a need identified on the resident's assessments.

After assessing individual needs, you take a more global view of the resident population as a whole. This is done by summarizing the individual programming needs of each resident and finding individual and group activities which help meet all the needs. While doing this, you can evaluate your current program offerings and make changes to meet the needs of your current resident population.

## Therapeutic Programming Levels

If the activity and social service programs are to truly meet the diversity of needs of the current population, the Activity and Social Service Professionals must design and provide programs which meet all levels of functional and cognitive needs.

Following is a table which gives you a visual reference from which to gauge the levels and programming categories. The levels are from one to eight, one being the most severely limited or regressed resident, to eight which could be an individual in the facility for a short term rehab stay.

Each level will have varying types of groups and goals. An individual may move from one level to another on an upward or downward path and consequently require different and specialized therapeutic programs to meet his/her current needs.

# Levels of Therapeutic Programming

**The levels are:**

1. Sensory Integration — Basic stimulation of multiple senses. These techniques can be incorporated into all levels.

2. Sensory Awareness Sensory Stimulation — Basic stimulation to elicit response and focus outside of self.

3. Validation Therapy — For a person who is very disoriented, whose goals are not focused on orientation.

4. Remotivation/Reminiscing — Stepping stone phase to and from sensory awareness. The resident is aware of self and motivated to seek out others.

5. Resocialization — Resident is socializing and is more oriented to person, time and place. Involvement with others is in a structured group and is crucial to maintain the current functional level.

6. Cognitive Stimulation Cognitive Retraining — Techniques used with a resident suffering from trauma to the brain and showing cognitive disorganization. These are rehab oriented groups.

7. Short Term Rehab — Programming which enhances personal goals worked on in physical therapy, occupational therapy, recreational therapy and speech therapy. Team approach involving use of leisure time.

8. Community Integration — Resident is preparing for discharge; focus on skills, resources and independence when back at previous living situation.

1 ---------------2----------------3----------------4---------------5--------------6--------------7---------------8
              LONG TERM STAY                | SHORT TERM STAY | DISCHARGE

Some residents will move from level to level. Use this with the Activity Needs Assessment (below) to be sure that you have programming which is appropriate for all of your residents. The chapter on activities uses these levels of cognitive functioning to divide activities into groups.

# Activity Needs Assessment

After you have assessed each resident to find out what needs each one has, you must design a program for your facility that meets the needs of the residents. To do that you need to know the current needs, interests, cognitive and functional levels of those individuals here today. An assessment of the current population is required. Perhaps the activity program was designed for what the residents' needs were last year and many of those people are no longer here. The activity program must be "*designed to meet, in accordance with the comprehensive assessment, the interests and the physical, mental and psychosocial well-being of each resident.*"[15]

Ask yourself how many residents benefit from the activity program. Does the program seem to cater to those able to attend large groups and classes? Are there a good percentage of residents uninterested in

[15] OBRA Tag F248.

attending? Are there a good percentage of residents in need of "supportive" activities (special needs and one-on-one programming)? Why do the alert, short-term rehab residents refuse to go to group activities? What do we offer to them as alternatives? Review the guidelines for the **Needs Assessment Form**, take a current census sheet and complete this form. The form and instructions are on the following pages.

# Guidelines for Completing the Needs Assessment Form

## Stage 1.

Each resident from the census sheet needs to be categorized in a single group. The group selected represents the level at which the resident functions most of the time. For example, if a resident is **MOSTLY** active but occasionally passively involved, s/he goes under "actively involved."

Place an asterisk (*) next to each man's name, as they also need to be addressed for specialized programs. Add the cognitive level after the name so you can be sure your mix of activities matches the cognitive functioning level of your residents.

This assessment form needs to be updated with names of newly admitted residents so every individual is reflected on the assessment. The form itself should be updated as often as the admission and discharge schedule demands it.

- Residents in **GROUP** 1 are active **to their own abilities** in group activities.

- Residents in **GROUP** 2 are present at group activities but passive observers — "fringe participants." (Ask yourself why.)

- Residents in **GROUP** 3 do not respond well to large group settings or they are in need of specialized one-on-one experiences or small specialty groups.

- Residents in **GROUP** 4 are alert and independent in leisure pursuits. They do not attend activities on a regular basis (at least 2 to 4 times a week). They do keep involved in individual leisure interests, have families and friends visiting and on occasion, attend events or special presentations.

- Residents in **GROUP** 5 refuse all activities. These individuals are alert but do not involve themselves in any individual leisure interests. They spend their days in their rooms or in the hall. They do not seek out companionship or activities.

- Residents in **GROUP** 6 wander. They do not stay in any location for more than 5 to 10 minutes and either walk or wheel themselves around the facility all day long.

- Residents in **GROUP** 7 are short-term rehab residents. These individuals are receiving therapy with the intent of being discharged as soon as possible. For the most part, they do not wish to enter into the world of a "resident" and avoid social settings and contact with most of the other residents. Their needs and goals are very different from those of an individual on long-term care.

- Residents in **GROUP** 8 may be young people, residents with NG tubes, residents with IVs or residents with a critical illness. Each facility varies greatly, so use this column as needed to keep track of residents who require mostly one-on-one activities.

- Residents in **GROUP** 9 have traumatic head injuries or are comatose. These two categories have separate needs but are grouped together in this form.

- Residents in **GROUP** 10 include other identifiable subgroups which have special needs including smokers and residents dependent on ventilators. They generally have a low attendance at group activities. They are usually alert and social within their own subgroups. These two groups are under the same column but obviously have nothing in common in terms of disabilities and program needs.

# Activity Needs Assessment Form

Activity Professional _____ Date _____

List the name of each resident in one column only.

| 1 | 2 | 3 | 4 | 5 | 6 | 7 | 8 | 9 | 10 |
|---|---|---|---|---|---|---|---|---|---|
| Residents actively involved in groups | Residents passively involved in groups | Special needs: hearing, visual and/or cognitive impairments | Alert and independent in leisure interests and choices | Refuse all activities and are not involved in leisure interests | Residents who wander | Short term rehab | Critically ill, Subacute, IV, NG | Comatose Head injury | Others: Smokers Younger Residents Ventilator Dependent *Add on to this list* |
| | | | | | | | | | |
| | | | | | | | | | |

# Guidelines for Completing the Needs Assessment Form

## Stage 2.

After the Activity Professional completes the needs assessment form s/he must now take a closer look at each category to further assess the population's programming needs.

**GROUP 1 ACTIVELY INVOLVED**
Individuals in this group attend and participate in leisure activities. Do they need to be better connected to functions out of the facility? Are they physically overexerting themselves by this high level of participation? (MDS 2.0 Section N )

**GROUP 2 PASSIVELY INVOLVED**
Individuals in this group choose not to initiate interactions and/or engage in leisure activities that require more skills or energy than they may possess. Determine why these residents are passively involved. Is it due to sensory losses or because they cannot tolerate a large group setting and shut down due to sensory overload? Is this passivity a long standing personality trait which would not be appropriate to change?

If these or other reasons make them poor candidates for group activities, their needs may be better met in Group 3. If they can be more actively involved, the ideal is to find ways to make that possible and therefore include them in Group 1.

Residents experiencing cognitive losses may be disoriented, but respond successfully to reality awareness and remotivation groups. Help facilitate their involvement to their maximum level of function and ability.

**GROUP 3. SPECIAL NEEDS**
Individuals in this group require specialized equipment, one-on-one attention and small specialty group work. On an average, this group will comprise a third or more of your population. The needs of this group are profoundly diverse. By reassessing this group into smaller cluster categories, you can offer not only the type of group to meet their needs and abilities, but also encourage social interaction. These may be for individuals with: hearing impairments, visual impairments, cognitive impairments, terminal illnesses, multiple sclerosis, language barriers, combativeness, cardiac and respiratory distress, etc. After you divide Group 3 into cluster groups, you will see what types of programs are needed to meet your current population needs. The next stage is to determine what level of programming is appropriate for the individual needs.

**GROUP 4. ALERT AND INDEPENDENT IN LEISURE INTERESTS**
Individuals in this group are able to and do participate in leisure activities of their own. If there is an activity of interest to them, they will usually join in, although this is usually not daily. These individuals are making choices about their leisure time. Be sure to clearly document their involvement in the activities which do not show up on the standard activity list so you can show that their leisure needs are being met.

**GROUP 5. REFUSE ALL ACTIVITIES**
Individuals in this group consistently refuse to engage in any leisure activity either facility sponsored or of their own choosing. These individuals may be involved in the same lifestyle they were accustomed to before admission. If so, be sure to document this and define how you came to this determination. Other causes could be depression, fear of groups, distrust or just plain lack of motivation. Obviously these people need a clear assessment to determine why they are making the choices that they are making. They may eventually become more involved in the development of a trusting relationship. They may be in need of specialized one-on-one programs. Or they may simply be making a personal choice not to be involved — which is their right. Be sure that programs are available for them and document their choice not to go.

**GROUP 6. WANDERING**
Individuals in this group do not participate in group activities due to their inability to focus and stay in one place for any amount of time. These individuals need supportive, one-on-one programming such as a Nature Walk & Talk group. Be creative in addressing their needs and uniqueness. Try to determine why

they wander. There are many messages within their mannerisms. Document clearly and concisely their needs, strengths and lifestyle.

## GROUP 7. SHORT TERM REHAB
Individuals in this group are hopeful about receiving necessary therapy and then discharge to a lesser care setting. Many of these individuals are too fatigued from intensive therapy sessions to attend groups. Others choose not to get involved because of the stigma attached to being a long term "resident" in the facility. The Activity Professional's role with these individuals will be more along the lines of a resource person or an adjunct therapy to enhance the rehab goals. Separate groups of activities designed for rehab residents may be very appropriate.

## GROUP 8. SUBACUTE, CRITICALLY ILL
Individuals in this group have a very high level of acuity. Many are unable to leave their rooms and/or become engaged in activity groups. These individuals' needs are very diverse and personalized. Many or most will be provided with services on a one-on-one basis. For Activity Professionals working in units in an acute care hospital, this is the major resident profile. The challenge is in creating a theme-oriented and individualized program which can be offered on a one-on-one basis or small group basis if there are a few residents up in the day room.

## GROUP 9. COMATOSE, TRAUMATIC BRAIN INJURY
Individuals in this group may eventually progress to leisure groups, but primarily will be in specialized one-on-one experiences. The individuals with head injury and in a semi- to full comatose state, are quite a challenge and demand a special understanding of what they can and cannot tolerate in terms of activity programming. Remember that these two groups are very separate with extremely different needs in programming. As with all residents, be familiar with the interdisciplinary approach and always feel comfortable asking questions of other team members to build on your understanding of the diagnosis.

For the resident in a comatose state, your interactions will vary according to which level of comatose state they are in. Residents with head injuries will usually be much younger people. According to the length of time since the injury and the physical healing of the injured area, this individual will need different types of programming interventions. Be sure to read the therapy notes and talk to the physical, recreational, occupational and speech therapists. They will be happy to help you link your time with the residents to specific therapy goals.

Cognitive retraining and cognitive stimulation are appropriate during progressive therapy and, again, need the team approach in identifying what is appropriate. In terms of group activities, be cautious with these individuals. A group may be over-stimulating for them, may cause agitation and combativeness or even seizure activity. It is normal for individuals with head injuries to have fluctuations in their tolerance level. Observe them closely and be aware of their reactions and tolerance to the stimulation. Keep them at a safe distance from commotion and other residents until they have been fully assessed and evaluated for this level of involvement.

## GROUP 10. OTHERS
Individuals in this group choose not to attend most or any of the groups but do spend most of their leisure time in a social network with others they feel comfortable with. (This may be especially true of smokers.) These individuals may not attend most or any of the other groups. Their attendance does not reflect specifics about them. Be sure to document their social connectedness within the group and all other pertinent information regarding interests, strengths and lifestyle.

When you have identified the needs of your residents from the list above, plan a set of activities which meets the needs of all of the individuals. Some ideas for activities are included in the chapter on *Activity and Social Service Groups*. When you have the activity plan, it is a good idea to check it against the OBRA Review forms on the following pages to see if it meets the OBRA requirements for activities.

# OBRA Review Forms

The purpose of these forms is to assure program compliance with the interpretations and terminology of the OBRA regulations. All of the following areas are within the regulations and should be a part of your program. After reviewing how to use the form for your department, take your monthly calendar and write down each activity in the most appropriate section. This is a quality review exercise to evaluate the programs you currently offer. (If you want to practice this evaluation on someone else's schedule, you can use the schedule in the section on *The Life of an Activity Professional* in the *Work Descriptions* chapter.)

*Stimulation Activities:*
Activities designed with the goal of offering input and stimulation to one or more of the senses.
Examples: Music, tactile activities such as pet visits, multi-sensory experiences such as themes that incorporate touching, tasting, smelling, seeing and hearing within the activity.

*Solace Activities:*
Activities which by nature provide solace. These are offered to residents who are critically ill, dealing with pain, have limited endurance and are spending most of the time in bed or in their room.
Examples: Relaxation tapes, pain management tapes, slides and videos, being read to, pet visits, memory book writing, creative and expressive opportunities.

*Physical Health:*
Activities which promote physical well-being. These should be offered to every resident.
Examples: Exercise class, movement to music, reinforcement of therapy goals, obstacle courses, wheelchair management, breathing exercises, walking and relaxation exercises.

*Cognitive Health:*
Activities which provide intellectual stimulation to maintain and enhance awareness and cognition. Cognitive activities should be provided for all levels of ability.
Examples: Current events, discussion groups, values clarification discussions, problem solving scenarios, life management skills, trivia, reminiscing, reality awareness, stress management techniques and orientation.

*Emotional Health:*
Activities which promote a sense of self, life review and empowerment.
Examples: All activities which bring out the individual either in a group or one-on-one situation, reminiscing, "this is your life" games, opportunities to discuss emotional concerns and needs in a supportive environment, socialization activities which assist in helping individual residents feel a part of a community or group.

*Self-Respect:*
Activities which support individual views and beliefs. Activities which promote respect in content and participation and at all levels of needs and abilities.
Examples: Cultural activities which introduce different customs and beliefs, all activities which focus on the individual and previous lifestyle and accomplishments, Resident Council.

*Male-Oriented Activities:*
Activities which are designed to meet the special interests and needs of the men living in the facility. These groups and activities are offered according to the percentage of men living in the facility.
Examples: See the *Resocialization* section of the chapter on *Activity and Social Service Groups* for 48 program ideas.

*Task-Segmentation:*
Activities which take into account a resident's need to have the task broken down into sub tasks in order to successfully engage in and complete the activity. Task segmentation is addressed on the MDS form and should be reviewed by Activity and Social Service Professionals.
Examples: Art projects, breaking the tasks down step by step; pick up the brush, dip brush into the paint, place brush onto the paper which is taped to the table, etc.

*Seasonal/Special Events:*
In order to enhance quality of life, staff need to be very aware of the normalization concept. Because many individuals cannot easily continue their previous lifestyle and routines after being admitted to a long term care setting, it is the responsibility of all staff members to assist in keeping life as normal as possible. Seasonal celebrations and acknowledgments of special events must be offered and reinforced in activities.
Examples: Birthdays, holidays, religious occasions, voting issues and elections, national, state, community and facility events.

*Indoor/Outdoor:*
Activities which are offered outdoors, weather permitting or indoors in different locations for variety.
Examples: Picnics and barbecues, outdoor walks, outings, opportunities for individuals to be outdoors in a safe and secured area.

*Community Based:*
Activities which help connect the resident with the surrounding community so they still feel a part of their community.
Examples: Outings into the community to the library, lectures, restaurants, fairs, stores. It is also important to provide the reverse so that community members, organizations and groups come into the facility to visit the residents.

*Cultural:*
Activities which identify and honor all cultures. These include activities that bring culture to the resident.
Examples: Museum docent visits, slide shows of famous painters and artists, painters coming into the facility to paint while residents watch or lead an art class for residents, special activities which honor other cultures and traditions.

*Religious:*
There should be a special group or presentation for all identified religious beliefs. These can be services, presentations, individualized room decorations which are theme specific, family involvement in sharing the event and beliefs.

*Adaptations/Special Needs:*
Activities which are adapted as required so that all residents can participate according to their individual needs and abilities. This could be an adaptive device, special seating arrangement, visual cues, an interpreter, etc.

*Activities for All Ages:*
Assurance that all age groups identified in the population have meaningful and age-appropriate activities available to them.
Examples: Special outings for young residents to concerts, restaurants, parks, intergenerational programs, staff involvement with activities so that there are people of all ages involved. This also refers to activities which are familiar to an individual according to his/her age, not the age of the staff designing the program. Involve the residents in identifying what would be appropriate.

*In Room Activities:*
Activities which are brought to the individual if they are not able or interested in joining into a group.
Examples: Bringing in a seasonal theme to the room along with decorations, providing specialized sensory programs to those in a semi-comatose state, residents who are ventilator dependent, including residents in their rooms on the resident council by discussing topics individually in the room after the meeting.

# OBRA Activity Program Review Form

**Tag F248 — Activities**
"... An ongoing program of activities designed to meet in accordance with the comprehensive assessment the interests and the physical, mental and psychological well-being of each resident."

**Facility** _____     **Date** _____

| Requirement | Activities Offered | Requirement Met |
|---|---|---|
| Stimulation Activities | | |
| Solace Activities | | |
| Physical Health | | |
| Cognitive Health | | |
| Emotional Health | | |
| Self-Respect | | |
| Male Oriented Activities | | |
| Task Segmentation | | |
| Seasonal/Special Events | | |
| Indoor/Outdoor | | |
| Community Based Activities | | |
| Cultural Activities | | |
| Religious Activities | | |
| Adaptations/Special Needs | | |
| Activities For All Ages | | |
| In-Room Activities | | |

# OBRA Activity Program Review Form — Part 2

**Questions to ask in reviewing the program (list examples for "yes" answers and ideas for the "no" answers):**

Yes/No

For residents who do not attend group activities, do you provide individual projects? ................... _____
Notes:

Do residents give input to the design of the program? ............................................................... _____
Notes:

Is transportation assistance by nursing staff allowing all interested residents to attend? ................. _____
Notes:

Are residents informed of opportunities? ................................................................................. _____
Notes:

Is the schedule of activities acceptable to the schedule of resident needs? ..................................... _____
Notes:

Do residents have a choice in regards to activities? ................................................................... _____
Notes:

Do you provide varied programming to meet the diversity of resident needs and abilities? ............. _____
Notes:

# OBRA Social Service Review Form

> **Tag F250 Social Services**
> "The facility must provide medically-related social services to attain or maintain the highest practicable physical, mental and psychosocial well-being of each resident."

| Requirements | Interpretation | + = Met<br>- = Not Met |
|---|---|---|
| Identify the need of medically-related social services and pursue provision of these services | Maintaining or improving ability to personally manage everyday physical, mental and psychosocial needs. | |
| Adaptive equipment | Assuring provision of special devices and equipment to enhance functional and emotional independence. | |
| Restraint reduction | Providing alternatives to drug therapy or restraints by understanding and communicating to staff why residents act as they do, what they are attempting to communicate and what needs the staff must meet. | |
| Clothing and personal needs | Assisting with identifying and purchasing needed supplies and items. | |
| Maintaining contact with the family about changes | Informing family about changes that occur in current goals, discharge plans and care plan meeting attendance. | |
| Referrals and outside services | Assisting with accessible transportation, talking books, absentee ballot forms. | |
| Financial and legal matters | Providing assistance with requests for attorney, pension information and updates, funeral arrangements. | |
| Health care decisions | Assisting residents with information about current health status and decisions pertaining to treatment. Requesting others to be a part of this decision-making process. | |
| Discharge planning | Assisting with living situations, home health services, transfer agreements with other facilities. | |
| Counseling services | Opportunity for residents to discuss concerns or assistance in obtaining outside counsel. | |
| Grief counseling | Meeting the needs of residents who are grieving. | |
| Support individual needs and interests | Keeping staff informed of individual interests and preferences to enhance a sense of self and self-esteem. | |
| Building staff and resident relationships | Inservice training to continually assist understanding and support of individual resident needs. | |
| Self-determination and choices | Empowering the resident to make his/her own choices about lifestyle in the long term care facility. | |
| Promoting staff awareness of dignity and individuality | Role modeling, inservice training, family council, resident council. | |

# OBRA Social Service Program Review — Part 2

**Questions to ask in reviewing the program (list examples for "yes" answers and ideas for the "no" answers):**

Yes/No

Do facility staff implement social service interventions to assist the resident in meeting treatment goals? ........................................................................................................ _____
Notes:

Do staff responsible for social work monitor the resident's progress in improving physical, mental and psychosocial function? ................................................................................ _____
Notes:

Has goal attainment been evaluated and the care plan changed accordingly? ............................... _____
Notes:

Does the care plan link goals to psychosocial functioning and well being? .................................. _____
Notes:

Have the staff responsible for social work established and maintained relationships with the resident's family or legal representative? ........................................................................... _____
Notes:

# Challenges and Techniques of Group Work

One of the most challenging and ever-changing roles that the Activity or Social Service Professional plays is that of group leader. Many factors come into play in determining the overall composition and capacities of the group and therefore, appropriate activities for that group. For example:

- When the majority of participants are frail and dealing with sensory and cognitive losses, the Activity or Social Service Professional must radiate confidence and fine tune activities to the capabilities of the group.
- When there is a high level of confusion or disorientation among group members, the leader will need to provide a high degree of structure and direction for the group.
- When the majority of the participants are cognitively aware and otherwise capable, the leader will need to be able to step back and allow the residents to assume natural leadership roles.

The following list presents some issues and needs that the Activity or Social Service Professional should consider when leading a group. Each requires a constructive and compassionate response from the leader whether through action or attitude.

| | | |
|---|---|---|
| passivity | lack of purpose | behavioral issues |
| anxiety | apathy | communication |
| confusion | dependency | disorders |
| anger | loneliness | embarrassment |
| lack of response | depression | regarding |
| feelings of | short attention span | condition |
| uselessness | sensory losses | wandering |
| low self-esteem | cognitive losses | hyperactivity |

Here are some tools and techniques that have proven helpful in working with groups:

- When setting expectations and goals for the group, be sure to be realistic about what this group of individuals can successfully achieve.
- Structure each member's environment within the group to enhance his/her abilities and thereby increase involvement in socialization, improve attention span and provide a positive and successful experience.
- Always focus on the group member *today* and the abilities that s/he has *today*.
- Acknowledge the efforts and accomplishments of each group member individually.
- Offer time within each session for individuals to share past memories and experiences.
- Verbally acknowledge any information acquired through conversation regarding past occupations, accomplishments and interests of group members.
- Introduce the familiar themes of family, pets, foods, holidays and nature regardless of group members' cognitive level.
- Remind the group of pleasurable experiences which are familiar to everyone.
- Allow opportunities to demonstrate what has been learned. Repetition and visual cues enhance learning.
- Remember that we all need to be needed. This can be a goal for a group — to be of help to others. Projects and gifts can be made for staff, visitors, entertainers and each other.
- Adults like to know that they are held accountable for their role in the group. Feedback from the leader is very important.
- Use touch to motivate and help to re-focus attention in the group. For residents who do not have family visiting regularly, their only touch may be during therapy or activities. Never forget how strongly one is affected and nurtured by holding hands, hugging or just touching another in a loving and appropriate way.

# 6. Activity and Social Service Groups

According to both federal and state regulations, and to meet the resident's needs, each long term care setting is required to provide a meaningful and purposeful program of activities. This program is for each and every resident regardless of ability or limitation. The intent is to assure that the leisure and recreation needs of people no longer living at home or in the community at large are being met. Therapeutic activities within a clinical setting are provided in order to meet specialized and individualized needs.

For most individuals the concept of leisure brings to mind *time* that is available to pursue hobbies and interests. The experience may be for relaxation or rejuvenation. It may be therapeutic or just recreational. Some individuals view leisure as a *state of mind*, having little to do with blocks of time. For these individuals, almost any activity, including work, can be viewed as a positive leisure experience. The way leisure is perceived is an important part of each person's personality.

The amount of free time available to individuals who are institutionalized is much greater than at any other time in their adult lives. In order to understand individuals, we need to understand their era and values. (This is known as the "cohort factor.") Many people, particularly those growing up in the early 1900's, give very little importance to this thing called leisure. Their work ethic usually made them value their work over the rest of their activities.

The importance of therapeutic activities is that they focus on individual interests and personalities and that they focus on *abilities* as opposed to *limitations*. If we can assist a resident in focusing on the strengths they still have, their limitations seem somehow more manageable. If you are working with an individual who feels that life is over because they have lost the ability to write due to a stroke, you can support them in their therapy goals, encourage trying something new or find another individual with a similar situation for mutual support. There are many options.

# Leisure Leisure Leisure

Leisure is a state of mind or an attitude.

Leisure motivates us to recreate.

Leisure is more the feeling experienced than the activity you are involved in.

Some elements of leisure are
1. antithesis of work
2. pleasant expectations and recollections (reminiscing)
3. minimal social role obligations
4. psychological perception of freedom
5. close relation to values of the culture (cohort factor)

## Important Factors Of Leisure For A Recreation Leader

1. You need to be aware of your own definition and attitude regarding leisure and its significance to quality of life.

2. Before you can promote leisure involvement in others, you should look inside and determine your personal motivation.

3. Leisure experiences are energizing, relaxing, stress reducing, challenging, playful, growthful and freeing. They can be experienced both in a **group** or **individually**.

4. The desire to be involved in a leisure pursuit is **innate**. Leisure itself is **learned**. So if you are interested in quality of life in your older years, you need to nurture this aspect of your life when you are young. **Start today**.

Many times, the importance of therapeutic activities is not measured by the activity itself, but rather in the value of the resident's involvement. Each activity has a purpose and a goal and within that activity each individual has a purpose and a goal.

For all residents in all facilities, the daily pursuit for quality of life and meaning is of profound importance. Sometimes, the only way to characterize this pursuit is as a struggle. Nevertheless, it is a most worthy struggle and one which the Activity and Social Service Professional carries on with dignity, courage, knowledge and professional expertise.

It is somewhat ironic that many Activity and Social Service Professionals in charge of planning the activities of others do not look to their own lives and choices for insights into leisure options and motives. Ask yourself the following questions:

- What is it that you do in your leisure?
- Do you enjoy being alone or with others?
- Do your interests vary or do you always seek out the familiar?
- Do you value leisure time as an important component of your own quality of life?
- If you were living in a long term care setting, could you still continue with your personal leisure interests? What help would you need from other people?
- Could these interests help you in dealing with new situations and problems?
- Could they bring meaning to your life? In what way?

# Activity Supplies

Certain equipment is required for running activity programs. We recommend that you have the following basic equipment somewhere in your facility which can be used for activities:

| | | | |
|---|---|---|---|
| Slide projector | Exercise balls | Pens, paints, | Word games |
| Bingo games | Bowling set | brushes | Trivia |
| TV & VCR | Large print books | Paper assortment | Cards |
| Stereo and Tape | Newspaper | Scissors | Scrabble |
| deck(s) with 4–6 | Reality orientation | Crossword puzzles | Pokeno |
| headsets | boards | Magazines | Musical tapes and |
| Parachute | Eraser boards | Puzzles | CDs |

Keeping track of your supplies is an important part of running activities. The chart on the following page shows one format for keeping track of supplies used for sensory stimulation that are distributed throughout your facility. Whether you use the Leisure Room concept discussed at the end of this chapter or not, you will still have some of your supplies in different parts of the facility. This form provides a way to keep track of where they are.

This is the kind of form that needs to be updated often if you are planning to use it to find out where something is. A white board that can be changed as supplies are moved or a computer program that is easy to use are ways to keep track of your supplies on an ongoing basis. This might be a good project for a volunteer.

If you really don't mind looking for supplies, then a form like this can be filled out every few months to be sure that you still have enough usable supplies where your volunteers, staff and/or residents can get to them easily.

(Please note that the numbers of items in the activity supply list are not recommendations about the number of items you should have in your facility. That decision comes from your analysis of the needs of your residents.)

# Activity Supply List

Date: _____

| Supply Item | Leisure Room | Station One | Station Two | Station Three |
|---|---|---|---|---|
| Tangle | 4 | 2 | | |
| Slinky | 3 | 1 | | 1 |
| Magnetic letters | 3 sets | | | |
| Frog Tac Toe | 1 | | | 2 |
| Sing a long radio | 2 | 1 | 1 | 1 |
| Stacking blocks | 2 sets | | | |
| Tape recorder | 2 | 1 | 1 | 1 |
| Tapes | 23 | 12 | 4 | 18 |
| Ring toss | 1 | | | |
| Parachute | 2 | | | |
| Dominoes | 2 | | 1 | |
| Large print cards | 4 | 1 | 1 | |
| Flash cards | 3 | 2 | 2 | 1 |
| Coaster sets for stacking | 3 | | | |
| Clothespins | 1 box | | 1 box | |
| Grooming items | | 2 | 2 | 3 |
| Writing materials | 3 | 2 | 2 | 1 |
| Trivia games | 2 | | | |
| Velcro catch game | 2 | | | |
| Pat mats | | 1 | 1 | |
| Scissors and paper | 1 | 1 | 2 | 1 |
| Checkers | 2 | | | |
| Plastic puzzles | 3 | | | |
| Koosh balls | 1 | 2 | 1 | 1 |
| Eraser board | 2 | | | |
| Safety locks and bicycle chains | 3 | | | |
| Maps | 6 | 2 | 2 | 1 |

Comments:

# Activity Analysis

Therapeutic activities are those which are provided and designed to enhance the individual treatment goals for each resident. When you have determined what the activity treatment goals will be, the next step is to analyze each activity. You can do so by using the form on the next page.

The purpose of this process is to separate the components of the activity and to determine what skills are needed in order to successfully participate and complete it.

Analyzing an activity occurs separately from assessing the individual. These are two separate assessment processes. By breaking an activity down into separate components, the Activity or Social Service Professional can recommend specific programs which will enhance interdisciplinary goals and can assist in adapting them to the needs and abilities of the individual.

The left side of the activity analysis form addresses the administrative components of an activity. Fill this in for each of the activities offered in your program. The right side of the activity analysis form focuses on the other components of the activity. Use this as a means of walking yourself through an activity experience to determine who it would be most appropriate for and also to determine what adaptations may be needed in order to offer it to more residents.

Each time that you design a new group activity, complete an activity analysis form. This documents your thoroughness and professionalism in designing a meaningful program.

In analyzing activities, you also want to recognize the type of social skills required to participate in the group. As the coordinator, you need to know what the purpose of the group is along with what type of interaction is expected of the resident. Will they be interacting with others, needing to work cooperatively, sitting with others but not required to socialize or share tools?

These are very important questions to ask. If you have a resident who you have assessed as being in need of stimulation, but unable to tolerate other people too close to him/her, you need to closely evaluate and determine what type of setting would meet his/her needs. S/he could handle an independent project at one table alone while other residents are seated at another table in the same room.

If you are interested in outlining the activity without the additional analysis, there is an excellent form in **The Album of Activity Policy and Procedures Manual** written by Recreation Therapy Consultants, (619) 546 - 9003.

# Activity Analysis Form

Activity _____    Type of Activity _____

### Administrative Aspects

Goal: _____

_____

Equipment & Supplies: _____

_____

_____

_____

Skills/Limitations of Participants: _____

_____

_____

_____

Procedures: _____

_____

_____

_____

_____

_____

_____

_____

_____

Length of Activity: _____

_____

_____

Precautions: _____

_____

_____

_____

Adaptations: _____

_____

_____

Date: _____

### Physical Aspects

**Body Position Requirements:**
sit _____ stand _____ walk _____
one handed _____ two handed _____
eye/hand coordination _____
gross motor _____ fine motor _____

**Sense Requirements:**
touch _____ taste _____ sight _____
hearing _____ smell _____

**Physical Requirements:**
endurance _____ speed _____
strength _____
cardiovascular activity needed _____

### Social Aspects

1:1 activity _____
small group _____
requires ongoing conversation _____
requires ability to share/cooperate _____
requires ability to listen _____
requires tolerance of close proximity _____
independent work within a group _____

### Cognitive Aspects

attention span _____
memory: long term _____ short term _____
thinking: abstract _____ concrete _____
sequencing skills needed _____
problem solving skills needed _____
time given for response: yes _____ no _____
object identification _____
directionality _____
amount of concentration needed _____
requires ability to follow _____ step directions

### Affective (Emotional) Aspects

use of past skills _____
use of past memories _____
highlights individuality _____
increases sense of self _____
promotes body awareness _____
fosters sense of belonging _____
experiences sense of success _____
anticipation, anxiety _____
requires use of new skills _____

Coordinator: _____

# Helping Them Be All That They Can Be[16]

## *Programming for Individuals with Cognitive Impairments*

If you have residents with significant cognitive impairments in you facility, you need to be especially careful to provide activity programs for them. OBRA requires that you develop programs which meet their leisure needs, too.

The basic goal of activity programming for residents who are cognitively impaired, as it is for any activities program, is to stimulate a person's response and to promote the highest level of functioning of which s/he is capable. Specifically, the goal is to continually simplify tasks so they remain within the individual's diminished abilities, thus allowing her/him to retain as much control over her/his life as possible and to maintain a sense of personal dignity.

Although these residents may have lost the ability to amuse themselves, because that requires memory capacity they no longer possess, they have not lost the ability to be amused or to feel good. Total inactivity is frustrating for anyone. Meaningless activity in which there is no sense of usefulness or challenge is deadly, even for the person who has memory loss.

In addition to memory loss, we are talking about programming for people who may also be experiencing increasing losses in judgment and initiative, the abilities to problem solve, attach meaning to sensory impressions, recognize familiar objects and express themselves. They may also exhibit aimless wandering, carelessness in their appearance, disorientation to person, time and place, irritability, personality and mood changes and compulsive repetition. Physical changes may include muscular weakness, gait changes, loss of balance and difficulties in performing Activities of Daily Living (ADLs). Cognitive deficits are often characterized by the decreasing ability to use past experience in the solution of current problems.

## General Activity Goals

1. To prevent or reverse the tendency to withdraw or deteriorate.
2. To retain or retrain recognition of articles once familiar.
3. To utilize physical and mental capabilities.
4. To accept the present surroundings.
5. To maintain or stimulate interests and social contacts.
6. To focus attention on own human worth or self-value.
7. To focus concentration away from physical condition.
8. To alleviate worry and distress.
9. To provide an outlet for irritation and resentment.
10. To promote speech.
11. To promote controlled fatigue and prevent excessive sleeping during the day.

---

[16] ©1991 Elizabeth Best Martini, MS, CTRS and Richelle N. Cunninghis, MEd, OTR, used with permission.

# Activities for Individuals with Cognitive Impairments[17]

These pages show a set of activities which are appropriate for individuals with cognitive impairments and the goals of the activities.[18]

| Type | Activity | Goal |
|---|---|---|
| **Reality Activities** | • Group/one-on-one sessions<br>• Review of day's activities<br>• Sensory stimulation | identity, socialization, improve/maintain memory, recognition, communication |
| **Art Activities** | • Filling in silhouettes<br>• Copying figures<br>• Collage<br>• Assembling pre-cut shapes<br>• Group murals<br>• Paint bag art<br>• Edible art | eye/hand coordination, recognition, sensory stimulation, creativity, accomplishment, follow directions, fine motor movement |
| **Activities of Daily Living** | • Tying shoes/fastening buttons<br>• Preparing vegetables<br>• Gardening<br>• Cooking<br>• Grooming | retain skills, sense of accomplishment, eye-hand coordination, object identification, memory, following directions, multi-step tasks |
| **Physical Activities** | • Fitness exercises (purposeful)<br>• Supervised walks<br>• Movement therapy<br>• Kick ball<br>• Bean bag toss<br>• Dice games | use excess energy, retain knowledge of body parts, competition, stimulation, socialization, maintain or increase range of motion, maintain or increase muscle tone, alertness |
| **Drama Activities** | • Musical plays<br>• Act out themes<br>• "Share a Face"<br>• Improvise with props<br>• Story telling<br>• Pantomime/charades | immediate enjoyment, socialization, cognition, communication skills, release of frustration, creative expression, problem solving |
| **Music Activities** | • Rhythm band<br>• Sing along<br>• Movement & music<br>• Follow the leader<br>• Old time dance steps | sensory stimulation, fun, exercise, reminiscence, coordination, following direction, socialization |

---

[17] ©1991 E. Best Martini, MS, CTRS and R. N. Cunninghis, MEd, OTR, used with permission.

[18] Two resources to find out more about working with people with dementia are *Wiser Now* (a monthly publication from Better Directions, PO Box 3064, Waquoit, MA 02536-3064) and Cunninghis, Richelle, 1995, **Reality Activities: A How To Manual for Increasing Orientation, Second Edition**, Idyll Arbor, Inc., Ravensdale, WA.

| Type | Activity | Goal |
|---|---|---|
| **Word and Quiz Games** | • Unscramble 3 or 4 letter word<br>• Hangman<br>• Categories<br>• Matching pictures<br>• Homonyms, synonyms, antonyms<br>• Old sayings, proverbs<br>• Discussion questions<br>• Trivia<br>• Spelling bees<br>• What's in a Name | improve cognition, sense of accomplishment, pride, socialization, increase memory, communication skills, competition, mental stimulation, problem-solving ability, attention span, increase self-esteem, reading skills, matching skills |
| **Group Activities** | • Discussion groups<br>• Reminiscence groups<br>• Simple card games<br>• Food & culture | decrease anxiety, encourage use of memory, socialization, past knowledge, creative expression, listening skills |
| **Individual Activities** | • Looking at photos<br>• Large puzzles<br>• Memory Box | past memories, manual dexterity, accomplishment |
| **Special Areas/ Undirected Activities** | • Opening/closing containers<br>• Opening/closing drawers<br>• Leafing through magazines<br>• Articles of clothing activity<br>• Art projects<br>• Tub of water with boats<br>• Fabric fold | exercise creativity, use past skills, coordination, use excess energy, meaningful activity, identifying use/purposes of common objects, fine motor skills |
| **Body Imagery** | • Sensory boxes<br>• Tactile experiences (e.g. hugging, touching)<br>• Movement exploration<br>• Drawing hands & feet<br>• Portraits of each other<br>• Writing name in the air | sensory stimulation, identification of body parts, cognitive awareness, socialization, increased awareness of tactile stimulation, range of motion, eye-hand coordination, spatial awareness |
| **Tactile Activities** | Scents, tastes, sounds, pets, children, nature, fabrics, lotions, etc. | sensory stimulation, environmental awareness, reminiscence, body imagery, tactile awareness |

# Activity Suggestions

This section of the chapter discusses the overall requirements for activities, the eight functional levels of activities in long term care facilities and then gives you some suggested activities for your facility in each of the categories.

If an activity program is going to be successful, it must provide all of these elements at the level appropriate for each resident:
1. Orientation and direction
2. Reassurance
3. Physical contact
4. Consistent routine
5. Choices which can be understood
6. Appropriate levels of stress
7. Verbal cues
8. Movement
9. Past identity
10. Socialization
11. Reminiscence

How do we accomplish this? Perhaps the best place to start is by modifying the environment. Decreased functioning can lead to situations in which the individual feels trapped in an environment that poses an apparently unsolvable problem and the person is unable to change or influence the situation.

1. Reduce noise and visual distractions
   a. Limit group size
   b. Limit number of people giving instructions
   c. Decrease background noises (TV, intercom, etc.)
   d. Show resident sound sources

2. Increase environmental clues
   a. Use color for identification (or shapes, animals, flower, food, etc.)
   b. Reduce glare (carpet floors, move light sources, seat residents with their back to light source)
   c. Eliminate prints and patterns on floors, walls and furniture
   d. Choose strong contrasting colors for backgrounds
   e. Allow time to adjust from outdoor to indoor lighting

3. Re-direct wandering behaviors
   a. Camouflage doors with barriers or room dividers
   b. Increase staff awareness of their own entering and leaving
   c. Try to schedule activities at shift change as distraction

4. Maintain each person's normal schedule as much as possible (helps person's sense of control)
   a. Clothing/dressing
   b. Bathing/showering time
   c. Reading/buying newspaper
   d. Church services

There are eight levels of activities which we can run. The particular ones we include for a particular resident depends on his/her level of functioning.

## Levels of Therapeutic Programming

1. Sensory Integration

Basic stimulation of multiple senses.
These techniques can be incorporated into all levels.

2. Sensory Awareness
   Sensory Stimulation

Basic stimulation to elicit response and focus outside of self.

3. Validation Therapy

For a person who is very disoriented, whose goals are not focused on orientation.

4. Remotivation/Reminiscing

Stepping stone phase to and from sensory awareness. The resident is aware of self and motivated to seek out others.

5. Resocialization

Resident is socializing and is more oriented to person, time and place. Involvement with others is in a structured group and is crucial to maintain the current functional level.

6. Cognitive Stimulation
   Cognitive Retraining

Techniques used with a resident suffering from trauma to the brain and showing cognitive disorganization. These are rehab oriented groups.

7. Short Term Rehab

Programming which enhances personal goals worked on in physical therapy, occupational therapy, recreational therapy and speech therapy. Team approach involving use of leisure time.

8. Community Integration

Resident is preparing for discharge; focus on skills, resources and independence when back at previous living situation.

The following sections talk more about these activity levels and give some examples of specific activities which we have found to be effective. Before we look at the activities as they are divided into the different levels, we want to discuss theme activities. The basic idea behind a theme activity is to create an experience which is appropriate for residents with many different levels of functioning. An example of an activity based on a mountain theme is shown on the next page.[19]

---

[19] An excellent resource addressing the issues of themes, special needs and programming for all levels is *Creative Forecasting*, PO Box 7789, Colorado Springs, CO 80933-7789. Phone: 719-633-3174, fax: 719-632-4721.

# Mountain Theme[20]

**Trigger Words:**      trees      streams      pine cones
                           log cabin     camping

**Environmental Enhancers:**

Gather bark, pine needles, pine cones, soil, rocks
Paint trees on butcher paper
Scent paper with wood musk perfume
Burn incense of pine
Play environmental tapes of the wind blowing, birds singing, thunder
Hang Christmas lights on ceilings to simulate stars
Use backpacks to hold supplies
Have a parachute with a fan to simulate clouds and wind
Wildflowers
Potpourri sachet
Pelts from furrier

**Activities:**

Create nature trails indoors or out.

Make group mural using pine needles for forest floor, tissue paper for leaves or dried leaves. Apply with spray adhesive.

Make bird feeders with pine cones, peanut butter and sprinkle bird seed on the peanut butter. Hang it outside.

Paint a tree branch on fabric (drapery size) and hang. Use it for hanging valentines, shamrocks, etc.

Create a campfire and sing songs.

Make toasted marshmallows or s'mores.

Invite SPCA to bring animals who live in the forest — rabbits, owls, birds.

Flashlight games/tracking.

Fishing game.

Storytelling.

Study objects with a magnifying glass.

---

[20] From Ann Nathan and Elizabeth Best Martini, used with permission.

# Level 1: Sensory Integration Activities

Each individual is born with the potential to organize input from their sensory system: proprioception, touch, hearing, taste, smell and vision. The sensory input needs to be "integrated," otherwise we experience a profound sensory overload on one extreme or deprivation on the other.

If everything that we felt, saw, heard and tasted at one time were processed in the upper brain simultaneously, we would be bombarded. Sensory integration is "the ability to organize all of the information that we process so as to better manage ourselves within our environment."[21]

As an infant, we make motor responses to the world around us. These responses are global as the entire body learns to move towards the stimuli. With integration of the senses, the motor responses become more coordinated and purposeful. Each component of the sensory system operates separately and also as a part of the whole system.

An experience incorporating all five senses leaves an indelible mark, much greater than with only one sensory input. It is as though the inner eye captures the experience so that all five senses can bring up the memory. How often do you smell a scent which reminds you of a past experience? The smell stimulated the memory but was not itself the focal point of the real experience.

When the developmental process has been altered in any way, individuals may not have the sensorimotor capacity to respond to their environment. They also may not have attained a normal cognitive level due to the sensorimotor deficits.

Individuals experiencing sensory losses or cognitive losses can use the rest of the sensory system to respond to their environment and also to rekindle past memories and learned responses. "A sensory integrative approach differs in that it does not *teach* specific skills — rather the goal is to enhance the brain's ability to learn to do these things."[22]

## Deficits in Sensory Integration

Any alteration in the developmental pattern of one's growth will impact the integration process and present one or many of the characteristics listed below:

1. Poor body posture, balance
2. Reduced visual discrimination
3. Short attention span
4. Irritability
5. Physical rigidity
6. Tactile defensiveness (lack of integration of the somatic sensory system)
7. Poor judgment skills
8. Limited cognitive function
9. Diminished tactile discrimination
10. Distractibility

---

[21] Ayres, A. Jean, 1971, **Sensory Integration And Learning Disorders**, Western Psychological Services, Pages 1-2.
[22] Ayres, A. Jean, 1971, **Sensory Integration And Learning Disorders**, Western Psychological Services, Page 2.

Many of your residents will exhibit 7 out of the 10 deficits listed above. Any resident who exhibits even a few of these will benefit from sensory integration activities because body and self-awareness are central components for participating in activity and social service groups.

# Goals Of A Sensory Integration Focus

1.  Use recreation and leisure to improve, habilitate or rehabilitate the physical, social, emotional and cognitive functional abilities of the individual.
2.  Educate toward quality leisure functioning regardless of level of functioning.
3.  Increase attention span.
4.  Build tolerance to physical prompts.
5.  Practice fine and large motor skills.
6.  Increase capacity for interactions.
7.  Increase tolerance to task levels of social and physical tolerance.

# Basic Introduction To Sensory Integration

As an introduction to Sensory Integration, we will look at some of the systems involved in an everyday activity. The components which are involved include:

> **Eyes (see)**
> **Proprioceptors (awareness of the position of the body)**
> **Vestibular System (balance)**
> **Tactile Systems (touch, feel)**
> **Olfaction (smell)**

These sensory nerve impulses are received and coordinated by the "brainstem" which in turn sends nerve impulses to our eye muscles so we can see; body muscles so we can sit, stand, walk, turn cartwheels and still maintain a sense of balance. It takes all of the parts of our body working together to successfully interact with things around us.

## A Stroll On The Beach

Imagine that you are walking on the beach barefoot. Your feet are being stimulated by their movement through the sand, your auditory system is processing the sounds of the ocean, you can taste the ocean on your lips and your eyes are guiding the way (along with enjoying the experience). Looking closer, you might ask, "How do my legs know how to maneuver in sand?" The sensory nerve impulses are responding to stimuli sent to the brainstem to be processed and sent back to the eyes to see, the spine to hold the body upright and the legs to move in symmetry with the arms for movement. Within each ear you have both your hearing mechanism (cochlea) and your balance center — the vestibular system.

> The vestibular system enables the organism to detect motion, especially acceleration and deceleration and the earth's gravitational pull. The system helps the organism to know whether any given sensory input — visual, tactile or proprioceptive — is associated with movement of the body or is a function of the external environment. For example, it tells the person whether he is moving within the room or the room is moving about him.[23]

The vestibular system is your organ of adaptability. This process carries over to cognitive functions. Sensory impulses bring about biochemical changes in the brain that are critical to the learning process.

---

[23] Ayres, A. Jean, 1971, **Sensory Integration And Learning Disorders,** Western Psychological Services, Pages 5-6.

The muscles, joints, ligaments and receptors associated with bones provide information to the brain stem about your relationship to the world around you. This is the proprioceptive system.

The relationship among the proprioceptive, vestibular and tactile systems gives you the ability to carry out the seemingly easy task of enjoying a stroll on the beach.

The vestibular system provides information about changes in your head position with respect to gravity. The objects you see around you and the surfaces you touch or stand on may be changing continually. When your head moves, a biochemical reaction occurs in your inner ear. This biochemical reaction enables learning, increases attention span and increases memory.

Tactile stimulation refers to the use of the nerves directly under the skin, "touching." Through experience you learn to identify textures, temperatures and hardness. Just like the muscles, all nerves need to be exercised. Because confinement in a long term care facility tends to decrease opportunities to touch and be touched, purposeful tactile stimulation should be planned.

The vestibular/ocular (eye-ear) nerve literally "holds" the image of what was last looked at. For maximum learning, an individual needs sensory stimulation and input into all sensory systems (vestibular, tactile, proprioceptive, visual and olfactory).

## Therapeutic Program Ideas

1. Encourage movement of the head in groups and individual interaction with an individual.
2. Create activities which encourage use of fingers and hands. (This movement allows brain to open up to new information.)[24]

   | | |
   |---|---|
   | clapping and rubbing hands | hand puppets |
   | string games | taffy pulls |
   | painting | window wiping |
   | hand holding | hand massages |
   | Velcro | |

3. Provide tactile discrimination activities (sand paper, soft, hard, cold, warm).
4. Always add scents to activity (scented objects, room sprays, scented pens). Try to avoid scents which are alcohol based. They actually stimulate a different set of olfactory nerves than a pure scent would. You reach more nerves if you use pure scents or oil-based scents instead of alcohol-based ones.
5. Create activities which provide body awareness experiences:

   | | |
   |---|---|
   | facial brushes | vibrators |
   | parachute games | rhythm balls rolled over joints of the body |
   | marbles and sand in a shoe box for foot and hand massage | |

6. Use art experiences with paint rollers. This activity moves the left arm across to the right and vice versa, which crosses the midline of brain hemispheres. By crossing midline you are helping to strengthen both hemispheres so the resident has a greater repertoire for responsiveness.
7. Create activities which encourage and promote body movements (leaning forward or with head leaning back).

---

[24] Adapted from Marsha Allen Workshop on Sensory Integration.

# Suggested Group Ideas[25]

## *Relaxation and Therapeutic Touch Group*

Ocean sounds can be the musical background for the activity. Each resident would receive a hand massage, a shoulder rub and the vibrator used after s/he is relaxed enough to accept the stimulation.

## *Body Awareness Musical Group*

Choose music such as Simon Says or songs which refer to noses, faces, hands, etc. The leader may touch the residents' hands for body identification.

## *Animal Assisted Therapy Group*

The tactile experience of holding an animal up to the resident, on their lap or in their hands.

## *Sensory Box*

Leader places resident hand or hands into a piece of soft furry fabric. This piece of fur could be of value with residents who are highly sensitive to touch.

## *Exercise Group*

Any exercise group or one-on-one experience can help a resident to be aware of a body part or to move that part.

A breathing idea is shown on the following page.

---

[25] A good book with 86 additional activities for residents with significant cognitive impairment is Parker and Will, 1993, **Activities for the Elderly, Volume 2, A Guide to Working with Residents with Significant Physical and Cognitive Disabilities,** Idyll Arbor, Ravensdale, WA.

# The Breath Experience

Regardless of the activity, incorporate breathing. Our breath not only enhances circulation and focused attention, but also encourages relaxation and a multi-sensory experience of self.

Begin each and every group with an awareness of body and breath in whatever way is possible.

**Activity Ideas**

1. (A E I O U) vowel repetition by all participants.

2. Blow a feather or Ping Pong ball across the table.

3. Party blowers, whistles, kazoos or pinwheels provide visual and/or auditory stimulation; then incorporate or reinforce the activity with use of one's breath.

4. Blow bubbles. Client touches falling bubbles and blows bubbles as they fall close to him/her.

5. Play a familiar (or just active) song and encourage humming along with movement to the music.

6. Play an environmental tape of the ocean and assist clients in stretching arms up and breathing.

7. As in all groups, let the participants know that the group has ended (closure) with a special song, hand shake, hug, clapping, etc.

# Level 2: Sensory Awareness/Sensory Stimulation Activities

The goals of Sensory Awareness and Sensory Stimulation Activities are to:
- elicit response or increase level of arousal
- prevent sensory deprivation
- encourage the individual to use the senses to respond to stimuli

The type of residents who need these activities include those who show problems with:
- severe disorientation
- cognitive and sensory deficits
- lack of ability to respond without sensory inputs
- self-stimulation
- deficits in sensory/perceptual integration
- rigid body and posture
- avoiding eye contact
- constant movement whether in wheelchair or not

The way you need to lead these activities includes:
- using touch
- being consistent
- being respectful
- expecting a response (self-fulfilling prophesy)
- speaking to the resident in an adult manner regardless of the lack of response
- using direct eye contact
- repeating, repeating, repeating
- letting them know you enjoy being with them
- being yourself
- using visual and verbal cues
- analyzing the stimulation level to avoid over-stimulation

## Importance of Sensory Awareness and Sensory Stimulation

One of the Activity Professional's most important goals is to provide each resident with a good quality of life in a long-term care setting. Obviously, this presents many challenges. One of the most critical and inclusive is that of providing adequate stimulation to each resident. The importance of *stimulation* (a human sensation and a response to one's environment) must not be minimized. If an individual fails to receive stimulation to his/her senses, the natural developmental process is thrown off track. In infants and very young children, for example, the lack of a loving human touch may produce a condition called "failure to thrive" which can threaten the very survival of the baby. This failure to thrive is also a critical risk to the very old if they no longer receive the most basic level of sensory stimulation that life requires.

Stimulation can be sensory, emotional, social and cognitive. When an individual at any stage in life is unable to reach out for stimulation, it must be provided through activity, environment and one-on-one interactions. Meeting these stimulation needs is one of the most crucial components that must be addressed when planning a resident's program.

This need should be addressed throughout the comprehensive assessment process. The Activity Professional's goal of providing each resident a high quality of life in a long term care setting can be furthered when an interdisciplinary approach is used. Notions that may seem abstract such as culture, individuality, autonomy and environment become real and down to earth when seen as opportunities for resident stimulation and growth.

Because people need a variety of sensory input and involvement to maintain their contact with reality, sensory stimulation is often an important aspect of long term care. Individuals who have not been responding for an extended period will often respond to changes in the sensory environment. All of the **feeling, hearing, seeing, smelling**, **tasting and moving** that an individual does during his/her waking hours makes up his/her sensory input; if this is limited, s/he will lose contact with reality.

Stimulation occurs when an individual interacts with the world and people around them. Stimulation helps one stay able to identify, process and then respond to stimuli and events. It is how we understand and interpret the experience of being alive. The charts on this page show the types of stimulation and sources of stimulation that are important for residents in long term care facilities.

# Categories of Stimulation

|  | sensory | emotional | social | cognitive |
|---|---|---|---|---|
| level of involvement | basic neurological stimulation — body responds at the basic nerve level | more complex reaction to stimulation— the interpretation and recognition of stimulation from the sensory level which is then interpreted by past memories | | |
| types of stimulation | touch proprioceptive smell sight vestibular taste hearing | anger insecurity pleasure desire | feed me, I'm empty desire for others need for friendship | memory (long and short term) problem solving sequencing |

# Sources of Stimulation

| Environment | People | Internal |
|---|---|---|
| Natural (uncontrolled) or controlled stimulation in the resident's environment which stimulates the basic senses as well as the higher senses of emotions and cognition | This is separated from environment only because we are so purposeful in the way we try to use ourselves (and tools) to make up for a lack of stimulation in the resident's environment | Stimulation originating within the resident him/herself. Includes proprioceptors and things like pain (e.g., from gas) or hearing voices. |

# Staff Involvement in Sensory Stimulation

In order for a sensory stimulation program to be successful, all staff members need to understand not only its therapeutic value, but also how they can use this type of stimulation in their work with the residents. The Activity Professional should provide inservice training and various tools and forms for staff use. Examples of the forms are shown on the following pages.

## Sensory Stimulation Supply List and Assessment Form

This form identifies supplies to be used in this program. Each item should be assessed for *all* possible types of sensory stimulation. As an example, "magnetic letters" would be assessed as a supply item which could be used for tactile and visual stimulation. It could also be a kinesthetic (body in motion) stimulation. If the staff person was requesting that the resident move the letters around and spell a name, this could be a cognitive stimulation tool also. The intent of the form is to be sure that all of the supply items have been assessed as to types of stimulation, safety issues and appropriate use. The comment section should be used to address safety and specific uses of the supply item.

We recommend that you have the following items available for a sensory stimulation program:

| | | |
|---|---|---|
| Tangles | Velcro catch game | Stuffed animals |
| Slinky (plastic) | Velcro strips | Name cards |
| Magnetic letters | Koosh balls | Cooking items |
| Ring toss | Writing materials | Busy boards |
| Parachute | Eraser board | Busy aprons |
| Dominoes | Water puzzles | Gardening items |
| Large print cards | Pat Mat (plastic pillow filled | Mystery box |
| Flash cards | with water and a sponge) | Fabrics & textures |
| Coasters to stack | Texture books | Musical instruments |
| Hankies to fold | Scratch & sniff | Etch a Sketch |
| Clothespins | Scents | Hardware trays |
| Maps | Pictures to sort | Wood working games |
| Grooming items | Photos to look at | |

We also recommend that each facility has at least one "Spinoza Bear" for use with residents. The Spinoza Bear is not only a soft, cuddly teddy bear. It is also a carefully designed, dynamically effective therapeutic tool that provides sensory stimulation. It comes with a library of tapes. You can order a Spinoza bear from Spinoza, 245 E. 6th Street, St. Paul, Minnesota 55101-1940. Phone: 1-800-CUB-BEAR.

## Sensory Supply Card

Each sensory supply item should have a separate card filled out on its use and goals. These should be available on a ring or in a binder attached to the supply box. We can never assume that everyone understands how to use a specific supply item. A photo of each supply item could be attached to the card describing it. It is a good idea to laminate the card.

## Resident Activity Cards

Each resident who has been assessed as in need of sensory stimulation should have a card filled out with specific and individualized information about his/her interests, responses and types of supplies which s/he has responded well to. Also include any activity which seems to decrease anxiety and elicit interest and focus away from an undesired behavior.

# Sensory Supply List

## Type of Sensory Stimulation Provided

| Supply Item | Tactile | Auditory | Olfactory | Gustatory | Visual | Kinesthetic | Cognitive | COMMENTS |
|---|---|---|---|---|---|---|---|---|
| | | | | | | | | |
| | | | | | | | | |
| | | | | | | | | |
| | | | | | | | | |
| | | | | | | | | |
| | | | | | | | | |
| | | | | | | | | |
| | | | | | | | | |
| | | | | | | | | |
| | | | | | | | | |
| | | | | | | | | |
| | | | | | | | | |
| | | | | | | | | |
| | | | | | | | | |
| | | | | | | | | |
| | | | | | | | | |
| | | | | | | | | |
| | | | | | | | | |

# Sensory Supply Cards

**Name of Supply Item:** _____

**How to Use It:** _____

_____

_____

**Goals:** _____

_____

_____

**Comments and Precautions:** _____

_____

_____

_____

**Date Written:** _____

**Author:** _____

# Resident Activity Card

**Resident Name:** _____

**Identified Leisure Interests:** _____

_____

_____

**What does this resident respond well to? Explain:**

_____

_____

_____

**What specific sensory supply items work best with this resident?**

_____

_____

_____

_____

**Safety Precautions and Interventions:**

_____

_____

_____

_____

**Additional Comments:** _____

_____

_____

_____

**Date Written:** _____

**Author:** _____

# Sensory Awareness Ideas[26]

Flashlight games to increase visual tracking. One game might be flashlight movement to music. Cover the light with colored cellophane to increase interest.

Glow in the dark balls and other materials can be used for games of toss and catch or hide and seek.

Straws to blow ping pong balls or paint across paper (group or individual) or cotton balls or whatever a straw can blow. Good for increasing lung power and speech skills.

Tearing newspaper or colored paper and playing freely as if they were Fall leaves. Then recycle into papier-mâché or stuff paper sacks of various sizes and play games of toss and catch or make a collage or seasonal decorations.

Use paper punches for activity similar to the one above. Increases hand strength and eye-hand coordination.

Matching a pile of shoes or socks or shirts. Teaches sorting and categories.

String painting with paint applied between two pieces of paper.

Milk cartons for bowling and building. They are inexpensive and lightweight.

## Shadow Design

| | |
|---|---|
| Equipment: | Slide projector or some similar light source. |
| Activity: | Aim projector light at wall or sheet or large piece of paper. |
| For: | Gross motor development and body awareness. To learn concepts; i.e., large and small, right and left. For increasing imagination/creativity. To have fun. |
| Examples: | Make yourself tall/small, move right or left, up or down pretend to be a bird, giant rock, move only your arms, for dancing and movement to music. |

## Hair Dryer Bubble Blow

| | |
|---|---|
| Equipment: | Old 1960's hair dryer or a fan and bubble soap. |
| Activity | Empty room of objects and start making lots of bubbles by holding bubble wand in front of blower. Touch the bubbles in free form movement. |
| For: | Increasing visual tracking skills as measured by following the movement of the bubbles, eye-hand coordination, enhancing imagination, for fun. |
| Cautions: | Bubbles make floors slippery. Use carpeted areas. |

---

[26] The ideas through **Tactile Finger Walk** are from Lois Herman Friedlander, RMT, MFCC.

## Free Form Ball Toss

| | |
|---|---|
| Equipment: | A dozen or more balls of soft texture in varying sizes. |
| Activity: | Empty the room of obstacles and throw balls at each other, kick balls to each other, roll them, kick backwards, etc. |
| For: | Increase body awareness through hand, eye and foot movements. Increase balance. |

## Free Form Pillow Toss

| | |
|---|---|
| Activity: | Variation on above ball activity but pillows have the advantage of being easier to manipulate for catching and throwing or kicking with feet. |

## Powder and Facial Scrubber Time

| | |
|---|---|
| Equipment: | As many Clairol Facial Scrubbers as necessary for your group. |
| Activity: | Put hypoallergenic powder on arms and "erase" it with the scrubber. |
| For: | Utilizing visual tracking skills, eye-hand coordination, enhancing imagination, for fun. |

## Tactile Finger Walk

| | |
|---|---|
| Equipment: | Peach packing materials from the local grocery or newspapers or mylar. |
| Activity: | Place materials on table. Have participants manipulate material. |
| For: | Utilize tactile awareness and discrimination, increase gross motor movement. |

---

### Humor

1. Humor has been defined as "A sense of joy in being alive." Humor should be incorporated in all activities. It creates a sense of playfulness and should be provided on an age-appropriate basis.

2. Individuals in stress and confusion oftentimes revert back to a happier time. We see this often in individuals who are no longer in touch with reality.

3. If we can offer a setting which is safe and playful — we may be providing a wonderful gift of not only reality but reminiscence to a happier time.

## Potpourri Sachet

| | |
|---|---|
| **Purpose:** | Olfactory Stimulation |
| **Skills Necessary:** | Verbal, fine motor coordination, ability to follow directions, moderate cognitive ability |
| **Goals:** | Utilize motor coordination (gross and fine)<br>Stimulate sense of smell<br>Complete a short-term task<br>Increase self-esteem by successfully completing the project |
| **Objectives:** | Each participant will make one potpourri sachet.<br>Each participant will participate in the use of a sachet. |
| **Materials:** | Cloth (to be cut into 4" to 5" square pieces)<br>Yarn or thin cloth ribbon<br>Fragrant dried flower petals (rose, lilac, gardenia or cedar chips)<br>Small bottle of fragrance oil |
| **Process:** | (Prior to activity pick and dry flower petals and treat with a few drops of fragrance oil — gardenia, rose, floral, etc.)<br>1. Seat participants around table.<br>2. Have prepared:<br>      cloth cut into 4" to 5" squares<br>      yarn or thin cloth ribbon in 4" to 6" lengths<br>      rubber bands<br>      mixed dried petals, enough for each participant.<br>3. Have each participant smell potpourri.<br>4. Have each group member:<br>      lay piece of cloth flat<br>      place dried petals in the center of the cloth<br>      fold edges up around the "potpourri"<br>      secure at top with a rubber band (may need assistance)<br>      tie ribbon in a bow around the rubber band.<br><br>optional — add string, yarn or thin cloth ribbon for hanging in room or bathroom or leave plain to freshen up drawers.<br><br>Provide closure for group. Thank each participant for attending. |

## Spice Kitchen

| | |
|---|---|
| **Purpose:** | Olfactory Stimulation |
| **Skills Necessary:** | Verbal, moderate cognitive functioning |
| **Goals:** | Promote/utilize stimulation skills<br>Practice interpersonal skills<br>Utilize discrimination skills<br>Access long term memory<br>Promote/utilize expression |
| **Objectives:** | Each participant will smell and identify at least one spice. |
| **Materials:** | Herbs and spices (cinnamon, anise, pepper, sage, cloves, lemon peel, orange peel, onion, chives, garlic, mint, oregano, horse radish, etc.) |

**Process:**

1. Gather participants around a table.
2. Give each participant an herb or spice (may have to distribute scents individually throughout activity to preserve group structure).
3. Choose starting participant.
4. Allow each group member to smell and identify his/her herb or spice.
5. Repeat process until all participants have had a turn.
6. Summarize participants' reactions related to herbs and spices.
7. Thank each participant for attending.

**Potential Problems and Solutions:**

1. If participant is nonverbal, s/he can identify scent through gestures and facial expressions or by group leader using questions in which responses are yes/no.
2. It is important to allow time for reminiscing between smelling of scents to allow "smell" sensors to become neutral.

| | |
|---|---|
| **Adaptation:** | Activity can be done on a one-on-one level and have participant identify several "kitchen" scents. |

# Sensory Stimulation Activities[27]

## Sight/Vision

Contrasting colors are most important to enhance visual stimulation. Colors such as red and orange are the easiest to see. Large cards and pictures of bright colors work well with residents who have poor vision. Other ways of using visual stimulation include showing slide pictures or using playing cards with pictures.

Play a game that increases visual experiences by placing a number of objects on a tray and having the participants name the objects. After the participants observe the tray for 3 minutes remove it and have the participants try to name all the objects on the tray. A variation would be to remove one or two of the objects and have the participants try to remember what was removed. Start with 6–8 objects and increase or decrease appropriately. Some other activities and objects to use for visual stimulation include:

| | |
|---|---|
| hiding activities | colorful objects |
| slides | tracking activities |
| electronic games | maps |
| mirroring/mirrors | different colored glasses |
| posters | TV |
| photos | flash lights |

Other ways to stimulate the sense of sight include:

1. Using a flashlight, move the light slowly in different directions for the individual to focus on and track.
2. Turn the light off and on slowly, then move quickly.
3. Shine light on different parts of resident's body.
4. Shine light on different people. If they are able to, ask the residents to identify or acknowledge those people in some way.

## Touch/Tactile

The fingers are filled with receptors that are stimulated by shapes and textures. The lips are also very sensitive to touch. The skin is the largest sensory organ of the body and touch is perceived differently in various areas of the skin. The entire surface of the body is capable of receiving sensory stimuli from the environment. Besides touch, the tactile senses also include pressure, temperature and pain.

Three of the most pleasurable tactile experiences include:
1. to be lovingly touched by another person i.e. hug, massage.
2. to feel the warmth of the sun on one's skin.
3. to hold an animal, i.e. SPCA visits or adopt an animal at the agency.

*Remember:*
1. Use tactile stimulation to arouse as well as to quiet.
2. Verbally describe activity or object, feel it, taste it. Ask about sensation received from a resident who is verbal, describe it for a resident who is nonverbal. Ask about preference and feelings. Describe the properties — soft, hard, rough, firm, warm, cold.
3. Introduce gradually. No more than three things at a time. Use it at least four consecutive sessions before introducing new things. Return when nine have been presented. Repeat set of nine 3 times before introducing new textures and sensations.

---

[27] This section (through the Surprise Bag Activity) was written by Ann Nathan, MS, CTRS and Elizabeth Best Martini, MS, CTRS, used with permission.

To stimulate an individual's tactile sense, objects may be placed in old socks, passed behind backs or under the table. Participants may try to determine what the objects are. A variation is to label paper bags with each letter of the alphabet, fill them with one or more items beginning with that letter and have the participants guess the object. Keep in mind that putting more than one item in a bag may be confusing to some individuals. Be careful with small items that could be put into the resident's mouth and cause choking. Rubber balloons are especially dangerous in this regard.

Some items that might be included are:

| | | | |
|---|---|---|---|
| apple | hair brush | oyster shell | sticky tape |
| balloon | harmonica | pipe | thimble |
| clothespin | ice tray | pliers | under shirt |
| cotton ball | jelly beans | quill | vegetable |
| cuff links | key | raisin | Velcro |
| dice | lemon | rubber ball | wishbone |
| eraser | marshmallow | softball | letter X |
| fork | nut | spool | yarn |
| golf ball | orange | spoon | zipper |

Another touching exercise is to give the participants a variety of objects to feel one at a time. If they are able to, the participants may be asked to describe one element of what they feel or they may guess the object. Some possible objects include:

| | | |
|---|---|---|
| cork | rope | sandpaper |
| corn silk | bird feather | grooming items: |
| leaf | candle | (shaving cream, |
| rubber glove filled with sand | styrofoam | powder puff, |
| velvet | thimble | make-up brushes, |
| peeled hard boiled egg | wet sponge | emery board, |
| flower | ice | lotions) |
| moss | raw potato, half peeled | |

The rubber puzzles that are manufactured commercially provide good tactile stimulation also. One can make his/her own game by selecting a shape such as a heart, circle or other geometric shape and cutting the pattern from materials with a variety of textures i.e. velvet, cork, card board, burlap, satin, plastic. Each shape is then cut into several pieces and all are put together in a box. Participants pick out the pieces and match them by their texture. When all pieces have been separated, the puzzles can be put together.

Sensory integration utilizes many of the same modalities. Refer to Sensory Integration for proprioception and vestibular stimulation activities.

## Taste

The sense of taste depends on receptors located on the taste buds which are on the tongue. There are four taste sensations; sweet and salt on the tip, sour along the sides and bitter along the back. After the age of fifty, there is an increase in the threshold of sensation for all four taste qualities. Because of these changes, those who are older need an increased amount of stimulation in order to get an adequate taste sensation.

Any experience with eyes closed increases taste awareness. It is interesting to see how many tastes one can identify with their eyes closed. Some tastes that they might identify.

| | | | | |
|---|---|---|---|---|
| allspice | honey | syrup | lemon | peanut butter |
| mocha | cinnamon | nutmeg | root beer float | |
| pickles | licorice | wintergreen | chocolate | |
| vanilla | berries | peppermint | orange | |

## Smell/Olfactory

A sense of smell seems to have an effect on emotions (i.e. pleasant, unpleasant, harmful etc.). Care should be taken to prevent the resident from tasting some of these items. Use sharp, distinct smelling substances (i.e. perfumes, colognes, soaps, flowers, herbs, food products, etc.). What smells are common to your environment? Refer to other segments of this chapter. A small amount of different substances may be put into jars and participants may guess the contents. Some suggestions include:

| | | | |
|---|---|---|---|
| vinegar | nutmeg | fresh cut grass | banana |
| vanilla | cloves | rose | almond |
| bay rum | coffee | sherry | tea |
| lavender | lemon | lilac | apple |

## Hearing/Auditory

To stimulate the sense of hearing, a leader or participant may make a series of sounds and may ask for identification and/or direction. The following are some suggestions:

| | |
|---|---|
| pouring water | balling up a piece of paper |
| common sounds in your particular environment | clinking ice in a glass |
| striking wooden matches | own voice on tape |
| rubbing two pieces of sandpaper together | jingling coins together |
| shaking a wind chime | slamming a door |
| rubbing wood against wood | banging an aluminum pie plate |
| ripping a newspaper, tearing paper | balling up dry leaves |
| hitting a spoon against bottles with different amounts of water in them | thumbing through a book |

Another suggestion to stimulate hearing is to drop different items and let the participants guess what was dropped. i.e.:

| | | | |
|---|---|---|---|
| book | marbles | coins | soft drink can |
| rubber ball | aluminum pie plate | keys | basketball |
| plastic dish | tennis ball | golf ball | ping pong ball |

Participants may produce their own variety of sounds by utilizing their voices and bodies. Body sounds of clapping hands, snapping fingers, stamping feet and rubbing palms together can be done by many people. Vocally, sounds may include: clucking, whistling, blowing air through loosely closed lips, coughing, crying, laughing, humming and using a variety of pitches and degrees of loudness.

Listening and identifying nature sounds and the everyday environmental sounds are also good listening experiences. Other ideas:

| | |
|---|---|
| indoor recirculating fountains | chanting |
| large bird cage | roving reporter exercise |
| symphony of emotions exercise | conversation |
| singing | radio/TV |
| tapes — personal ones made by family, friend, therapist | |

See the activity description on the next page for one way to run this activity.

# Auditory Discrimination/Sequencing

**Skills Necessary:**　　Verbal/nonverbal, functional attention span, moderate auditory functioning, moderate cognitive functioning

**Goals:**

To promote/enhance auditory awareness
To promote/enhance memory recall
To promote/enhance socialization
To maintain/increase sequencing skill
To maintain/increase attention span
To maintain/increase discrimination ability

**Objectives:**

1. Each participant will differentiate between at least two different sounds played by group leader.
2. At least 50% of group participants will appropriately sequence more than two sounds (i.e. sticks, bell, drum, snap, clap, hand swish).
3. Each participant will verbally identify (or point to flash cards for) two sound producers.

**Materials:**

- Variety of sound-producing instruments or objects (not exceeding more than five per activity).
- Hide sound producers in a box, under the table, behind chalkboard, etc.

**Process:**

1. Seat participants around a table.
2. Explain to participants that various sounds (hidden to them visually) will be produced for them to listen to and identify.
3. Begin by having the group identify the individual sounds which you have selected.
4. Choose a starting participant.
   a. Produce a sound and have the participant identify it; or turn toward the sound or respond in any way possible.
   b. Produce a second sound and have participant identify it.
5. Repeat process with each participant.
6. Select a participant.
   a. Produce three successive but different sounds.
   b. Ask participant to identify them in the order that they were produced.
7. Thank each participant for attending.

**Problems and Solutions:**

1. Try to use sounds that are distinctly different. Some sounds may be too similar for participants to differentiate.
2. If a sequence of three sounds is too difficult, encourage the group to help or cut back to two.
3. If three sounds are too easy, add more sounds.
4. Flash cards of each sound can be made to assist those with verbal limitations.

**Adaptation:**

Sounds could be categorized by certain themes (i. e., air sounds, animal sounds or sounds in the facility).

# Paint Bags

**Skills Necessary:**          Verbal/nonverbal, minimal fine motor skills, low cognitive skills

**Goals:**                     To maintain/increase fine motor dexterity
                               To maintain/increase direction following
                               To promote/enhance creativity and self-expression

**Objectives**                 Each participant will move finger, hand, foot, etc. along bag creating a design.

**Materials:**                 zip-lock bags
                               various colors of tempera paint

## Process:

1.  Group leader makes bags taking each zip lock bag and filling it with one color of paint (medium consistency). Use just enough paint so that bag is fully covered but can still lie flat.
2.  Gather participants around one table, if possible, or two pushed close together.
3.  Place a paint bag in front of each and explain (while demonstrating) that it is to be used like a writing tablet.
4.  Suggest simple designs, letters or numbers to be drawn on the paint bag with finger. Allow time for participants to comply, repeating and assisting when needed.
6.  Explain and assist participants in smoothing design off bag front.
7.  Repeat process 5 and 6 using various suggestions according to group skills.
8.  End the activity by having participants sign their names or make a hand print in the paint bag.
9.  Thank each participant for attending.

## Problems and Solutions:

1.  Participants who are lower functioning may not be able to independently move fingers or to follow directions. Provide assistance while allowing participant to utilize maximum capabilities.
2.  Suggest more complex designs for participants who are higher functioning or allow them to create pictures of their own choosing.

## Adaptations:

1.  Various liquid mediums could be used (i.e., colored vegetable oil, colored sand, etc.) to provide a variety of tactile stimulation.
2.  More than one primary color can be used for some residents.

# Sand Hide 'N' Seek

**Skills Necessary:**   Verbal/nonverbal, minimal fine motor skills,
low to moderate cognitive skills

**Goals:**   To promote/enhance memory recall
To promote/enhance visual and tactile stimulation
To maintain/increase fine-motor coordination

**Objectives:**   Each participant will attempt to find an object in the sand at least once.

**Materials:**   Plastic tub, bucket or box filled with sand and/or cornmeal
Ten small objects of various sizes and shapes (i.e. comb, ball, blocks)

## Process:

1.   Arrange group around table (if group is large, use two tables and two tubs).
2.   Group leader will identify objects being placed in the sand.
3.   Place tub next to starting individual.
4.   Place five objects in tub and bury in sand.
5.   Request participant to put hands or foot in sand to become accustomed to its texture.
6.   Request participant to find one object with hand and remove it from the sand.
7.   Replace the chosen object with one not yet used, always keeping the same number of objects in the tub. When all ten have been used, repeat process.
8.   Thank each participant for attending.

## Potential Problems and Solutions:

1.   Participants who are low functioning may attempt to eat sand. Cornmeal may be used as a substitute.
2.   For participants who are nonverbal, promote the use of physical gestures (such as head nods, simulation of object use) as responses to questions asked by the group leader.
3.   If participants are unable to follow directions, use hand-over-hand method.

## Adaptations:

1.   Use shapes and colors rather than actual objects.
2.   Use large puzzle pieces. Each member pulls one piece from sand and, when all the pieces have been removed, the group attempts to put the puzzle together.
3.   Place marbles in sand and move hand or foot over them.

# Scented Group Mural

| | |
|---|---|
| **Skills Necessary:** | Verbal/nonverbal, minimal fine motor ability, minimal cognitive functioning |
| **Goals:** | To promote/enhance olfactory stimulation<br>To promote/enhance visual and tactile stimulation<br>To maintain/increase fine motor skills<br>To encourage cooperation within a group |
| **Objectives:** | 1. Each member of the group will contribute 1–2 pieces of yarn to the picture.<br>2. Any group members who are verbal will contribute at least one statement each concerning the scent of the yarn and its relation to the picture. |
| **Materials:** | Large cardboard sheet<br>Various colored yarn (cut in 1" strips)<br>Scissors<br>Glue<br>Oils or perfumes to pre-scent yarn according to the theme<br>(Could also use fresh fruit juices) |

**Preparation:**

1.   Group leader adds scent to the yarn the night before by dabbing yarn with various oils or perfumes of flowers, fruits, etc., according to chosen theme. Allow the yarn to dry.
2.   Group leader draws items from theme on cardboard, for example: fruit (apples, watermelon, grapes, etc.).

**Process:**

1.   Gather group participants around table.
2.   Group leader explains theme and the project, displaying the cardboard drawing.
3.   Give each participant yarn strips.
4.   Have group participants choose a strip.
5.   Put glue on small area of cardboard and demonstrate putting yarn on the board.
6.   Have first participant choose strip of her/his choice; glue the chosen area and place yarn on area.
7.   Repeat procedure for each participant.
8.   Discuss finished picture.
9.   Thank each participant for attending.

# Texture Collage

| | |
|---|---|
| **Skills Necessary**: | Verbal/nonverbal, minimal fine-motor skills, low to moderate cognitive functioning |
| **Goals:** | To promote/enhance tactile and mental stimulation<br>To promote/enhance socialization and awareness of others<br>To promote/enhance group cooperation<br>To promote/enhance self-expression<br>To increase eye-hand coordination |
| **Objectives:** | Each participant will place 2–3 objects on the collage. |
| **Materials:** | Large paper or cardboard piece<br>Textured items preferably centered around a theme<br>Glue |

**Process:**

1. Place participants around table.
2. Discuss already chosen theme (i.e. nature, spring, flowers, sports, games).
3. Spread out items that the group leader brought in related to theme. Have each participant choose at least 2–3 items that s/he will place on collage.
5. Place large cardboard in front of starting individual.
6. Have participant point or express where s/he would like to place the first item.
7. Assist participant to put glue there.
8. Ask/assist participant to place item on glued area.
9. If able, participant pushes cardboard to next individual.
10. Repeat steps 6–9 until all participants have placed their items on the collage.
11. Discuss finished collage.
12. Thank each participant for attending.

**Potential Problems and Solutions:**

Some participants may try to eat the items. Hold back stimulation item until time to be used or implement close supervision.

# Surprise Bag

| | |
|---|---|
| **Skills Necessary:** | Verbal/nonverbal, finger sensation to feel objects, moderate cognitive function |
| **Goals:** | To promote/enhance tactile stimulation<br>To promote/enhance mental stimulation<br>To promote/enhance memory recall<br>To maintain/increase fine motor skills |
| **Objectives:** | Each participant will touch and may identify (if able) at least one object in the grab bag. |
| **Materials:** | Bag(s) (preferably cloth)<br>Ten small objects of various shapes and sizes |

**Process:**

1.  Seat participants in a circle.
2.  Explain to participants that there is a bag of objects in which they are to:
    a.  Reach in the bag.
    b.  Feel for an object that they can identify (if able).
    c.  Remove the object from the bag to confirm their identification.
3.  Choose a starting participant.
4.  Repeat process #2 with each participant.
5.  Optional: Reminisce about objects.
6.  Thank each participant for attending.

**Potential Problems and Solutions:**

1.  The group leader may need to give verbal clues to assist in identification.
2.  Flash cards of each object could be made in advance for participants who are nonverbal or for easier identification.

**Adaptations:**

1.  Objects can be based thematically such as kitchen items, babies, environmental themes, holidays, seasons, vocations, etc.
2.  Objects can be based on various shapes or colors.

# Therapeutic Use of The Vibrator[28]

*Always request physician approval for vibrator stimulation.*

The use of a vibrator is an excellent tool to be used in conjunction with other sensory awareness experiences.

Values of this tactile experience:
- To assist resident in body awareness and specific body parts.
- To stimulate sensory receptors and the kinesthetic/proprioceptive sense of self.
- To experience the sense of touch in a safe and relaxed setting; this is especially helpful in work with tactile defensive residents.
- To encourage a sense of exploration and curiosity of the world around them.
- To facilitate the experience of "feeling rooted" in one's body — even if only for a short duration of time.

Techniques for the use of the vibrator:

- Always tell the resident what you will be doing and what s/he will be experiencing. If possible, let the resident touch and feel the vibrator both on and off.
- Approach slowly to determine tolerance to touch and to the vibrator.
- Stop use of the vibrator if you sense the resident is experiencing any pain or discomfort — you want the experience to be pleasurable.
- Begin to touch resident on shoulders, arms or hands; avoid extremities if you are unfamiliar with the resident's medical condition.
- Vibrator use is most beneficial and successful with drug free participants; some medications will decrease one's sense of touch and awareness.
- The average amount of time to use a vibrator is 2–3 minutes per resident.
- Literature indicates that 10 seconds on and then 5–10 seconds off may be the most effective way of building sensory receptivity.

---

[28] Ross, Mildred, OTR and Dona Burdick, CTRS. **Sensory Integration**, p. 72, 1981, Slack, Inc., Thorofare, NJ.

# The Sensory Box

The sensory box is a concept created to stimulate the Activity Professional's imagination in working with residents who are limited in sensory and cognitive abilities. This can either be a box, a tray, an apron or any other idea that you create to reach out to those most in need.

This box or tray will be designed, used and adapted as you work with it. Design new changes or additions to meet individual needs. When designing it, design it so that it is easy to clean between sessions with different residents.

## Description

When working with residents who have regressed, a leisure goal could be to elicit focus, curiosity, response and involvement in a sensory experience — if possible. This would be through a multi-sensory experience. The response may be movement of the eyes or tracking of an object (visual), reaching to touch a bright object (proprioceptive, tactile), moving to music (auditory), tasting a piece of fruit (gustatory), recognizing or responding to a familiar scent (olfactory).

## CURIOSITY = EXPLORATION = LEARNING = RECREATING

### Creating the Sensory Box

The sensory box or tray can be created with almost any safe non-toxic, non-edible objects. Use a variety of objects to elicit responses to as many of the senses as possible. Determine if the box or tray is for:

> An initial sensory curiosity experience where the resident is not directly touching the objects, but receiving auditory and visual stimulation
>
> *OR*
>
> A hands-on sensory experience.

Create a box or tray which can be used as part of your inventory of supplies for special needs. Be sure to include a written picture and description of your creation.

### Some Sensory Box ideas:

A gift box with scarves to fold and tie together. Scarves can also be attached to Velcro to attach and remove.

Musical instruments in a box. Some of the smaller items can be Velcroed on to the box sides. A resident can touch them or pull one out and use it.

A box of familiar items to rekindle memories. It could be a box of ties, socks, chains, a wallet, a pocket watch or photos.

A television tray with magnetic letters and magnets attached which can be used as a communication board, color sorting or letter identification experience. (Remember, never place your magnetic letters near a computer or computer disks.)

A basket of balls of all colors, sizes and shapes.

A bed rail cover with Velcroed objects to stimulate a resident on bedrest during a one-on-one visit.

A plastic shoe bag with twelve pockets. Add gloves of different types and fabrics. They could be gardener gloves, evening gloves, plastic gloves, bicycle gloves, etc. This could be a visual experience or a tactile and sorting experience.

Different scents and oils on cotton balls. Each cotton ball can be placed in a zip lock bag with pin holes in it or in a nylon stocking kept in a plastic container.

Musical gloves. These are commercially purchased in a toy store. They are battery operated and make music when touched on the finger tips. They are also great for teamwork.

## Closing a Sensory Stimulation Session

In order to close the Sensory Stimulation Session, any of the following may be used:

1. a song
2. a poem
3. a story with a theme
4. a story book with moveable parts for group members to try or
5. a review of the time spent together in the group sessions.

Always reassure members that it was good to have shared the time together. Offer a handshake or a hug. Holding hands increases attention span. The day and date should be reviewed. A reminder statement should be given regarding the next group meeting time.

# Level 3: Validating Activities

The goal of validating activities is to validate the memories and feelings of individuals who are very disoriented. They do not focus on orientation but rather on the resident's perception of what happened in the past and his/her memory of this at the present time (correct or incorrect — it doesn't matter). For more on validation see Naomi Feil, 1993, **The Validation Breakthrough**, Health Professions Press.

Use these activities with residents who have the following characteristics:
- Moderate disorientation
- Time/place confusion
- Unawareness of environment
- Lack of rational thinking
- Locked into fantasy (as if to embrace a safer, happier time)
- Feelings are mirrored in body movements
- Distractible

Some of the things you need to do to make these activities work include:
- Use touch with approval
- Maintain eye contact
- Communicate with clear and repetitive conversation
- Acknowledge feelings
- Mirror movements
- Validate verbally both their feelings and fantasy
- Use active listening. If s/he needs to go home to feed the children:
  a.   acknowledge his/her thought
  b.   acknowledge his/her experience as a father or mother
  c.   state: "You must have very special children" or "What is your son's name?"
- Use age appropriate themes
- Encourage laughter and humor
- Be yourself

Some programming ideas which promote the validating process include:
- Name Games — to increase identity and sense of self
- Music — can be used as an opening and closure of group for structure
- Movement — body awareness and identification activities
- Hand/eye coordination exercises
- Parachute games
- Hand gesture games
- Ball games
- Trivia, simple matching games
- Pet programs
- Show-and-tell to stimulate feelings
- Visual cues
- Intergenerational programs
- Discussion groups which rekindle fond memories of different themes (kids, work, school, home, pets, food, holidays, travel)
- Unravel the meaning behind the responses you receive in conversation and body language
- Use simple creative/expressive program ideas

Another program idea is shown on the following pages.

# What's In A Name?

Giving someone back the memory of their name — *especially if they have forgotten it* — is giving them the gift of self. Our name not only represents ourselves, but the history of our family and a personal interest story about the people who named us.

**Purpose of Activity:**
1. To provide reality
2. To introduce each participant by name
3. To stimulate reminiscence of family and self
4. To encourage social contact within group
5. To learn the history behind different names
6. To provide a discussion-oriented group to participants who can respond successfully to direct questions regarding their names
7. To feel pride in oneself
8. To be recognized for yourself as the accomplishment
9. To be part of an enjoyable and sometimes humorous experience
10. To respond to the expectations of others
11. To reduce feelings of being disenfranchised

**Type of Appropriate Participant:** This group has been successfully offered to both alert and responsive participants as well as a group comprised of participants with cognitive losses.

**Duration:** 30 to 40 minutes

**Supplies Needed:**
Name tags (optional)
Library resource books **What to Name Your Baby, Origin of Names, Popular Names According to Years**
Famous First Names — Quiz
Family stories of names/nicknames
List of nicknames
Pictures of famous people (optional)
Well known records (to name famous singer) (optional)
Who Am I?

**Procedures :**
1. Place your participants in a circle facing one another.
2. You should be seated with the group, but able to move about and directly assist or respond to any of the participants.
3. **Begin the activity with yourself** — state your name and give a personal story about your name, family names, nickname, etc.
4. It is recommended that you add humor to your story since this will set a playful mood for the group.
5. After you share the story of your own name, go around the circle to each person.
6. Have each participant state their name, ask if they ever had a "special" name that their parents called them, etc.
7. Mention their last name and country of birth.
8. If one of the participants, upon hearing his/her name, becomes anxious and hesitant to respond, reaffirm the name and mention that you find it to be especially pretty or unique. This will help decrease his/her anxiety regarding the need to respond to you.

9.  Depending on how well the activity is received, you may begin the Famous First Name quiz. You name a first name and ask the participant's to call out a last name which comes to mind.
10. Using all the names of the group members, the leader may also design an art project displaying the names on a mural, a poem, a picture as a closure to this group or a future group.
11. **To close this group** the leader could go around the circle stating all the names and have each individual hear their name being spoken one last time.
12. Go around the circle and while stating each name, have the group member write the name in the air as an exercise.
13. End with a round of applause for the group.

**Other related program ideas :**

- Use this group as a progression towards a "beginning writing" group — where the participants write their signatures as a first exercise.
- When leading adults through any group process, add the element of education and human interest. This piques their interest in the topic and provides a sense of pride and dignity to the participants.
- Once an individual feels respect for you as facilitator, s/he will be more receptive to respond appropriately because *you* have that expectation of them.

# Level 4: Remotivating/Reminiscing Activities

Remotivation is a bridge between the time a resident is concerned only about his/her own problems and the time when s/he is ready once again to help others in the community. It is important for each of us to think of ourselves as an important, contributing member of a community. These activities are designed to help the resident see that they have contributed by looking at past achievements. The activities also help to point out that even if the resident has lost some level of functioning, s/he is still able to make a contribution.

The goals of remotivation activities are to:
- Start the process of bringing the individual back into the community
- Stimulate thinking about the real world
- Stimulate and revitalize individuals who have shown interest or involvement in the present or future
- Increase a sense of reality
- Begin practicing healthy roles
- Maintain present functional level

Use these activities with residents who have the following characteristics:
- Fearful of decreased cognition
- Short term memory loss
- Forgetful
- Passive
- Able to follow directions
- Good potential for progress

Some of the things you need to do to make these activities work include:
- Consistency
- Clarity of communication
- Encouragement
- Ability to facilitate responses
- Reinforcement of strengths and abilities
- Reinforcement for individuality and life
- Humor and laughter
- Touch and eye contact
- Being yourself
- Giving immediate feedback for involvement and response

The activities in this section are usually done one-on-one or with small groups, but notice that it is very possible to have both people in the one-on-one session be residents. The activities for remotivating and resocializing work together. A resident who is remotivated and is now working on resocializing can help you with another resident who is ready for remotivation activities.

With the right group of people you can create activities that run themselves with little effort on your part. Just make sure that each of these activities is documented to explain how and why it was beneficial to each of the residents.

Some ideas which are appropriate for Remotivation Groups include:
- Name Game
- Sharing stories of yourself with another resident or a group
- Gardening

- Cooking
- Pet Programs
- Familiar Themes (family, pets, work, food)
- Creative writing
- Exercise/movement/breathing
- Trivia
- The question book
- Life review

An interesting idea is shown on the following page.

# Food and Culture Class

**Description:**  Food and Culture is a class emphasizing social interaction and reminiscing, utilizing culture and food as a theme.

**Materials:**  Food to be prepared
Music, slides and visual aids to enhance the cultural theme

**Content:**  Use geography and culture as the basis for the class. Discuss:
1. music
2. dances
3. geography
4. memories

**Set Up:**  Have food, music and decorations set up in the activity or dining room. Also be sure to include residents who are confined to their rooms by taking decorations and food to them. Perhaps participants could have name tags with their names both in English and Italian.

**Activity Process:**
1. Welcome.
2. Introduction to theme "ITALY."
3. Movement to Italian music.
4. Geography and description of life in this country (slides, maps, photos, costumes, flags, weather, houses, families, customs).
5. Reminiscing/discussion. Discussion topics may include; travel, vacations, family heritage, people we know who are Italian, famous people who are Italian.
6. Class participants receive some token to wear which represents the country (flag, paper flower in country colors, name tag, copy of familiar setting in that country).
7. Social exchange with conversation to complement theme.
8. Food preparation or cooking experience (after lunch so as not to decrease appetite). Example: Bring in a pasta machine, explain how it works, pass out lengths of fresh pasta for tasting.
9. Discuss other Italian food experiences such as prosciutto ham and melon. Slice melon with a hint of ham for taste. Talk about where the melons are grown, etc. This section can be very adventurous and fun.
10. *Closure of class.* Using a few Italian phrases, thank participants and look forward to next week's class on: Morocco — exotic land of spices.

# Level 5: Resocializing

When an individual has participated and met the goals as a member of a remotivation group, s/he will be encouraged to build onto these social skills and continue to successfully interact with others. This is known as Resocialization. Resocialization can be considered step two in the process of bringing the individual back into the facility community.

The residents who are able to participate in resocialization activities are also likely to be able to engage in other thoughtful activities. The activities in this section encourage the resident to explore his/her feelings, as well as interact with others in a meaningful way.

The goals of resocializing activities are to:
• Finish the process of bringing the individual back into the community
• Stimulate and revitalize interest in other people
• Practice healthy roles
• Promote greater level of independence
• Encourage social interaction
• Build social skills
• Increase ease in social encounters with others
• Build relationships with other residents

Use these activities with residents who have the following characteristics:
• Able to follow directions
• Interested in socializing
• Interested in the concerns of other residents
• Good potential for progress

Some of the things you need to do to make these activities work include:
• Consistency
• Clarity of communication
• Encouragement
• Ability to facilitate interactions
• Reinforcement of strengths and abilities
• Reinforcement for individuality and life
• Humor and laughter
• Touch and eye contact
• Being yourself

You will also need to coordinate groups of residents who are willing to work together to help each other regain the ability and desire to socialize with others.

Some ideas which are appropriate for Resocializing Groups include:
• Sharing stories of yourself with another resident or a group
• Problem Solving Groups "What would happen if ... "
• Resident Council
• Creative expressive experiences
• Drama/role playing
• Life review
• Creative writing
• Helping others

- "Who Am I?" quiz
- Dear Abby

Other ideas follow. Many of these ideas are considered social service groups, often run by Social Service Professionals. There is no requirement about who should be in charge of them. As with all team situations, the person with the time and understanding of the goals and concerns should be responsible for creating and supervising the groups.

One good thing about these groups is that they involve residents who are able to function well enough cognitively to be part of a group. In many cases these groups provide a pleasant change of pace for the Activity or Social Service Professional. They allow group members to re-explore emotions that they may have felt they needed to check at the door when they came in. In a well functioning group, you will be able to have fun, too, as you explore the past and present through the eyes of people with significantly different experiences than your own.

**There are five important aspects to the design of a resocialization group:[29]**

1. "Climate of Acceptance" Use introductions to create accepting environment.
2. "Bridge to Reality" Read article aloud to develop a group theme.
3. "Sharing — The World We Live In" Develop topics through questions and visual aids to encourage responses.
4. "Appreciation of the Work of the World" Think of work in relation to selves.
5. "Climate of Appreciation" Take time to express pleasure with group and plan next meeting.

---

[29] Robinson, A. M. "Remotivation Techniques."

# Let's Talk![30]

## Fifty topics guaranteed to get discussion started

*Do you want to improve your residents' self-image, decrease their boredom, increase interaction among staff and residents, decrease negative resident behaviors and reinforce positive ones, plus stimulate verbalization? Group socialization sessions may be the answer. Conducting weekly group sessions just takes a little planning. Limit meetings to 30–45 minutes, have a definite structure and only include residents who are not disruptive in a group. Begin each meeting by asking residents to give the date. Next have members recite the names of others (to encourage memory and socialization). Then introduce new residents.*

*Now you're ready to move on to the topic. The session topics listed here are varied and have all been used successfully at a veterans' nursing home. They are designed to stimulate the senses. This is important because the elderly, whether institutionalized or at home, can become progressively nonverbal as the aging process diminishes vision, hearing and mobility. These 50 topics are general. By personalizing them you can boost your residents' verbalization and feelings of self-worth. Plus, leading a weekly group can be challenging and rewarding for you.*

## *WHAT TO TALK ABOUT*

### *Sensory Sessions*

**1. Colors:** Have residents name the colors of construction paper as you hold up the sheets. Ask if the color makes them feel hot or cold, sad or happy. Then name objects indoors and outside that are this color.

**2. Puppets:** Ask residents to tell stories, express feelings and portray fears, using the puppets.

**3. Wildlife:** Borrow stuffed animals from a museum or arrange for an animal expert to come to talk. Discuss habitats, mating, foods, pets and nature facts.

**4. Famous Lady For A Day:** Distribute wigs, hats and scarves to female residents and have each devise a costume and talk about whom she is portraying.

**5. Barnyard Visit:** Arrange with a local animal shelter or youth group to bring in various animals. Then have the residents discuss proper care for the animals; allow hands-on contact.

**6. Surprise Bag:** Give each resident a shopping bag containing a variety of small, common objects. Ask the residents to select an item and discuss how it is used.

**7. Botany:** Bring in fresh leaves or flowers. Ask residents to touch and smell them. Then talk about gardens and favorite plants.

**8. Halloween:** Let the residents "dress up" pumpkins with paint, glue and glitter. They can reminisce about dressing up as a child and maybe read aloud Washington Irving's *Legend of Sleepy Hollow*.

**9. Stuffed Animals:** Have residents give the animals names and tell where they might be found in nature or fiction. Discuss the toys the residents had as children.

---

[30] This section is by Harriet Berliner, RN-C, MSN, ARNP, geriatric nursing service at Harborview Medical Center, Seattle, WA.

**10. Ladies' Day:** Arrange with a cosmetics company to demonstrate products geared for elderly skin care. Discuss how residents used to dress up when they were young, fashion changes and different hair styles.

**11. Fashion Show:** Ask a local clothing store or specialty shop for the disabled to put on a fashion show. The residents can act as models and you can discuss fashions from powdered wigs to grunge.

**12. Art Critique:** Bring in sculptures and artwork in different media. (These can often be borrowed from a library or museum.) Discuss different art forms, likes and dislikes and favorite artists and their works. Let the residents touch the artwork and discuss the different textures and effects.

**13. Touch Stimulation:** Have each resident reach into a bag, close his or her eyes and try to match samples of various fabric swatches and sandpaper by touch.

**14. Architecture:** Using large sheets of paper and markers, draw simple house types and discuss them.

*Music Sessions*

**15. Favorite Music:** Get a tape player and cassettes of music from different time periods like the Big Band era. Residents can sing or clap to the music and reminisce about dates and dancing and favorite singers and groups.

**16. Sing Along:** Have someone play piano or guitar and then you can all sing "old favorites."

**17. Percussion "Jam":** Borrow instruments or make them using common items like combs. Let the residents "play along" to piano or taped music. This is especially fun at holiday times.

*Reminiscence Sessions*

**18. War Stories:** Talk about wartime job changes, hardships, rationing and loss of loved ones.

**19. Birthdays:** Discuss the ages of participants, who's the oldest and who's the youngest. How did they celebrate in the past? How would they like to celebrate now? Ask what age they would like to be again and why. How old would they like to live to be?

**20. Holidays:** Each month, discuss holidays and how residents used to celebrate them.

**21. Memories:** Use tapes or videos of old radio or television comedies and humorous old commercials. Have the residents name all of their favorite comedians and programs, tell some old jokes and discuss vaudeville versus the comedians of today.

**22. Home Cooking:** Bring fresh home-made bread. Then talk abut the residents' favorite meals, their own best recipes and helpful hints and their special cooking talents.

**23. Advertising:** Borrow old newspapers or magazines from a library and discuss old versus new products. How have things changed? Compare old and current prices.

**24. Home Remedies:** What did their mother give them when they were sick? Discuss advances in medicine, country doctors and home remedies.

**25. Presidents:** Have the residents name all of the presidents, then discuss old campaign slogans and different parties and platforms.

**26. Sports:** Show old sports films and talk about the residents' favorite athletes, "superstars," the Olympics and artificial turf.

**27. School Days:** Ask residents about their favorite teachers, schools, types of discipline, grading systems and best subjects.

**28. Occupations:** Discuss careers and jobs and how they've changed over the years, salaries, equal pay, women in the job market. Ask if they would work for a woman boss.

**29. Idols:** Have the residents talk abut the most influential people in their life. Then ask: Do you think you have emulated them? Whom do you feel you have had an effect upon? Can you name some famous world leaders?

**30. Old Cars:** Pass around photos of old automobiles. What was the resident's first car? What part has the auto played in their life (weddings, rushing to the hospital to give birth)?

## General Discussion

**31. Astronomy:** Hang up a large poster of the solar system. Then residents can name planets, describe their sizes and compositions and discuss space travel, astronauts and inventions. Ask if they would like to be astronauts and where they would go. What will future life in space be like?

**32. Geography:** Use a large map of the US or the world. Have residents show where they were born and have lived. Tell travel stories.

**33. Favorite Dinner:** Ask residents where they would go. With whom? What would they eat if they could go anywhere in the world?

**34. Let's Make A Meal:** Use pictures from diet or nutrition posters. Serve sliced fruit and iced tea or punch during discussion. Talk about proper nutrition, the food pyramid and plan a full day's menu. Have residents comment on how they feel about the food pyramid versus the four (or seven) food groups.

**35. Love:** What does love mean? Should everyone marry? Discuss weddings and families and today's morals versus the past.

**36. At The Movies:** Have the residents name all the cowboys, comedians, male and female stars, animal stars, villains, movie monsters and silent film stars they can.

**37. Plan A Picnic:** Plan the menu, date and time and enlist volunteers to barbecue or arrange for box lunches indoors. Discuss past family picnics.

**38. Ethnic Day:** Talk about ethnic souvenirs, photos and costumes brought by residents or their families. With the help of families and staff, this can be expanded to include ethnic music, food and decorations.

**39. Politics:** Use current events materials like newspapers and magazines. Discuss present world and national events. Talk about different political systems and how they're changing.

**40. Travel:** Choose a specific country and use slides, posters or film to start a discussion of dress, customs, foods, products and travel. Staff can also show vacation films.

**41. Guest Speakers:** Use the local college and hospital speakers' bureaus, which are often free.

**42. Values:** Ask the residents what beliefs and values are important to them. If they had their life to live over, what would they do differently?

**43. Shipwrecked:** Ask what three things the residents would pack in their suitcase if they knew they were going to be shipwrecked on a desert island.

**44. Literature:** Discuss favorite authors and books, story types and forms of writing the residents like best. Taping their stories to start a "living library" might be a good idea.

**45. Poetry:** Choose a poem and read it as a group or have a member read or recite one of his or her favorites. Discuss what it means, other poems remembered and poems they had to memorize as a child.

**46. Clowns:** Put up posters of clowns or circuses. Talk abut the types of clowns they remember, their favorites and circus memories. What makes people laugh?

**47. Life After Death:** What are the residents' religious beliefs, concepts of heaven and hell? Do they fear death? Do they believe in reincarnation?

**48. Inventions:** Discuss the first inventions made by man, the most significant ones, the most harmful. What would the residents like to see invented? Is man's life easier or harder today and why?

**49. Pen Pal Club:** Contact the local school or Scout troop and ask that they send letters and photos to the residents to be read and answered as a group.

**50. Alphabet Soup:** As you say each letter of the alphabet, have residents call out people, places and things that begin with that letter.

# Creating a Living History Group

One of the most difficult tasks of a leader working with people who are frail is to spark interest, generate conversation and discussion and keep them involved and curious in the events of the day.

**Why is Living History important?**

*"No one wants to be a footstep planted in the sand near the rushing sea, a footprint to be washed away into eternal waters, a sign seen for an instant and then erased forever. The sense of identity with other loving creatures, a sense of belonging to the human endeavor or being a part of creative movement, a realization that one's life has counted to someone else have to be realized by persons growing older."*
    *— author unknown*

Realizing that one's life has counted to someone else by having experienced something, shared this with others and made their lives richer and easier is giving life purpose. This purpose is important at all ages, but especially for people who are in the process of life review.

**How to develop a Living History group:**

The most important elements are personal interest, thought provoking questions and topics which can be "brought home." An example would be a headline of an air disaster. Instead of referring to this event as frozen in time, personalize the event with other events that some of your group may have experienced. "Do you recall when the Hindenburg blew up in 1937? How about the problems with the Apollo 13 flight to the moon? How did those affect you and your family?"

Then bring the group back to the present event. Now they have shared personal experiences and the facilitator should take this energy and direct it into discussion of current events. By incorporating the past and present, you are validating the importance of personal experiences and acknowledging that we all play significant roles, not only in our own lives, but in the lives of those around us.

**How to Begin a Living History Group**

Begin with a small group of approximately seven to eight individuals. It would be ideal to combine some people who are avid news readers and television watchers with those less involved but curious. This creates a good mixture.

Start with a few items on the news or in the paper to start off the class. Also mention the dates and weather conditions in your city and the home towns of group members.

Take the theme that you started the group with, such as, "The unemployment rate is increasing across the United States." Then bring the national issue closer to the group with: "What was your first job and how much did you make? How did Roosevelt's CCC program assist those troubled years?"

The group should now be in discussion, remembering years past and connecting them to events taking place today. It is rewarding for someone to feel proud in sharing personal anecdotes, taking pride in their citizenship and feeling that they are still involved in their world.

**Responsibilities of the Living History Instructor**

Be aware of your group member's special interests and backgrounds. Refer to this information and to the individual to acknowledge their accomplishments or experiences.

Have your materials prepared with at least three topics to work around. Avoid reading from the newspaper itself. If one topic shows little response, leave it and start another one immediately. Any lapses of time create distance with your group.

Feel comfortable in directing specific questions to a group member and asking for his/her opinion.

Encourage the group to get involved with voting issues and writing letters to the local Congressional Representatives regarding pertinent issues.

Take topics of interest from the group and incorporate these into future classes.

Share personal experiences which are taking place in your life and within the day-to-day confines with your class. Have them get involved with solving dilemmas which you are experiencing. This type of interactive problem solving and discussion among the group creates the ultimate goal of all groups: concern and involvement in a continually changing world.

# Pen Pals

**Goal:**            To provide a structured opportunity for residents in a long term care facility to write to residents in another long term care facility.

**Objectives:**
1. Establish a relationship with residents in a similar, yet distant, environment.
2. Compare emotional and physical likenesses in life styles in the two facilities.
3. Relieve the isolation created by living in a self-contained environment.
4. Re-use social skills (letter writing) not often employed after entrance into a long term care facility.

**Residents' needs/problems**:

For many residents who enter a long term care facility, the world outside seems to fade away as their world becomes more and more centered in the facility. Many also forgo the social skills they had used routinely. Even shopping and church-going provided some outlets for these skills. This group will provide an opportunity for the expression of social needs which an enclosed community cannot meet and will, hopefully, stimulate the ability to "reach out." It will also be a forum for comparing coping skills with others who are hospitalized.

**Number of residents involved:**            3 to 7

**Number of sessions:**            Optional

**Length of sessions:**            30 – 40 minutes

**How often:**            Weekly

**Agenda ideas:**
1. How do we initiate new friendships?
2. What is it about our everyday lives that we wish to communicate through letters?
3. Can we become interested in someone that we will never see and only know by way of written communication?
4. What can we say that will offer comfort/support to a new friend who is reaching out to us?
5. Do we really have the energy and need to expand our environment?

# Using Relaxation to Address Anxiety

**Goal:** To learn relaxation techniques in response to anxiety produced by living in a community environment and to share relaxation techniques that work for individuals who are participants in the group.

**Objectives:**
1. Offer a quiet, stress-free environment which will allow maximum participation in this activity.
2. Provide visual and word cues for use as personal focal points to initiate the relaxation process.
3. Exchange personal coping mechanisms with other group members.

**Residents' needs/problems**:

The group will begin each session with a series of exercises to relax the participants. Individuals will be given attention to ensure that everyone participates. After this portion of the class is completed, there will be group discussion and experimentation with ideas elicited from group members.

**Number of residents involved:** 6 to 12

**Number of sessions:** Optional

**Length of sessions:** 20 – 30 minutes

**How often:** Weekly

**Agenda ideas:**
1. What visual/auditory images do you use to separate yourself from your surroundings and begin to relax?
2. What are the barriers to relaxation that you currently experience?
3. What is the most effective way to create a stress-free environment in your present situation?
4. Drawing from your past, paint a verbal picture for the group of the most relaxing memory you can think of.
5. What relaxation techniques have you used successfully in the past?

# Living in an Institutional Setting

**Goal:**             To provide a special time in the week for participants to express feelings regarding loss of autonomy, to discuss replacements for losses and to provide a support network for participants by allowing them to share experiences.

**Objectives:**       1.  Stimulate discussion regarding issues of life change.
                      2.  Discuss coping mechanisms which have been adapted to a changing life style.
                      3.  Share feelings of loss and restructuring.
                      4.  Support change as an enabler.

**Residents' needs/problems**:
                      The basic group method will be discussion/sharing. Feedback will be given each week by participants, especially if anyone has tried a new coping skill.

**Number of residents involved:**      3 to 8

**Number of sessions:**                Optional

**Length of sessions:**                20 – 30 minutes

**How often:**                         Weekly

**Agenda ideas:**
                      1.  List the range of feelings you have experienced since you started living here.
                      2.  What facet of your previous life do you miss the most?
                      3.  What things can be brought from home to give you a feeling that you are living in a place that is more like you want it to be?
                      4.  Has there been any substitute person or thing in your current environment to help you cope with your lost autonomy?
                      5.  Do you find solace in accepting the fact that you are receiving care that you need?

# Life and Times in a Long Term Care Facility

**Goal:** To provide a structured opportunity for participants to express their feelings and concerns about living in a closed society, i.e. the long term care facility.

**Objectives:**
1. Discuss loss of personal freedom: what is the most significant loss for your?
2. Explore choices/options that are available in the long term care facility.
3. Relate successful/unsuccessful coping skills with others in the group.

**Residents' needs/problems:**
When living in our own homes, totally independent or with help, we are in control. Options are taken away when hospitalization becomes necessary. Some may never fully adjust to this lack of independence and limited choices. This group may provide a forum for involving residents more fully in their environment and giving them an opportunity to problem solve some of the obstacles to freedom of choice.

**Number of residents involved:** 3 to 7

**Number of sessions:** Optional

**Length of sessions:** 30 – 40 minutes

**How often:** Weekly

**Agenda ideas:**
1. What loss has been the most significant for you?
2. What do you do when the facility staff wants one thing and you want another?
3. What coping mechanism do you use to make it okay for you while you're here?
4. How do you assert your right to choice as provided by federal regulations?
5. What gain has been the most significant for you?

# About Music and Memories

**Goal:**            To provide a structured opportunity for participants to reminisce about music and the part it has played in their lives.

**Objectives:**      1.  Divide the decades between 1920 and 1960 into segments and focus on the most popular music of each era.
2.  Provide historical information which coincides with the music being presented.
3.  Identify memory associations of the music and history for each person who is able to express this.
4.  Interact within the group to stimulate memory and orientation.

**Residents' needs/problems**:

This group was formulated as an outgrowth of the weekly sing-along sessions, which attracted a cross section of residents, probably because of the high energy it provided and also because of the memories it seemed to stimulate. Residents who are not communicative and/or oriented in other areas are often able to sing along with the old songs or even dance. This group is an intellectual extension of that emotional experience.

**Number of residents involved:**          5 to 10

**Number of sessions:**                     Optional

**Length of sessions:**                     45 – 60 minutes

**How often:**                              Weekly

**Agenda ideas:**
1.  What is it about music that stimulates your emotions?
2.  Which music memory has the most significance for you?
3.  How does music influence your mood?
4.  Is there an era in music which reflects the time in your life when you were happiest?
5.  Have you created any music memories since you became a resident here?

# Cooking Class — Incredible Edibles

**Goals:**
1. Provide an opportunity for involvement in a familiar pastime
2. Achieve success in a short term activity project
3. Encourage socialization and team effort in a group
4. Reminiscing
5. Rekindling of a past interest
6. Opportunity to achieve success
7. Provide a time of enjoyment
8. Provide a nutrition-related activity to meet needs of residents and enhance self-care skills

**Equipment Needed:**
- Recipe
- Handiwipes or wet towels
- Big bowls
- Plates
- Measuring cups and spoons
- Electric skillet, toaster oven or convection oven
- Pot holders and hot pads
- Supply of spices, sugar, flour, etc. (these really enhance the group)
- Blender
- Utensils to serve and eat the finished product
- Some of these supplies may already be available through the Dietary Department. Be sure to plan these classes with the Dietary Supervisor to schedule times which work out for both departments.

**Length of Activity:** 1 hour

**Number of Participants:** 8 to 12

**Precautions and Adaptations:**
1. Be sure to place participants according to equipment proximity and helpful partners (i.e. a resident who is blind should be next to someone who will be willing to help him/her).
2. Check the bowl sizes so the resident will be able to reach inside easily.
3. Use utensils which are large and easily manipulated by hands with arthritis.
4. Be careful of all electrical wires, hot pans and placement of oils, liquids, etc.
5. CHECK SPECIAL DIETS BEFORE THE ACTIVITY BEGINS!
6. Create jobs for participants which will be success oriented, choice producing and achievable.
7. Be sure to praise each participant's efforts.
8. As often as possible, have the participants be responsible for decision making and choices of recipes and procedures.

**Procedures:**
1. Be sure that all participants have clean hands before beginning.
2. Pass Handiwipes to each participant to clean hands before each session begins.
3. Have the room all ready and prepared to begin. All ingredients, pictures of finished product and recipes should be on the table.

4.  Explain the recipe and procedures to the group. Detail special jobs that you will be delegating.
5.  Be sure that the recipe entails jobs for many hands. (If the recipe is made for individual servings, this is not a problem.)
6.  Find a recipe which can be completed within an hour's time.
7.  If this involves cooking/baking time, have something planned for the interim.
8.  Include nutrition and a discussion of the ingredients involved. Try to cook and make things which are nutritious and a supplement to the diet, if possible.
9.  Have the cooking group share favorite recipes with the group and try to schedule some of these into future classes.
10. When they are experienced enough, have the group make special hors d'oerves for a Happy Hour or prepare treats for staff recognition.
11. Don't forget your camera!

**COOKING CLASS IDEAS**

1.  Miniature pizzas (English muffins, cheese, mild sauce)
2.  Guacamole and chips
3.  Finger sandwiches (bread, cream cheese, olives)
4.  Blender fruit drinks (bananas, milk, yogurt, vanilla)
5.  Cookies and hot chocolate
6.  Melons, their history and differences
7.  Cold blender soups (tomato, cucumber)
8.  Pita bread with a variety of stuffing (taco style)
9.  Pigs in a blanket (small Hormel sausage in white bread)
10. Coleslaw
11. Club sandwiches
12. Quiche
13. Stir fried vegetables

# Men in a Women's World — Discussion[31]

When a man enters a long term care facility, he may suddenly become aware of an unusual phenomena. For the most part, he has entered into a world of women, where less than 30% of the population are men. That in itself is unusual; but what is more unusual is the fact that 80% of the staff are women, the majority of visitors appear to be women and that the main group of volunteers are again, women. It is not that he doesn't like women; it's a problem of being so grossly outnumbered and unrepresented in his male differences.

Another consideration for the new male resident would be the limited ability of other males to relate to him. More than 1/3 of the 30% of male residents appear to be mentally incapable of communicating or relating because of their medical and/or mental conditions.

It is interesting to note that the number of boys born makes for a greater population of males than females until the age of 18. The shift begins at this age, due to accident, suicide, war, lung cancer, emphysema and industrial accidents. By the time middle age is reached, the trend is to a greater female population.

For an Activity or Social Service Professional whose responsibility is to meet the needs and interests of each resident and to develop individual activity care plans, it has become an ever-increasing problem to plan successfully for men in long term care facilities. The majority of activities offered are oriented towards the majority population of women and it is women who attend the predominant number of activities offered.

> *One experience with a facility planning for a men's activity consisted of an afternoon special event where 15 men were brought into a small dining room. A woman wearing a coat entered the room, set down a tape recorder, removed her coat and began to belly dance for the men. The dancer was well endowed and wore enough veils to create a suggestive appearance. The veils were slowly removed. For some men, the movement and closeness of the dancer offended their religious beliefs. Others were well entertained. The staff was entertained, too, peeking in to see the men's reactions. After 15 minutes and 3 dances, the music stopped, the dancer was thanked, beer and chips were served and the men were taken quietly back to their areas. The belly dancer was the only program offered to the men.*

Our planning and scheduling of men's activities has got to involve more depth, consideration, balance and variety. Here are some basic concepts and recommendations for your consideration in planning activities for the men in your facilities.

The first step is vital and involves assessment of leisure interests. Without an individual assessment of each man's interests, you are not doing justice to their special needs. Review your assessment and activity check sheet and note the types of activities you review with the male residents. Most of the assessments being used have detailed and specific female-oriented activities. An approach to a male-oriented assessment is to include activities where you need to probe for more detail and specifics in discussing both likes and dislikes. For example, following the questions of whether a man enjoys fishing there should be details of what kind, where, when, with whom and how often. It would be most important in the interviewing and assessment process to concentrate on the individual and his background, rather than the content of your prepared activity program. (Besides, you are not meeting the requirements of OBRA if you gear your assessment to activities that you offer instead of activities that the residents are interested in.) There will be plenty of time to orient the resident to the existing activity program. Discussing only the existing program may act as a barrier to his opening up to express his particular interests and background.

---

[31] **Men in a Women's World** is by Michael Watters, CTRS. Used with permission.

The lack of leisure skills or mastery of specific activities in earlier life can cause problems in involvement later. Men are embarrassed to start a new skill with the fear of not being competent or appearing to be unsuccessful. Activity and Social Service Professionals will need to consider the fear of failure, self-consciousness or public showing of self with a disability as deterrents to a man's participation. Any one of the above mentioned situations can be enough to cause withdrawal or resistance to participation. It was also found that if a person had a positive view of himself earlier in life, that is generally carried over to later life skills. The same is true of a negative view of self and feelings of low self-esteem.

Another interesting fact appears to be that the blue collar worker engages in fewer leisure activities than those in white collar jobs and professions. The white collar and professional tended to work outside the home, in the community and with many different people. Their leisure activities tend to be more diverse and of an active nature. The blue collar workers tend to engage in more family-centered, home-based activities. Reasons were based on income, educational level, home locations, peer expectations and access to leisure areas. There appears to be a definite relationship between the man's job role and his use of leisure time. Consideration needs to be given to the elements of technical work, selling, manual labor, the number of hours worked, job isolation, the reading required for a job, the use of tools and specialty tools used, sociability on the job and overall responsibility which can be useful in developing a creative care plan.

Another major area of concentration and interest appears to be a man's family, especially the children. In a California facility, the Activity Professional asked a group of men meeting for the second time, what they were most proud of and each individual responded with glowing stories about his family. Men appear to talk a great deal about how proud they are of their families and can go into detail of the history of each child and grandchild.

Activity and Social Service Professionals should begin to make a concerted effort to recruit male volunteers, both group and individual, to provide the meaningful relationships which are otherwise lacking in other areas of the facility.

In one San Francisco facility there was a man who had been a union organizer for the garment industry. After entering the facility, he had reduced his activities to staying in his room and wearing only his bathrobe. Due to his long history as a San Francisco resident, he was asked to make a presentation for a special earthquake survivor party. He arrived, wearing his blue suit with a flower in his lapel and made a warm and sincere welcome to the gathering. This was the beginning of his continued role as the host and emcee at parties and special events for the facility.

If you search your facility, you will find duties, responsibilities and roles which give male residents some of those roles that have been lost or re-invest them in duties and activities which they have long since put aside.

For example: The Adopt-a-Grandparent program plays into the role of confidant, friend and family member which many have lost as their own family has diminished. Maintenance personnel may become involved by supplying ideas, materials and leadership for tinkering with projects which many of the men used to enjoy. Adapted setups for tools and work benches can give back a sense of work and productivity. Barbershop quartets, choirs, sports events and discussion groups can give some of the camaraderie which has been lost with the reduction of male social contacts.

In summary, although men represent a small minority in a world of women, their needs and interests should be given careful consideration, planning and timely involvement in the overall activity program. Being left out of the activity program services should not have to be another loss in the series of life's disappointments. Sincere efforts, specific programming ideas, recruitment of volunteers and groups, plus a commitment to involve men in dynamic programming can make a change in the life of a facility.

**Some specific program ideas include:**

- Making or repairing toys and children's furniture
- Construction of wooden animals
- Coin collecting
- Animal care and feeding
- Bone and horn polishing and engraving art
- Brass crafts
- Bonsai
- Printing
- Rope tying
- Contests and non-cash gambling
- Story telling of special events in history
- Cooperation games and events
- Films of famous men who may have had an effect on their lives
- Sport quizzes, trivia, records and events, personalities
- Men's group singing
- Activities sponsored by men's groups (social clubs, fraternities)
- Debate, Toastmaster speaking groups
- Mime and theater groups
- Walking club — wheelchairs included
- Metal smith work
- Wire work — soft wire sculpture
- Electrical work — tinkering with small appliances
- Soap carving
- Sawdust craft — relief maps
- Monthly breakfast speakers
- Speakers and visits to service equipment: fire station, ambulance, police station, farms, construction sites
- Hardware store owners who show the latest in tools
- Tournaments
- Liar's contest
- Lunch at a local men's club
- Fishing outings
- A day at the races
- Big Brothers sponsorships
- Adopt-a-Grandparent programs
- All male play readings
- Talent show
- Wood making projects
- Readers for the blind
- Teaching specialized subjects — computers
- Pool and billiards
- Bocce ball
- Bird watching — field identification
- Men's fashion show
- Rock collecting
- Stamp collecting
- Radio equipment
- Gold panning

# Men in a Women's World — Activity

**Goal:**        To provide a structured opportunity for men to discuss their lives in a society of women; i.e. the long term care facility.

**Objectives:**
1. Compare and contrast life in a long term care facility and life in a society as a whole: Who is in control — men or women?
2. Discuss individual adaptations to dependence on women for most care.
3. Interact in a group of mostly men to provide relief from the women's society.

**Residents' needs/problems:**

The men now living in long term care facilities have, for the most part, lived their lives with the assumption that men are dominant in society. It is assumed that they are the decision makers, the ones in control of their life situations. When long term care becomes necessary due to physical limitations, however, the status of men changes, as does the amount of their perceived control.

What effect does this have on the male ego, this loss of control and this entry into a society dominated and controlled and mostly populated by women? This group explores these issues with men in long term care facilities.

**Number of residents involved:**        3 to 5

**Number of sessions:**        Optional

**Length of sessions:**        30 – 60 minutes

**How often:**        Weekly

**Agenda ideas:**
1. What is it like to be in a matriarchal society?
2. How do you see your role?
3. How has this changed since you were "out in the world?"
4. What have you learned to do in this environment to enable you to assert yourself as an individual?
5. Is there any way you could have prepared yourself to live in this new "society?"

# Level 6: Cognitive Stimulation and Retraining Activities

Cognitive Stimulation is a term coined for techniques used in therapy to stimulate cognitive function and assist in retraining an individual to his/her optimum level of function. These techniques may also give an individual memory tools and strategies to compensate for a memory loss s/he has experienced.

There are many excellent resources in this field to draw from. Activity ideas may vary from concentration games, completion of simple tasks such as puzzles, color and shape sorting, connecting dot-to-dot puzzles, hand water games which involve sensory motor skills, analogies, trivia games, problem solving situations, etc.

Other valuable resources for memory retention and cognitive stimulation activities are the speech therapist, occupational therapist, recreational therapist and psychologist under contract with your setting. Each of these specialties will offer ideas specific to the immediate needs of the resident.

Memory and cognitive function techniques can also be utilized with residents who are there for short term rehabilitation even though they are generally focused on therapy goals and not interested in most of the other programs that are offered.

## Memory

In nearly all of the cognitive stimulation programs offered through the activity department, memory techniques and interventions will play an integral part.

Memory loss can occur for many reasons. Some of these may be related to depression, nutritional imbalance, medications and changes, emotional losses and significant transitions. Other reasons for memory loss are more organic such as a head injury, stroke, cerebral tumor or a progressive degenerative disease such as Parkinson's disease, Alzheimer's disease and other dementia disorders.

Memory takes place as three separate processes:

1. From our earliest experiences, we not only explore and learn new things — but, in addition, our brain registers this information. This is the first process of memory — Input.

2. The next function of memory is to store this new information in such a way that it relates to the experience. This is the second process of memory — Storage.

3. The final and most important function is the ability to retrieve and use the information experienced and learned before. In the retrieval process, the brain is able to dip into its bank of information and retrieve information specific to the current need. This is the last process of memory — Retrieval.

Memory is quite a miraculous feat and, of course, there are things that can go wrong in all three processes.

In addition to the three processes of memory there are also three types of memory:[32]

1. **Sensory Motor Memory:** From the physical and sensory experience, we use visual, auditory, tactile, proprioceptive, olfactory and gustatory senses. An example of this would be a smell that brings back a memory associated with it, the proprioceptive experience or whole body experience of walking on sand at the shore. This sensory motor memory seems to predate all other memory and leaves an imprint on us forever. Sensory stimulation is an intervention to restimulate and remember through this process.

2. **Short Term Memory:** The short term memory is the ability to experience and replay new information. Short term memory is exactly as stated, short term. If we read a map and go in that direction, we have processed the new information and applied it to the current task. If we are learning a new card game, we need to understand the rules and process them in order to successfully participate in the game. This is our working memory.

3. **Long Term Memory:** Long term memory is information which was stored a long time ago. It is our secondary memory. Some residents may not remember who you are or what their own names are, but they will be able to sing all the words of an old song. A similar example would be the ability to recite, word for word, a poem that was learned 60 years ago.

The more that one has memorized in their lives, the stronger the memory. In the early 1900's, education was based on memorizing material and reciting it in class. Because of this method, many of the individuals living in long term care settings can successfully recite and engage in activities which focus on long term memory skills.

Programs we develop need to include all three types and processes of memory. According to the individual's health issues, you can determine what type of memory intervention is most needed.

# Brain Function

The types of cognitive stimulation and retraining activities that are required depend on the diagnosis of the resident. Sometimes there is known damage to some part of the brain (as with a stroke). The chart below provides a brief summary of the functions of different areas of the brain and should help you understand which skills have been lost.

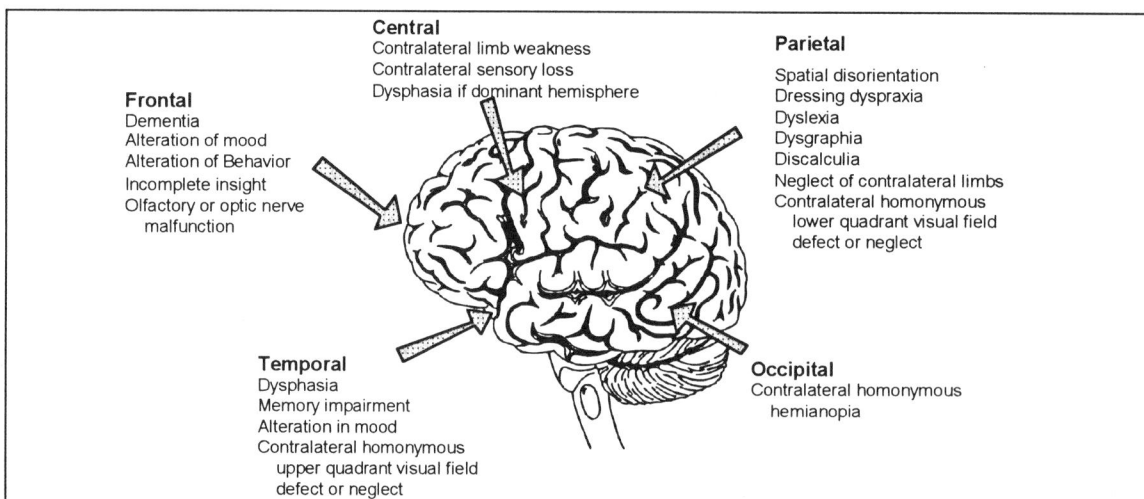

**Central**
Contralateral limb weakness
Contralateral sensory loss
Dysphasia if dominant hemisphere

**Parietal**
Spatial disorientation
Dressing dyspraxia
Dyslexia
Dysgraphia
Discalculia
Neglect of contralateral limbs
Contralateral homonymous
    lower quadrant visual field
    defect or neglect

**Frontal**
Dementia
Alteration of mood
Alteration of Behavior
Incomplete insight
Olfactory or optic nerve
    malfunction

**Temporal**
Dysphasia
Memory impairment
Alteration in mood
Contralateral homonymous
    upper quadrant visual field
    defect or neglect

**Occipital**
Contralateral homonymous
    hemianopia

---

[32] Atkinson, R. C. and Shiffrin, R. M., 1971, "The control of short-term memory and its control processes," **Scientific American**, 225, 82-90.

# Popular Games for Cognitive Stimulation[33]

The following is an alphabetical list of games that are commercially available which could be used in a cognitive stimulation program. This list is by no means comprehensive. The manufacturer of the game is provided after each entry (unless the game is available through several manufacturers) along with a listing by number of the cognitive skills required. The number coding of cognitive skills is as follows:

1. Perceptual accuracy — All games require perceptual (usually visual) accuracy to some extent but some focus on accuracy as a goal.

2. Spatial organization — Games requiring, as a basic focus organization of material in two or three dimensions are given this designation.

3. Perception-motor functioning — This entails fine motor functioning or motor speed when it represents a primary component of the game.

4. Verbal skills — Games addressing the generation of words or other verbal material.

5. Math skills — Games in which basic arithmetic plays a central role, including the handling of money.

6. Convergent problem solving — The emphasis here is on piecing together solutions in a step-wise fashion, an essential component to effective strategy.

7. Divergent problem solving — Flexibility in approach is the hallmark. In other words, diverging from step-by-step solutions to generate new strategies.

8. Sequencing — This is often a component of convergent and divergent problem solving but, in some cases, is a goal in itself.

9. Memory — All games require ongoing monitoring and recall as part of the game process but some games focus on memory itself, that is, the ability to retrieve information from long-term storage.

The complexity of the games varies a great deal and is very difficult to rate in a consistent fashion. However, even complex games can be made more simple by altering rules, such as by removing special cards and liberalizing time constraints. For instance, the game Uno (International) can be simplified by removing all special cards, such as Draw Four and Reverse.

---

[33] Williams, J. M., 1987, "Cognitive Stimulation in the Home Environment," **The Rehabilitation of Cognitive Disabilities**, Center for Applied Psychological Research, Memphis State University, Plenum Press, New York, NY.

# Games for Cognitive Stimulation

Aggravation (Lakeside) — 6
Backgammon — 2,5,6
Bargain Hunter (Milton Bradley) — 5,6
Battleship (Milton Bradley) — 2,6
Bed Bugs (Milton Bradley) — 3
Bingo — 2
Boggle (Parker Brothers) — 4,7
Checkers — 2,6
Chess — 2,6,7
Clue (Parker Brothers) — 6
Connect Four (Milton Bradley) — 1,6
Dominoes — 1,2
Erector Sets — 2,3,6
Etch-A-Sketch (Ohio Art) — 2,3
Foursight (Lakeside) — 2,7
Gridlock (Ideal) — 1,2,6
Lego — 1,2,3
Life (Milton Bradley) — 5,6
Lincoln Logs (Playskool) — 1,2,3
Lite-Brite (Hasbro) — 1,2,3
Lotto (Edu-Cards)
   Farm Lotto — 1,6
   Object Lotto — 1,6
   Go-Together Lotto — 1,6
   The World About Us Lotto — 1,6
   Zoo Lotto — 1,6
Luck Plus (International) — 1,5
Mastermind (Pressman) — 2,6
Memory Original (Milton Bradley) — 2,9
   Animal Families (Milton Bradley) — 2,9
   Fronts & Backs (Milton Bradley) — 2,9
   Step by Step (Milton Bradley) — 6,8

Mhing (Suntex) — 6,7,8
Models, plastic replica — 1,2,3,8
Monopoly (Parker Brothers) — 5,6
Mystery Mansion — 6
Othello — 2,6
Paint-by-numbers — 1,2,3
Parcheesi (Selchow & Righter) — 6
Password (Milton Bradley) — 4,6,9
Pay Day (Parker Brothers) — 5,6
Pente (Parker Brothers) — 2,6
Perquacky (Lakeside) — 4,7,9
Picture Tri-Ominoes (Pressman) — 1
Pic Up Stik (Steven) — 3
Racko (Milton Bradley) — 8
Rage (International) — 6,8
Risk (Parker Brothers) — 2,6,7
Sabotage (Lakeside) — 6,7
Scotland Yard (Milton Bradley) — 2,6,8
Scrabble — 2,4,7,9
Smath (Pressman) — 2,5,6
Sorry (Parker Brothers) — 6
Think & Jump (Pressman) — 2,6
Toss Across (Ideal) — 3
Tri-Ominoes (Pressman) — 1
Tripoley — 1,8
Uno (International) — 1,8
Verbatim (Lakeside) — 4,7,9
Whodunit (Selchow & Righter) — 6
Word War (Whitman) — 4,6,7,9
Word Yahtzee (Milton Bradley) — 4,7,9
Yahtzee (Milton Bradley) — 5,6

# Memory Book

This activity is for an alert resident interested in documenting their lives for family and friends in a life review process. The use of a memory book is valuable for individuals who remember, recall and reminisce; and also for individuals who can utilize these memories and reinforcers to feel safe, enhance long term memory, reduce anxiety and promote safe, acceptable social responses.

A memory book highlights the individual and increases a sense of self and self-esteem. This book can be experienced both on a one-on-one basis or in a small group setting. Family and friends are invited to share stories and memories of this individual and perhaps bring in photos to bring the stories to life.

There may be pages with reinforcement statements. Many individuals dealing with memory loss issues become easily agitated and upset with the loss of words and memories. Each person needs their own pages of reminders that will be individualized to their needs and concerns.

The book can be filled with art and writings from its owner. This book should always be available and accessible for the individual to find or keep around.

| | |
|---|---|
| **Goal:** | Opportunities for resident to reminisce about his/her life; to reexamine past experiences, beliefs, values; to recall happier times; to socialize with others. |
| **Equipment Needs:** | Memory Book — blank book with questions from master list. (See the following pages for a sample Memory Book.) Photos, drawings and stories from the resident or his/her family and friends which can be placed in the memory book. Pen. |
| **Length of Activity:** | 30 – 45 minutes |
| **Number of Participants:** | 1– 6 |
| **Adaptations:** | Move chair up close to bed; possibly use tray table to write on. |

**Procedures:**
1. Greet resident; catch up on recent events (briefly).
2. Sit down; ask resident next question from the list below or other questions that have been suggested for this resident. (You can briefly review last session if you like.)
3. Be patient — give resident plenty of time to answer. Ask helpful questions to stir memory.
4. Do not be too aggressive — this is not a quiz! Be kind, helpful. Keep an open mind — you will hear all kinds of things — funny, heart-warming, aggravating, very sad.
5. Thank resident; read next 1–2 questions for next time.
6. Resident presents completed book to loved one(s).

**Questions For A Memory Book About Your Family:**
1. From what country or countries did your family ancestors emigrate? When was this and where did they settle?
2. What are your parents' names?
3. When and where were they born?
4. What was your mother's maiden name?
5. What do you remember most about your mother from your childhood?
6. What do you remember most about your father?
7. What work did your parents do?
8. What is your birth date?
9. Where were you born?
10. Was there anything unusual about the circumstances of your birth?
11. Were you born in a hospital or at home?
12. What is your full name and how was it chosen? Does it have a special meaning?

13. Who in your family do you most look like?
14. How many brothers and sisters did you have? (List them in the order they were born and include children who may have died early in life or at birth.)
15. Where did you fit among them?
16. To whom did you feel closest?
17. How did you spend your time together?
18. Did you ever take trips or vacations with your family? Where did you go? Tell about a favorite one.
19. Was another language besides English spoken in your home? What was it?
20. Did your family attend a church or synagogue? Was religion an important part of your family life?

# *My Memories*

## by

# My name is

# My spouse's name is

I was born on

My hometown is

Places I lived

# Occupation

# Hobbies, interests

# I currently live at

# My favorite photos:

# FAMILY STORIES

I have _____ children.

Their names are:

_____

_____

_____

_____

# My favorite memories to share:

My room number is

#_____

My roommate's
name is

_____

Lunch is served at
_____ P.M.

Dinner is served at
_____ P.M.

# *Some reminders:*

## My purse is in my room.

## My children know where I live so I don't have to worry.

## When I smile, I feel better.

I don't have to worry because all of the bills for staying here are taken care of.

Everyone here knows my name and who I am.

I am very safe here with people who care for me.

# Some of my favorite things to do are:

_____

_____

_____

_____

_____

_____

# Level 7: Short Term Rehab Activities[34]

One of the current issues of Activity and Social Service Professionals in long term care facilities is how and what to do with the short-term or acute rehabilitation residents who prefer not to get involved in activities and who have very specific and different needs.

This section will look at working with residents who are in your facility for rehabilitation treatment. Some of the important questions include:

- What is rehab? What is the team? Who are the players?
- How do you help rehab succeed?
- How do you work with consultants vs. facility employees?
- How do you coordinate care after specialized therapy (PT, OT, RT, Speech Therapy) has occurred and the resident needs to stay in the facility?

The goal of rehab activities is to help the resident get back to the target level of functioning as quickly and easily as possible.

Some of the things you need to do to make these activities work are

- Realize the differences between the rehab resident and the long term care resident.
- Provide activities that are coordinated with the goals of other members of the rehab team.
- Understand if the resident is too tired to participate in your activities.

## The Rehab Team

### Rehab, a slang abbreviation for rehabilitation
The definition of rehabilitation is to restore to good condition, to make suitable again, to reestablish on a firm sound basis.

### The Team Players
Working in rehab in a long term care facility may include working with the following members of the rehab team: Doctor, Nurses (licensed and aides), Physical Therapist, Occupational Therapist, Speech Pathologist, Respiratory Therapist, Recreational Therapist, Hospice Workers, Clergy, Dietitian, Social Service Professional, Activity Professional, Psychologist, Psychiatrist, Administrator.

Each facility addresses the resident on rehab in a team approach. Facilities hold meetings on a regular basis to design a specific plan for each individual. The content of these meetings may be resident progress, discharge planning, coordination of services, eligibility for current insurance coverage, eligibility for programs, services in the future, planning for family conferences, resident care plan and sharing of information and techniques that may or may not be working.

It is important to get to know the therapists in your facility and their individual roles as part of the team. Some therapists are consultants under contract and are in the facility specifically to work with an individual resident. They need to be approached directly so that they can understand your role and willingness to help follow through with their treatments. On the other hand, some therapists are full time employees within the facility. They may be available for additional support for the activity and social service departments regarding specific residents and their therapy.

---

[34] This section is by Lauren Newman, OTR. Used with permission.

# The Role of Activity and Social Service Professionals

## When the resident is actively involved in therapy

When a resident is newly admitted to a long term care setting and is receiving therapy on a daily basis, his/her primary goal is to regain strength and independence and be discharged. Because the focus is short term and centers on returning home, this individual is usually not interested in activities which are offered. For some, the experience of socializing with residents who are confused and disoriented is a hard and constant reminder that they may also need to remain long term and possibly begin to experience further declines in function. Because of this, their choice is often to go to therapy and then spend the majority of the day in their room. Some residents in rehab will seek out other participants in rehab programs for support and contact because of their common challenges and goals.

The Activity or Social Service Professional needs to listen closely at the rehab meetings so that s/he understands clearly what the therapy goals are and how the resident is progressing with them. At this stage, you should discuss with the therapists how activity staff can reinforce and align themselves with the current therapy goals. If the therapist encourages the resident to work with you, there is a greater chance for either involving the resident in a group or in working with them on a one-on-one basis. Therefore, it is important to make agreements with the therapists regarding the non-therapy time the residents may have.

## When assisting with the therapists' treatment goals

The following set of goals are examples of ways that activities can help residents make progress toward their therapy goals:

When the therapist has given approval for independent ambulation, the Activity Professional can assist with *"increasing endurance of walking."* This can be done with the help of a walker or other device. Activities such as mail delivery and assistance with resident transportation to and from activities may be appropriate.

*"Increase endurance in time out of bed in wheelchair from 1 to 2 hours per day."* The Activity Professional can find activities that will not only challenge but engage the resident in meaningful activity which can at the same time be enjoyable.

*"Increase strength in upper extremity."* This could be incorporated into an exercise group, bean bag toss, balloon volleyball, parachute game and movement to music.

*"Increase endurance and accuracy in upper extremity."* This could be stacking and sorting activities, sewing or weaving, bingo, checkers, puzzles and many other activities.

*"Improve visual scanning skills."* This could be done through bingo and flashlight tag.

*"Improve conversational skills: auditory comprehension, intelligibility of speech, word finding."* This could be done in social service discussion groups or as part of an activity where conversation goes on between the participants.

*"Improve reading and writing skills."* This could be done with current events groups, through discussions of literature or by writing down life histories.

*"Improve skills in ADLs: grooming and dressing."* This could be helped with various grooming activities (including fixing nails or hair) and activities involving period clothes.

## When the resident stays after formal therapy has ended

When residents are discharged from formal therapy services and need to stay in the facility for additional convalescence or long term stay, the need for activity involvement becomes crucial. Many residents feel a sense of failure and loss when they have not been able to achieve their therapy goals. They often develop close and significant relationships with the therapist. This therapist plays a pivotal position in refocusing the resident's goals and establishing a new framework. By encouraging work with the Activity and Social Service Professionals with goals similar to the ones previously established, the therapist assures the resident a better chance of not "giving up" and continuing his/her work towards a higher functional level.

In determining the best and most realistic discharge plan for a resident, the interdisciplinary team works closely with the physician to assess the resident's level of independence. The Activity Professional can help assess this level of independence and orientation by including the resident in a "helper" or a volunteer role and closely observing him/her in group settings and projects. Things such as mail delivery or requesting the residents' assistance with special projects and events help not only to assess their abilities, but also to give them a sense of usefulness and self-esteem which are paramount to their continued progress.

### When the resident is in need of long term stay

The Activity or Social Service Professionals may be the most helpful staff members facilitating the transition to long term care and daily routine. After acute rehab is completed, there is usually a room change for the residents. This means new roommates, new orientation to the area of the facility and sometimes different staff members attending to their needs. The activity and social service staff may be *the* point of stability for these residents.

## Trends

The profile of the resident in a long term care facility is as diverse as the services provided. What once was a setting created for individuals who were frail or elderly has evolved into a setting which provides for a profoundly differing resident population. Today a resident may be young or old. S/he may be receiving treatments such as chemotherapy, wound care, IV therapy and head injury treatment, previously offered only in acute care settings. Along with these specialized treatments, we may be seeing residents needing special care from ventilator dependent services and tracheotomy units. There will also be an increase in the numbers of residents of all ages who are HIV positive.

As the acuity level increases, so does the need to clearly understand medical diagnoses and how Activity and Social Service Professionals play an integral role in quality of care and quality of life issues.

# Level 8: Community Integration Activities

At times it may be vital, prior to discharge, for the resident to be escorted into the community on short outings. Not all residents can adjust immediately to a new (usually lower) health status. They may need a therapist to venture into the community with them, helping to solve problems along the way. Such help from a therapist (and the rest of the team) involves preparatory activities which take place both inside and outside of the facility.

Some of the activities involve the use of standardized integration programs such as the **Community Integration Program (CIP)**[35]. Others involve the use of activities in the facility for the development of skills such as working, communicating and the basic ADLs. One important element of community integration activities is to never let the community get too far away from the resident's day-to-day life.

Activity and Social Service Professionals work with the interdisciplinary team's goal of discharging residents ready to leave the facility. Some of the ways that Activity and Social Service Professionals can assist in this process are

- Identify and list community resources for leisure activities in the community.
- Assist resident in contacting support groups or recreational groups s/he has expressed interest in joining.
- Create a "map" of the community with names and addresses attached to the map or reference.
- Offer resident the name of a resident or staff person to call if s/he has any questions or needs to talk after discharge and during integration into community.
- Identify transportation systems which resident may need to contact in community.
- Touch base with family briefly by phone or during discharge to offer them support in and after discharge.

Much of this process is discussed in more detail in the *Discharge* section in the chapter on *Resident Care*.

As a step toward a return to the community, you can establish programs such as the Intergenerational Program (see the next page) to reconnect your residents with the community outside the facility. Even if the residents need to stay in a long term care facility for medical reasons, they can still be an integral part of the community outside.

---

[35] Armstrong, Missy and Sarah Lauzen, 1994, **Community Integration Program, 2nd Edition**, Idyll Arbor, Inc., Ravensdale, WA.

# Intergenerational Programs[36]

"People of all ages can be friends," Daisy answered when I asked her why she, an eight-year-old girl, enjoyed participating in an intergenerational program.

"My own children, even my grandchildren, are grown-ups now. An adult is not nearly as interesting as a bright, young child. I enjoy sharing ideas with them and hearing about their lives," explained Ted, a former college professor, when asked the same question.

These simple statements contain the components for a successful intergenerational program. These components are: 1. acceptance and enjoyment of each other's differences, 2. sharing ideas and 3. caring. The task is to provide an atmosphere that will allow these characteristics to flourish.

In 1989 we wanted to start a program that would provide a framework for children's and senior's natural affinity to blossom. There wasn't a lot of information available on the sort of program that we envisioned, so the learning process has been through trial and error. We have had a few disasters and many high points. As our awareness of our strengths and limitations has grown, along with our ability to trust the process, our program has become a happy event for all of us.

## Know Your Participants

However, don't assume that all seniors will enjoy children and that all children will enjoy seniors.

A new woman in our group was a retired school teacher. Because of this we assumed she would be ideal for our intergenerational program. It soon became apparent she felt that children were just one step above slime on the evolutionary ladder. Fortunately, we discovered this before she joined the program or her presence would have caused a few tears and nasty comments.

Another woman, Esther, was also a retired school teacher. On our visits with the children there were always at least four little girls hovering around her. She was able to hold an audience of 20 seniors and 30 children listening in rapt attention to her stories. (She must have been a fabulous teacher). The rule we learned from this is to know the seniors in the program and not to push anyone. Don't assume that because a person was a school teacher s/he loves children. Conversely, don't assume that a well-worn Merchant Marine won't melt when s/he is around the kids. Children bring out qualities in seniors that will surprise you!

## How to Get a Program Started

The ideal situation is if you have a school-aged family member or a friend who can introduce you to a teacher. Most teachers are open to having an intergenerational program. If you don't know someone who is a teacher, make an appointment with the principal of the grade school closest to your facility. Discuss your program idea. They will tell you which teacher would likely be interested. (Usually it is a teacher with an interest in history.)

Set up an appointment with this teacher. Ask him/her the level of the children's writing and reading abilities. We've done this program with preschool, second, third and fourth graders. Our personal preference is the fourth grade. Nine and ten year-olds are young enough to be openly creative and harbor fewer preconceived notions than adults while possessing good verbal and writing skills.

Our favorite teacher has the qualities that work best for our program. She is flexible and organized. You may have very different needs. What is important is to determine your needs and find someone who will fulfill them.

---

[36] **Intergenerational Program** is from Marcia Weldon. Used with permission.

## The Seniors Who Are Involved

Having tried this with both the frail elderly and with those who attend adult day health centers, our preference is for the latter. However, if you have a stable population of high-functioning adults in your residential or long term care facility, this activity could be perfect for them.

If your seniors will forget the children's visits or if you have a largely fluctuating population due to death, your program will be of a different sort than the one described here. The seniors and children will still enjoy each other's company, but they might not experience connections that are as deep or lasting.

## The Time Involved

1.   1 – 1½ hours of group work each week, reading and responding to children's correspondence.
2.   One visit every 1½ – 2 months, alternating between the school and your facility.

## Your Facility

Please don't invite children to your facility if you have a lot of people sitting in the halls, people screaming or strong odors. One of the positive aspects of this program is to familiarize children with the elderly and to those people with physical disabilities. Ideally, they will take this comfort into their adulthood. Scaring them will have the opposite effect. If your facility sounds like the one above, meet the children in a park or only go to their school.

## Introduction — A Beginning

After finding a teacher and a classroom, you can begin your program a few weeks after school begins. We start the program by taking photographs of our participating seniors. We mount them on a poster board. When that is completed, we spend an hour asking the seniors in our group to dictate an introductory letter for us to take to the children's classroom. (They might include anecdotes, jokes, their philosophy of life, etc. How they describe themselves as a group is enlightening.) We take the letter to the children's classroom and read it to them.

We leave the poster with our pictures in their classroom and take pictures of the children to hang on the wall of our facility. We use the pictures as a stimulus for the seniors to discuss the activities they'd like to participate in with the children. We make lists.

Remember: You build the frame, let the seniors and children paint the picture. This is their project!

## First Visit

Before the first visit we have exchanged several letters and/or drawings. (As group leader it usually works best to let the seniors dictate what they want to say. You write it down in one joint letter.) This creates a discussion group and the seniors get to learn things about each other they never knew before. Also, it allows participation for everyone, regardless of dexterity with a pen.

The children enjoy sending separate letters and drawings. Resist the temptation to tie specific children and seniors together in a pen-pal, one-on-one situation. If someone is sick during a visit or drops out of the program, their pen-pal will be very disappointed. It's best to let friendships develop naturally.

Halloween is the perfect time for a first visit. If the children come to your facility, ask the teacher if they can wear their Halloween costumes. The seniors can also wear costumes, hats and/or makeup applied at the facility or at home. Get your staff involved. We have made trick-or-treats and created a spook house in a bathroom.

Throughout the school year, every month and holiday will suggest a project. Here are a few ideas we have enjoyed sharing with each other. These are a sampling of the activities our children and seniors have participated in together. You are limited only by your imagination and the excitement of your participants.

1. Letters on construction paper leaves: "What I'm Thankful For."
2. Letters at Christmas, i.e. "My Favorite Christmas."
3. Making and exchanging Christmas gifts.
4. Hopes, fears and wishes for the New Year
5. "The First President I Remember." (Some seniors remember hearing a president speak in their home towns when they were children, etc.)
6. Making Valentines.
7. Making a huge paper quilt (1–2 children and 1 senior per square); collage forms.
8. Seniors begin story/poem, child finishes it.
9. Child or senior tells dream, child or senior illustrates it.
10. Trading riddles and jokes.
11. EAT LUNCH TOGETHER!!!
12. Overlaid and printed hand prints.
13. Sock hop.
14. Compile a book of all the stories, poems, etc., you've created. Give a copy to all involved and present one to the school library during a visit to the school.
15. Time capsule.

## Final Visit

Two weeks before school ends, make your final visit to the school. Eat together. With the teacher, plan a closing ritual. **This is the best day of the year!!!** Some kids cry, some seniors cry and even some activity staff members get teary-eyed. Take your camera or, better yet, bring a friend to film for you. You'll want to have pictures for your bulletin board and scrapbook. A videotape is nice for starting off your next year.

## Everyone Wins

Seniors and children have a natural bond. Both groups of people get tired of being bossed around by middle-aged members of society. Both groups are willing to have fun, relax and enjoy simple pleasures.

The benefits of an intergenerational program for seniors are numerous. Children are not only willing to listen to their stories, they listen with enthusiasm. The children's attentiveness and genuine respect raises the senior's self-esteem. Sometimes the children bring books and read to seniors on a one-on-one basis. In this activity the seniors are able to provide a real and valuable service to the children. We have seen children read to seniors who were unable to read aloud in the classroom.

"The children are so well-mannered, polite and considerate." We cannot tell you how often we have heard this after our first visit. The program provides the seniors a sense of peace, safety and satisfaction by letting them know there are good children in the world despite what they hear and read in the media.

Seniors also benefit from an intergenerational program, because when they are with the children they absorb their energy like a sponge. We have seen elders who shuffle around the facility swinging on swings, playing tether ball and doing the hokey-pokey. **Proximity to youth is a powerful medicine.**

The children derive a sense of history and continuity from the seniors. The seniors let the children fuss over them and worry about them. This sort of nurturing empowers the children and gives them a positive role model to carry into their adulthood. They lovingly push the elderly who are in wheelchairs. They walk slowly with those who are able to walk, taking their arm. We have seen several classroom "bad boys" surprise their teacher with their tenderness and compassion.

The old adage, "You get as much out of something as you put into it" aptly describes an intergenerational program. It takes work and planning, but the rewards are enormous.

Everyone wins. The children gain a feeling of stability; the seniors are given the gifts of energy, meaning and purposefulness. Both gain a sense of community and fun. During your final visit when the children and seniors are hugging each other, when people are smiling and crying simultaneously and you have witnessed small miracles of health and communication — you may feel the biggest winner is the group leader. You created a garden where love and understanding could grow. It doesn't get any better than that!

# Leisure Room[37]

While working as Activity Professionals, we realized there was a need to have resources more readily available and accessible to residents and staff.

We felt that the answer was a room containing supplies and resources for a diverse population of residents. The room would be available during the day and scheduled, with supervision. This leisure resource room would provide independence, access, creativity and learning opportunities both on a one-on-one and group basis.

The Resource Room provides a vast variety of tools for reality orientation, sensory stimulation, reminiscing, exercise, educational growth, musical tapes, equipment and games. Pets can be brought in for visits and pet care.

The resources and supplies can constantly change as resident needs change. Newer equipment can be added and new ideas tried. Work stations can be developed and redeveloped. Residents and families will add new ideas and be a good resource for future equipment needs.

In one area of the room, an individual with dementia may be engaged in a sensory stimulation activity, while another individual may be watching a movie with a headset on. People may come in to watch others or to see the promotions for the book of the week.

The table space can be used for small sensory awareness groups along with special events such as birthdays, showers and outside speakers.

This room is a wonderful space for those with busy therapy schedules during the day and who would like to be involved in leisure events after dinner. The hours for this room would depend on resident needs and schedules.

## How to develop this idea:

The first step is a review of your budget. What is the monthly budget for activities? How is it spent? Divide the budget money so as to continue purchasing needed monthly items and begin to add new items and supplies for this new area. Each month you should be purchasing educational, musical and creative equipment which can be used for many reasons and with a variety of individuals.

If your budget does not allow for new capital expenditures, seek out donations, discounted merchandise and items found in garage sales.

## Finding a room:

Look around and reassess space usage in your facility. Do your residents have a large open area that they spend time in? Are there chairs, a table, a TV? Does it have potential for this type of resource room? If so, you could have cabinets made which can be locked when staff leave for the day.

Many older facilities have a large living area off of the front entrance. Perhaps there is potential in this area. People usually congregate in the front anyway and this would be bringing the activities to them.

These changes do not have to occur overnight. Begin by building onto what is already there. Add to this with activity supplies and equipment.

---

[37] by Pat Hubbard, AC, SSD and Elizabeth Best Martini, MS, CTRS, ACC. Used with permission.

Use volunteers, family members and scheduled assistants to occupy the room throughout the day, facilitating small groups and assisting independent leisure pursuits.

Incorporate nursing assistants and staff to bring residents to the resource room. A few minutes of encouragement will make a difference.

This room could also be interdisciplinary in nature. The occupational therapist or speech therapist are always looking for a stimulating environment in which to work and the supplies are all accessible for ready use.

## Who uses the room:

All residents use the room. Now you have an area where all activity equipment is available for use. There will be no more running around to store and retrieve materials.

Think of the possibilities in helping to meet individual needs and provide a safe and structured environment for staff to bring their residents. The possibilities are as endless as the imagination in developing activity goals and programs.

Of course you need to let the rest of the staff know about the room. At the end of the section is a suggested flyer to give to other members of the treatment team.

## What to purchase:

Since the Resource Room is locked up when activity staff are off duty, you now can purchase valuable equipment that can be seen and kept for repeated use. Educational books and equipment are no longer kept in boxes or storage to be brought out on special occasions.

The equipment used in this room should meet the needs of the majority of residents. Is there a larger population of residents diagnosed with Alzheimer's or dementia related disorders or are there alert residents who are physically unable to be fully independent? The population dictates purchasing needs.

Create a wish list of supplies and keep a file of supply items and ideas for future reference. The next page has a list of ideas to start with.

# Leisure Room Supplies

## Supplies need to be :

*Safe, stimulating, purposeful, colorful, age appropriate, accessible and used as a resource by all staff.*

## Equipment and Supplies:

- VCR and tapes
- TV
- Slide projector
- Encyclopedias
- Typewriter
- Pens and paper
- Adult coloring books, art projects
- Poetry books, short stories, books on art, history, health
- Sensory supplies such as soft puzzles, stuffed animals
- Auditory discrimination games, sorting games, mirrors
- Adaptive devices for writing, hearing and seeing
- Trivia questions
- Etch-A-Sketch
- Mystery box to place hands in and guess object
- Exercise equipment and supplies of all sizes and shapes
- Rhythm sticks
- Tangle game
- Pictures sorted according to objects and themes
- Record player/CD player/tape deck with good speakers, head sets
- Records, tapes and CDs
- Guitar
- Casio player

- Aquarium
- Bird cage
- Large print books, fabric sample books, greeting card books, carpet samples
- Miscellaneous games and large puzzles
- Colorful posters
- Sorting games
- Collection of balls (large and small of various textures)
- Sensory boxes according to theme
- Magnetic letters and board
- Grooming kits (need to be individualized)
- Makeup mirror
- Familiar items such as kitchen utensils, hats, gloves, hankies, ties
- Large dominoes, cards, checkers
- Magazines and pictures to sort through and look at
- Homemaking tasks — folding napkins, sorting silverware in a container, counting paper money
- Large blocks and dice to move and stack
- Sensory apron
- Laundry baskets for storage
- Scarf collection
- Olfactory stimulation kit
- Wood working ideas: hardware trays, sanding projects, key collections
- Velcro games

# The Leisure Room Concept

*The leisure room is designed to provide available leisure activities and supplies to residents with varying levels of needs. The supplies and equipment are accessible for use by all staff to enhance interaction, socialization and a multi-dimensional sensory stimulation experience.*

Because this room is created to encourage active participation at all levels, the supplies are kept in this room and need to be supervised and protected by all staff members. This is a room designed to enhance quality of life to residents. It belongs to all of us and needs to be watched over by all of us.

Supplies will be kept in clear bins which are marked according to level of cognitive and functional abilities. If a CNA brings a resident into the room and provides them with one of these supply items, s/he must return to the room within a short time to reassess how the resident is doing.

The activity staff will schedule times when the room will be supervised by staff and volunteers. These hours will be posted. When there is no structured supervision, the responsibility lies with the CNA for both supervision and proper management of the materials. (i.e. placing supplies within reach, introducing new activities and putting away supplies in appropriate places).

Any comments, recommendations and requests in regards to the room and supplies should be discussed with the Activity Staff.

# 7. Documentation

What is a health record? Why are health records kept? Who owns the health record? Are there rules to follow when making an entry in a health record? Are there mandated forms and content to the health record? These questions and more will be answered in this chapter.

First, an introduction to the basic requirements of clinical record keeping as defined in the federal regulations (483.75l 1–5, Tag F514 Clinical Records). The health record is owned by the long term care facility and kept for the benefit of the resident and the health care team. The record is used for primary resident care, for continuity of care, for quality assurance — proof of care given, for research and for reimbursement or billing. The health record must be protected from loss, destruction or unauthorized use. The record must be kept for the period of time required by state law; or five years from the date of discharge if there is no requirement in state law; for a minor, three years after the resident reaches legal age under state law.

All information in the health record must be kept confidential. No information may be released without authorization from the resident except when it is required by law, third party contract or transfer to another health care institution. The facility must permit the resident to inspect his or her records within 24 hours of request and must provide copies no later than 2 working days after notice from the resident. All records are kept in accordance with accepted professional standards and practices. Records must be complete, accurately documented, readily accessible and systematically organized. These are the minimum requirements for record keeping.

Every state will have requirements as well and facility and corporate policy may also require additional record keeping practices. The wise practitioner will be familiar with all regulations and policies. If copies of the federal and state regulations are not readily available in the facility, they may be reviewed at the local county law library.

Let's look again at the purposes of the health record.

1. Primary care. The record gives the information the health care team needs to deliver direct care — orders for medications, treatments, diet and nursing care as specified in the treatment plan for the resident.

2.    Continuity of Care. The record provides a means of communication among members of the health care team and gives a report of assessments, interventions, evaluations of the resident's progress and response to the treatment plan.

3.    Quality Assurance/Proof of Care. The record documents care and services provided. The record can be examined by outside reviewers for evidence of appropriate care and intervention. The record is a legal document and can be used as evidence in defense of claims of providing inadequate care and intervention. (If a treatment *isn't* documented in the health record, the legal assumption is that it *wasn't* given.)

4.    Research. The record can be used by health care professionals for research in many fields.

5.    Billing/reimbursement. The record is reviewed by third party payers for proof that services, supplies and equipment were provided as claimed.

Because there are so many purposes for the record, including that of evidence in legal proceedings, standard documentation principles have been established. Following these principles assures that the record can be used for all of the purposes listed above. Failure to follow the principles may render the record useless.

# Documentation Principles

Entries into the record must be permanent, legible, timely, accurate and authenticated. Let's examine each of these principles.

1.    Permanent. All entries must be made with an indelible ink pen. Do not use pencil, erasable pen or a felt tip pen which may run when wet. Your entry should not be erasable or alterable once in the record. Pages of the record should never be destroyed before the legal time requirement nor should the record be modified by crossing over or using correction fluid.

2.    Legible. Write clearly. If your penmanship is poor, try printing. You and others must be able to easily interpret what you write. Do not use short hand or other personal abbreviations. (A set of generally recognized abbreviations is shown on the next page.) Use a pen dark enough that the entry is capable of being photocopied or faxed. Black ball point pen is best.

3.    Timely. Document as events occur noting the complete date: month, day, year and time. Don't rely on your memory and don't document actions in advance. Never backdate, tamper with or add to notes previously written. Never write between lines or squeeze in words after the fact. It should never appear that the record has been altered with the intent to mislead.

4.    Accurate. Entries should be factual and describe only events that you know to be true through direct observation. Entries should be objective, describing what you can see, hear, smell or touch. Subjective entries — hearsay, statements from others, opinions or feelings — should not be used unless they are documented in the form of a direct quote from a resident or family member.

It is also important that the entries are within the scope of your education, training and, if applicable, your professional credential. Entries should be specific to your discipline and appropriately express your clinical opinion. Use only words which you understand. Don't attempt to diagnose or assess a resident's psychological or physical condition unless you have the appropriate training. Never speculate about possible causes or interpret a resident's behavior unless it is your legal responsibility as a credentialed therapist or social worker to do so. For an example, a resident's weeping may be caused by many factors, both internal and external. Unless you are trained to assess the causes with assessment tools or observation, you must wait for the resident to tell you what is

# Abbreviations

| | |
|---|---|
| c̄ | with |
| s̄ | without |
| AC | Activity Coordinator |
| ADL | activities of daily living |
| AKA | above the knee amputation |
| aka | also known as |
| am | morning |
| amt | amount |
| ASHD | arterial sclerotic heart disease |
| AV | audio visual |
| B&C | board and care |
| bid | 2x daily |
| BKA | below the knee amputation |
| bp | blood pressure |
| BRP | bath room privileges |
| c/o | complain of |
| CHF | congestive heart failure |
| COPD | chronic obstructive pulmonary disease |
| CPR | cardiopulmonary resuscitation |
| CTRS | Certified Therapeutic Recreation Specialist |
| CVA | cerebral vascular accident |
| d/c | discontinue |
| DD | developmentally disabled |
| dme | durable medical equipment |
| DON | Director of Nursing |
| DSD | Director of Staff Development |
| dx | diagnosis |
| ETOH | alcohol |
| fx | fracture |
| GI | gastrointestinal |
| gm | gram |
| H&P | history and physical |
| HBV | Hepatitis B Virus |
| HIV | Human Immunodeficiency Virus |
| HOH | hard of hearing |
| I | independent |
| IDT | interdisciplinary team |
| ie | such as |
| IM | intramuscular |
| IV | intraveneous |
| L | left |
| lb | pound |
| LE | lower extremity |
| MDS | Minimum Data Set |
| mg | milligram |
| MI | mentally ill |
| MI | myocardial infarction |
| MS | multiple sclerosis |
| noc | night |
| NPO | nothing by mouth |
| ∅ | no/none |
| OBRA | Omnibus Budget Reconciliation Act |
| OOB | out of bed |
| OT | Occupational Therapy |
| pm | afternoon, evening |
| PO | by mouth |
| PoC | Plan of Correction |
| prn | as necessary |
| Pt | patient |
| PT | Physical Therapy |
| q | every |
| qd | every day |
| qh | every hour |
| R | right |
| r/t | related to |
| RA | rheumatoid arthritis/restorative aide |
| RAP | Resident Assessment Protocol |
| rehab | rehabilitation |
| res. | resident |
| ROM | range of motion |
| RT | Respiratory Therapist, Recreational Therapist |
| s/p | status post (after) |
| SNF | skilled nursing facility |
| SOB | shortness of breath |
| SP/ST | Speech Pathologist, Therapist |
| SSC/SSD | Social Service Coordinator/Director |
| Stat | immediately |
| T-22 | Title 22 (California) |
| THR | total hip replacement |
| TIA | transient ischemic attack |
| tid | 3x daily |
| tx | treatment |
| UE | upper extremity |
| URI | upper respiratory infection |
| UTI | urinary tract infection |
| w/c | wheel chair |
| WFL | within functional limits |
| wk | week |
| WNL | within normal limits |
| wt | weight |
| X | times |

causing the weeping before you state a reason. Even then the reason should be documented as a quote from the resident.

Document only what you do. Do not document actions of other members of the health care team. Do not document actions or interventions that you aren't legally allowed to perform (and don't perform them in the first place!).

5.     Authenticated. Sign all entries with your name and title. First initial and full last name with title is acceptable. Example: M. Smith, AC. In signing with your title, you let the other members of the health care team know your background and training.

All of this may make the documentation process look intimidating. You may be saying to yourself, "But I'm only human! Humans make mistakes!" You're right. Because you are only human, there are methods for correcting honest mistakes. It is important that corrections look like corrections and not deliberate attempts to mislead or defraud. Simple errors in charting, the wrong word, date, name may be corrected by drawing one line through the error, dating and initialing it. The time is sometimes recommended.

Example:

The first part of an entry was correct but then ~~the words that were here originally were not correct.~~           error SW 3/16/96

Omissions in charting, forgetting to record an event, may be made as late entries to the record. The current date and time is entered, then the phrase "late entry for _____" entering the date and time for the missed event.

Example:

4/5/96 2:00 PM Late entry for 4/5/96 10:00 AM.

Late entries should not be made long after the event and are generally recommended to be made no longer than 48 hours after the missed event. Some states will only allow late entries if they are made in 24 hours or less. Check with your medical records professional or legal counsel. If a late entry is not allowed and the information is felt to be important to the record of resident care, an addendum may be made. This is done on a separate page of the record. The current date and time is entered, then the phrase "Addendum to the record for _____" entering the date and time for the missed event.

Both late entries and addenda to the record should be used sparingly. The impression created (and it is an accurate impression) is one of inaccuracy and lack of timeliness in record keeping. Late entries and addenda cast doubt on the reliability of the entire health record. In all documentation, remember that many people, including the resident and family, may look at the record.

Claims for slander and defamation of character may be avoided by describing events factually, avoiding blaming and finger pointing and by avoiding personal opinions. Do not document an observation in the record that you would not support in public. Entries into the record should be objective as stated above. Instead of describing a resident as a "nasty old man," the description could be a "99 year old male dissatisfied with facility routine."

Be aware of residents rights when documenting and remember that the resident and the family should be a part of the decision making process. Statements of problems and concern about resident and family behavior should be discussed openly and should not be discovered by the resident or family only upon reviewing the record.

# Introduction to Required Documentation

Activity and Social Service Professionals are responsible for five types of documentation about the resident. Each one must be written carefully to be sure that it reflects the actual state of the resident and meets all federal and state regulations. The documents include:

## 1. Initial Assessment

Each department is responsible for conducting an initial assessment on every new resident. The activity assessment includes identification of needs, interests, strengths and lifestyle. The social service assessment includes psychosocial needs, interests, strengths and lifestyle.

Within 14 days after a resident is admitted, the Activity or Social Service Professional (in the United States) must transfer his/her findings to the relevant parts of the Resident Assessment Instrument (RAI). The Activity Professional is responsible for the Minimum Data Set (MDS 2.0) Section N. The Social Service Professional is responsible for Sections E and F. Activity and Social Service RAPs also need to be completed if one of the relevant triggers is set off. You may decide to include the RAP interventions in your programming or you may decide not to include them. Either way the RAP note describes *how and why* you come to the conclusion to proceed or not proceed with a care plan.

## 2. Resident Care Plan

A resident care plan is required within seven days (Medicare) after the RAP is signed off. The plan must describe how the facility intends to care for the resident, including interventions to help the resident reach and maintain his/her fullest potential for well-bring.

Each intervention is documented in three parts. First there is a statement of a problem, need or strength. Then there is a goal which says what the team hopes to achieve, either solving a problem or building on a strength. The final part is the approach that will be used.

The Activity and Social Service Professionals need to be careful of two important points in the resident care plan. First, the issues listed on the resident care plan must be issues that have already been identified on the assessments. Second, the resident and/or his/her legal representative have the final say on whether the care plan is adopted. They have the right to refuse any proposed treatment.

## 3. Discharge

The Social Service Professional is responsible for writing a discharge plan for residents who have the potential for discharge or for documenting why discharge is not an option for the resident. These plans should be updated quarterly and whenever any significant change occurs.

## 4. Monitoring Documentation

This set of documentation is used to keep track of the resident's progress. We recommend that both the Activity and Social Service Professional do a 30 day re-evaluation note to reassesses the initial care plan. Review the earlier assessment and state any changes that need to be made. This is not required but we recommend it because a resident may change significantly in the first 30 days.

The Activity Professional needs to document participation in activities to verify the approach and plan. For many residents a bedside log will be necessary. Be sure to show type, frequency, length of visit and response to visit. One of the most important pieces of information is to record when the resident refuses to go to activities. This can be used to document that activities were available and to help the treatment team find patterns so that they can offer activities and other interventions which better meet the needs of the resident.

The Social Service Professional needs to keep a log documenting services and counseling provided to the resident. This could be either in the progress notes or in a separate log. Be sure to identify date, nature of service and the follow-through that is required.

Any time a positive or negative change in the resident's abilities is noticed or when milestones of the care plan have been reached, the Activity or Social Service Professional should write in the resident's progress notes to document the change.

The final piece of monitoring documentation is the quarterly progress note. This is your opportunity to give information on the activity plan including any progress or changes during the last three months. Be sure to address, as appropriate, the resident's mental status; family and resident involvement; any health issue which may impact psychosocial health, needs and interests; therapy involvement; previous leisure and lifestyle information; customary routines and interests; potential for falls; psychoactive medication (if any); mood disturbances; behavioral issues; and need for task segmentation. End with a goal for the next quarter. The quarterly goal should be the same as on the care plan. The Social Service Professional should also update the discharge plan quarterly for residents who display a potential for discharge to lesser levels of care and annually for long term care residents.

## 5. Update Documentation

There are two times when the care plan must be updated: whenever a significant change occurs in the resident or, if no change has occurred, at least once a year.

A change of condition note should be written whenever a change occurs. If a major change which involves two or more potential risk factors has occurred, a new MDS must be completed and consequently a new activity treatment plan. If there has been a minor change which affects the level of involvement, write a note describing exactly what this change is. Also include any new emphasis or information for the Activity or Social Service Departments.

More detailed information about each of these types of documentation, including examples, will be found in the next chapter on *Resident Care*. A summary of documentation, in chart form, is shown on the next two pages.

# Activity Documentation

**1. INITIAL ASSESSMENT FORM**
Assessment and identification of needs, interests, strengths and lifestyle. Design of Activity Plan within 7 – 14 days of admission.

**2. MDS FORM**
Complete Section N within 7 – 14 days from admission and at least once a year. To be reviewed quarterly. Activity RAP to be completed if a trigger is set off.

**3. RAP SUMMARY SHEET**
Activity Professional either gives the information to RAI Coordinator or completes Activity section as needed. PROCEED or NOT PROCEED with care plan and additional information. RAP note describes *how and why* you come to the conclusion to proceed or not proceed with a care plan.

**4. RESIDENT CARE PLAN**
Problem/Need/Concern, Goal, Approach. The information regarding these concerns must be issues already identified on the activity assessment. This must be prepared within 7 days (Medicare) after the RAP is signed off.

**5. 30 DAY RE-EVAL NOTE**
Reassesses initial plan. Review and state changes, if any. This is a *recommended* addition to the requirements as a resident may change significantly in the first 30 days.

**6. ATTENDANCE**
Document participation at activities to verify above approach and plan. Bedside log, if necessary. Be sure to show type, frequency, length of visit and response to visit. Also code if a resident refuses.

**7. QUARTERLY PROGRESS NOTE**
This is a narrative note which gives information on the activity plan (progress, changes, etc.) Address: mental status, family and resident involvement, previous leisure and lifestyle information, customary routines and interests, potential for falls, psychoactive medication (if any), mood disturbances, behavioral issues, need for task segmentation, any health issue which may impact activity involvement, therapy involvement and goals and needs and interests. End with a goal for the quarter. The quarterly goal should be the same as on the care plan.

**8. CHANGE OF CONDITION NOTE — Document when a change occurs**
If a major change which involves two or more potential risk factors has occurred, a new MDS is required to be completed and consequently a new activity treatment plan. If there has been a minor change which affects the level of involvement, write a note describing exactly what this change is. Also include any new emphasis or information for activities.

# Social Service Documentation

**1. INITIAL ASSESSMENT FORM**
Assessment and identification of psychosocial needs, interests, strengths and lifestyle. Design of Social Service Plan within 7 – 14 days of admission.

**2. MDS FORM**
Complete within 7 – 14 days from admission and at least once a year. There are varying dates for completion related to state requirements. To be reviewed quarterly. Social Service RAPs to be completed if any triggers are set off.

**3. RAP SUMMARY SHEET**
Social Service Professional either gives the information to RAI Coordinator or completes Sections E and F. PROCEED or NOT PROCEED with care plan and additional information.

**4. RESIDENT CARE PLAN**
Problem/Need/Concern, Goal, Approach. Same as on assessment form. The information regarding these concerns must be issues already identified on the assessment. This must be prepared within 7 days (Medicare) of when the RAP is signed off.

**5. 30 DAY RE-EVAL NOTE**
Reassesses initial plan. Review and state changes, if any. This is a *recommended* addition to the requirements as a resident may change significantly in the first 30 days.

**6. SOCIAL SERVICE LOG**
A record documenting services and counseling provided to the resident by the Social Service Professional. Be sure to identify date, nature of service and the follow-through that is required.

**7. QUARTERLY PROGRESS NOTE**
Your opportunity to give information on the psychosocial issues and plan. Address: mental status, family and resident involvement, any health issue which may impact psychosocial health, needs and interests, goal for the quarter. This should be the same as on the care plan. You should also update the **discharge plan** quarterly for residents who display a potential for discharge to lesser levels of care and annually for long term care residents.

**8. CHANGE OF CONDITION NOTE — Document when a change occurs**
If a major change which involves two or more potential risk factors has occurred, a new MDS is required to be completed and consequently a new treatment plan. If there has been a minor change which affects the level of involvement, write a note describing exactly what this change is. Also include any new emphasis or information for social services.

# 8. Resident Care

Planning resident care is a five step process. It starts with the initial assessments that you and the rest of the treatment team make. After all of the assessments have been made, the team meets to create a care plan which is designed to meet the needs of the resident, the goals you will be working on for the next quarter and the progress you expect to see. The third step is implementing the care plan and monitoring the progress the resident is making. The fourth step is updating the care plan based on your observations of the resident or because the resident's condition changes. The final step, which may not be appropriate for all of your residents, is discharge planning. The discharge plan summarizes the current condition of the resident, the care s/he has received and the continuing care that will be needed.

This chapter will look at what needs to be done in each of these steps, especially showing the documentation required to demonstrate that each of the se steps was done correctly.

## Initial Assessment

The first step in resident care is to assess the resident. Assessment is the process of discovering who your resident is and what his/her physical and psychosocial needs are in terms of optimum care and functional status. You use that information to create the care plan for the resident.

The assessment process begins with the first information that you receive about a new resident. During the first few days after admission, you should introduce yourself to this individual in an informal visit. At this time you will be making observations in areas such as appearance, understanding and comprehension, orientation to person, time and place, understanding of diagnoses and any personal possessions or items in his/her room which give information on past lifestyle and interests. You may or may not have had a chance to review this person's medical chart before meeting him/her the first time. With the information gathered from this initial visit, you proceed to the medical chart for more information specific to past social and medical history, primary and secondary diagnoses, rehabilitation issues and goals, etc.

As you get to know the resident better, you will make updates to your information about the resident. The original assessment and the updates provide important information for making program plans. Planning programs for individuals requires making plans based on what the person is like now and making adaptations when the resident changes. That is what the ongoing resident care process is designed to let you do.

# Assessing a New Resident

The assessment process employs a variety of techniques to reveal as complete a picture as possible of a resident's situation and condition. On the next pages are forms for gathering the information you need on a new admission.

Usually there is an initial assessment or screening form. The information you gather using this form will be used to fill out the MDS and the RAPs. This assessment should be done within the first seven days after admission.

The assessment of new residents is the key to individualizing and understanding residents' needs. Meet with them informally to introduce yourself. Offer support and welcome them without too many questions during this first visit. Make your visit short unless they ask you to stay longer.

During the first informal visit, you are in the first stage of the assessment process. Keep your eyes open and listen carefully to the conversation. There is some factual information that you need to find out during the initial assessment process. Some you will be able to get from talking to the resident and his/her family. Other information will come from the medical chart. The information includes:

| | | |
|---|---|---|
| date of birth | lifestyle | level of alertness |
| marital status | leisure interests | orientation |
| children | hobbies | hearing |
| religion | talents | vision |
| occupation | political interests | adaptive devices |
| physical history | social history | compensatory skills |
| language(s) spoken | voter registration | language |
| communication skills | communication deficits | |
| | | |
| allergies | emotional health | attention deficits |
| special diets | dependency issues | short term memory loss |
| grooming issues | mental attitude | long term memory loss |
| | | |
| diagnoses | prognosis | discharge plan |

But what is more important to creating an appropriate care plan is understanding the resident as a person, not as a set of facts. When you complete this part of the assessment form, do it outside of the resident room so this person will not feel anxious about the answers that s/he gives you.

- Discover who this person is!
- Be aware of cognitive and functional levels.
- Be aware of sensory deficits.
- Be aware of ability to communicate needs and interests.
- Be aware of personal possessions in the room.
- Be aware of previous lifestyle issues and interests.

We have included forms which you can use to gather information about new residents. The forms, as they are presented, include information that we feel is most important, but you may need to modify them to meet the needs of your facility. Following the forms are some additional tools and techniques to help you gather information for the initial assessment.

# Activity Assessment

This form is designed for the Activity Professional to complete the initial activity assessment on a new resident. This is an example of an assessment (intake) form. There are many variations and styles available. The form will be completed before the MDS and used in conjunction with the MDS assessment process.

## Voting Status:
Is the resident registered to vote? Is s/he interested in voting? Does s/he have an absentee ballot? This question is not asking for political party preference but whether a resident is interested in registering or completing a change of address form.

## Communication and Cognitive Patterns:
In this section, circle the most appropriate answer. Feel free to write specific information next to the answer if needed.

## Mobility Information:
This area addresses any mobility issues, assistive devices or transfer information regarding a resident who can ambulate but also spends a certain amount of time in a wheelchair. Add any information which assists you in the assessment process. Mobility is important in addressing how functional and independent a resident may be. You also need to know whether this resident needs assistance to and from activities or whether their therapist will be encouraging them to propel themselves to and from groups.

## Identified Leisure Interests:
List any leisure and lifestyle information which has been gathered by family, staff or previous medical notes. Only list interests which have been identified. Do not add areas which *you think* would be of interest to this resident.

## Levels of Programming:
When you reach this part of the assessment, you have not only reviewed the medical record, but also interviewed and possibly observed the resident on a one-on-one basis or in a group activity. This is your assessment of what level of activity programming s/he needs. Circle the types of programs from the list. If you need to add to the list, be sure to do so. *Remember: for each level circled, you must document involvement and response to this type of program. So, when you circle two areas, you must document on these two areas in the progress notes also.*

## Cognitive and Sensory Deficits:
If the resident is assessed with significant sensory and/or cognitive deficits, use this section to signify appropriate activity programs.

### Sensory Stimulation:
For the resident who is regressed. Sensory Stimulation is a therapeutic intervention and program which provides multi-sensory experiences to residents who otherwise would not reach out or respond to stimuli. Although all of us need stimulation, this specific program is for a resident with minimal to no response unless presented in a structured program.

### Reality Orientation:
Reality Orientation is a therapeutic intervention and program in which the staff members *reinforce* reality and remind the resident of person, time and place. This is appropriate for residents dealing with memory loss. The goal of this type of program is to orient them to reality. It takes consistency and structure and must be goal oriented. In Reality Orientation, most of the one-on-one and group sessions follow the same format for consistency and are the same each session.

**Reality Awareness:**

Reality Awareness is a therapeutic intervention and program which creates an awareness of the world and people around the resident. The goal of Reality Orientation is *to orient* and the goal of Reality Awareness is *to be present in the moment,* to be aware of people and environment while receiving stimulation in a pleasurable group setting. The activities of these groups vary with familiar themes and seasonal topics.

If the resident who you are assessing meets any of the above descriptions, circle the program and whether this will be on a one-on-one basis or a group setting or both.

## Assessment Comments and Treatment Plan:

- This section of the form is to be completed for every assessment. If a resident is identified as having sensory deficits, specify what *type* of sensory stimulation that you will be starting with (Auditory, Tactile, Gustatory (taste), Visual, Olfactory (smell) )

- If there are any identified behavioral issues that need to be addressed, indicate specifically what they are. Some examples would be: hitting, screaming, eating inappropriate objects, poor judgment skills which may be safety issues, etc.

- This section should also be used to record any other areas that you feel need to be addressed. Be specific about the treatment plan and goal.

# Activity Assessment

**Resident Name:**_____ **Room No.**_____

**Admit Date:**_____ **Date of Birth:**_____

**Former Occupation:**_____ **Voting Status:**_____

**Religion:**_____ **Marital Status:**_____

**Diagnosis:**_____
_____

**Diet:** _____ **Diet/Fluid Restrictions:** _____

**Communication and Cognitive Patterns: (circle most appropriate answers)**

| | | | | |
|---|---|---|---|---|
| **Hearing** | Good | Fair | Poor | Deaf – Hearing Aid L R |
| **Vision** | Good | Fair | Poor | Uses Glasses |
| **Oriented to:** | Person | Time | Situation | Object |
| **Short Term Memory** | Good | Adequate | Poor | |
| **Long Term Memory** | Good | Adequate | Poor | |
| **Behavioral Concerns** | Agitated | Combative | Screams | |
| **Decision making ability** | Independent | Needs assist w/new situations | | |
| | Moderately Impaired | Severely Impaired | | |
| **Makes self understood** | Usually | Sometimes | Never | |
| **Ability to understand others** | Usually | Sometimes | Never | |

**Mobility Information:** _____

**Identified Leisure Interests:** (Information gathered by interview, family, previous history)

_____

_____

**According to this activity assessment and in addition to the MDS, the following level of programming is identified as appropriate for this resident's leisure needs and interests: (Circle)**

| | | |
|---|---|---|
| Social Interaction Activities | Religious Activities | Creative/Expressive Activities |
| Relaxation and Solace Activities | Group Games and Projects | Physical Activities |
| Community Outings | Outdoor Activities | Resident Council |
| Intellectually Stimulating Activities | Task Oriented Activities | One-on-one |
| Rehab Oriented Activities | Work Related Activities (with physician's orders) | |

**For residents with Cognitive and/or Sensory Deficits: (Circle)**

| | | |
|---|---|---|
| Sensory Stimulation | Group | One-on-one |
| Reality Orientation | Group | One-on-one |
| Reality Awareness | Group | One-on-one |

**Assessment Comments and Treatment Plan for Resident:**

This section needs to be completed for each resident regardless of program level. (Indicate senses which will be the target of initial sensory stimulation activities — if assessed as a need. Indicate behavioral problems which would require precautionary action — if any.)

_____

_____

_____

_____

_____

**Date:**_____ **Activity Professional:**_____

# Social Service Assessment

The social history of the residents: who they are and were, where they lived, who they lived with, their occupations and the kinds of community support they received prior to admission describe the patterns of previous lives. These patterns help you tailor treatment plans to match each resident's individual and unique needs.

Typically, gathering this information for the rest of the team is the responsibility of the Social Service Professional. That person should ensure that an accurate picture of the resident's social history is presented as inaccuracies could lead to inappropriate treatment goals from the rest of the team.

Two methods of obtaining the information are presented. On the next page are a set of questions you can ask to help you write a narrative social history. The following two pages show a more structured form for gathering much of the same information. We suggest using the structured form while using the questions to help you fill in the narrative sections on the second page, but adapt the forms as required to meet your particular needs.

A note of caution: do not allow yourself to be constrained by these intake forms. These forms are simply tools to provide a skeleton of selections to be used during the assessment process.

When you have made all the appropriate checks and notes on whatever from you choose to use, consider taking a blank progress note and developing a narrative statement based on the material you have gathered during the interviews you conducted to obtain your data. Focus on the personality of the resident; describe actions and reactions and important relationships. Use your skills everyday; no one's assessment is ever finished, even the most ill resident continues to evolve within the boundaries of the facility.

Identify changes because change is what we are always alert for: it drives our care interventions. But do not stop with the identification of change. Chart it. Make sure that the rest of the care team also knows about the change. Be assertive; do not wait to react. Act on behalf of the resident every day by assessing, documenting and keeping all information current.

# Social Service Assessments for New Admissions
## Psychosocial Information

## I. Reason For Admission To A Long Term Care Facility At This Time
- Where was resident living previously?
- What were precipitating factors?
- How was admission decision made? Was resident involved in the decision?
- Were family or friends involved in the decision? Did they help with moving in?
- Who is primary contact person for the resident?

## II. Social History
- Where did the resident live?
- Where was the resident born?
- What was his/her occupation?
- Why did s/he stop working?
- Was s/he married? Length and quality?
- Did s/he have children?
- What other important relationships did s/he have in the past or present?
- What were the most significant life events and/or losses? How did s/he react to these events?
- How does s/he feel about them now?
- What is the ethnic, cultural and religious background? How important to resident?
- Has s/he seen a psychiatrist or other similar professional? Why? How long?
- What are his/her current relationships with family or friends like?
- Who provided this information?

## III. Current Psychosocial Functioning
- Does the resident have the capacity to make decisions regarding individual needs and wishes?
- How does the resident present her/himself to other people?
- Is s/he well-groomed? Is there anything striking about his/her appearance?
- Does s/he have any idiosyncratic mannerisms?
- What is his/her general behavior like? (e.g., nervous, clingy, sad, quiet, content, etc.)
- What is his/her cognitive functioning like? Is s/he oriented to person, place and time?
- Is s/he forgetful of recent or remote events?
- What does s/he talk about most of the time?
- What are his/her fears?
- How does s/he cope with physical and emotional losses?
- What is his/her sense of humor like?
- What achievements is s/he proud of?

## IV. Psychosocial Care Plan Recommendations
- What difficulties is this resident likely to experience in adjusting to a long term care facility?
- What can be done to ease his/her adjustment?
- How can specific departments in the facility be of help?
- Will family members also need assistance? How?
- Will family members participate in resident care? How?
- Should this resident be encouraged to attend group activities or be left alone?
- Should this resident be referred for social work assessment?

## V. Discharge Planning Assessment
- Why is skilled nursing required?
- Under what conditions will this resident be able to leave?
- What social or environmental supports would be required?
- What is the projected timetable?
- Does resident agree with discharge plan?
- Does family agree with discharge plan?
- What difficulties can be anticipated in implementing this plan?

# Social Service Assessment

*Medical Record #* _____  *Admission Date* _____

*Room #* _____  *Admitted From* _____

*Readmit*     *Yes* _____ *No* _____  *Date of Birth* _____

## I.  Identifying Information

Name: _____  Age: _____  Sex: M ____ F ____

Religion: _____  Contact: _____

Diagnosis: _____

Marital status:  Never Married _____ M _____ W _____ D _____ Sep. _____

Financial Resources:  Medicaid _____ Medicare _____ Private _____ Other _____

Responsible Party or Conservator: _____  Relationship: _____

## II.  Mental Status

|  | Yes | No | At Times |
|---|---|---|---|
| 1. Oriented to: | | | |
| Person | _____ | _____ | _____ |
| Facility/Room | _____ | _____ | _____ |
| Season | _____ | _____ | _____ |
| Staff | _____ | _____ | _____ |
| 2. Long Term Memory Problem | _____ | _____ | _____ |
| Short Term Memory Problem | _____ | _____ | _____ |
| 3. Problem Behavior: | | | |
| Wandering | _____ | _____ | _____ |
| Verbally Abusive | _____ | _____ | _____ |
| Physically Abusive | _____ | _____ | _____ |
| Socially Inappropriate | _____ | _____ | _____ |
| Indication of Delirium | _____ | _____ | _____ |
| 4. Quality of Life: | | | |
| Makes Own Decisions | _____ | _____ | _____ |
| Uses Telephone | _____ | _____ | _____ |
| Manages Own Money | _____ | _____ | _____ |
| Takes Own Medication | _____ | _____ | _____ |
| Sets Own Goals | _____ | _____ | _____ |
| 5. Has Verbal Expression of Distress | _____ | _____ | _____ |
| 6. Has Observable Signs of Mental Distress | _____ | _____ | _____ |
| 7. Receives Psychoactive Medication | _____ | _____ | _____ |

|  | Yes | No | At Times |
|---|---|---|---|
| 8. Emotional Status: | | | |
| Moods Interfere With Daily Activity | _____ | _____ | _____ |
| Aware of Diagnosis | _____ | _____ | _____ |
| Participates in Care Plan | _____ | _____ | _____ |
| Accepts Facility Placement | _____ | _____ | _____ |
| Expresses Upset Over Lost Roles/Status | _____ | _____ | _____ |
| Unsettled Relationships: | | | |
| Family Member | _____ | _____ | _____ |
| Other Residents | _____ | _____ | _____ |
| Staff | _____ | _____ | _____ |

## III. Personal Data:

A. Family Relationships/Emotionally Supportive Persons:

| NAME | HOW RELATED | PHONE |
|---|---|---|
| _____ | _____ | _____ |
| _____ | _____ | _____ |
| _____ | _____ | _____ |
| _____ | _____ | _____ |
| _____ | _____ | _____ |
| _____ | _____ | _____ |
| _____ | _____ | _____ |

B. Birthplace_____ Education_____
   Lifetime Occupation_____

C. Cultural Background _____
   Interests/Hobbies _____

D. Adaptive Aids Used/Needed:
   Hearing Aid _____ Glasses _____ Dentures _____
   Clothing _____ Special Eating Equipment_____
   Ambulation Equipment _____

E. Information Received From _____
   _____

## IV. Identified Psychosocial Problems/Needs/Concerns:

Areas include: psychosocial, family, financial and social

_____
_____
_____
_____
_____
_____

Discharge Plan: _____

Social Service Professional _____ Date of Assessment _____

# Assessment Box — For Less Responsive Residents

There are many reasons that a resident may not be as responsive to some facets of the assessment processes as you might wish. The assessment box is a therapeutic tool to assist the resident in taking a more active role — to participate more fully in the initial assessment process.

The box should include both familiar and unusual items. Some of these items should be leisure related. Some should be orientation objects. Others should be unique and unexpected in order to stimulate the senses.

## Some items found in an Assessment Box could be:

| | |
|---|---|
| paint brush and paints | wallet |
| various types of small balls | deck of cards |
| sand paper | sports equipment |
| camera, view finder | binoculars |
| whistle | egg beater |
| pictures of familiar things | maps |
| sheet music | music box, tapes |
| coins, keys, silverware | scarves, gloves, ties |
| mirror, lotion, make up | gardening tools |
| potpourri | newspaper |

## Assessment Procedures:

1.  Eliminate as many distractions as possible.
2.  Sit across from the resident at a distance where there is close eye contact and s/he does not need to strain to hear you.
3.  Place the objects either on the table in front of the resident or leave them in the box and place the box on the table.

At this stage of the assessment, the goal is to create curiosity about the objects and then to assess the resident response to the objects. The goal is for the resident to identify items that appear familiar to him/her. This tells you what is familiar to the resident from his/her long term memory. These may become leisure activities or games created for this individual because of *his/her* response to them.

There are a multitude of observations you can make. You are most often looking for response to either familiarity or interest. For example, if there is positive and immediate response to a picture of a dog, this could indicate a past and also present interest and affection. If further indications confirm this observation, animal related programming would be a good idea. Remember, curiosity can initiate involvement and growth.

Puzzles with more than one shape that require the resident to place a piece in the correct outline, could indicate that s/he recognizes and processes the steps necessary to engage in this leisure pursuit.

Some individuals have experienced cognitive and sensory losses. Visual cues may assist them in participating more fully in the assessment process. Regardless of the functional level, you should strive to make the assessment experience an empowering one and the Assessment Box is an ally in this effort.

Some specific questions you may seek to answer through observation include:
*   Does resident seem most interested in bright objects? small objects?
*   Does s/he appear to recognize the object presented?
*   Does s/he use the objects as intended (e.g., does not try to eat the photograph)?

- Can s/he repeat the name of the object or acknowledge recognition with a yes/no or a nod of the head?
- Is there any differentiation between positive or negative responses?
- Does s/he look for an object that has been removed?
- Is s/he unwilling to return an object to you?
- Does s/he refuse to respond to this entire experience?
- Is s/he able to use small motor/fine motor movements to pick up and examine objects?

Focus to task and success in involvement can hopefully be nurtured and expanded with information gained through this assessment activity.

# Standardized Assessment Tools

Some Activity and Social Service Professionals may decide to use a standardized testing tool in addition to the forms shown here to obtain more information about a resident. Some assessment tools have been written using ideas and information obtained from rigorous research. Examples of standardized testing tools include both reality orientation scales and life satisfaction scales. Two books which provide greater information on the subject are **Assessment Tools for Recreational Therapy** by burlingame and Blaschko, 1990 and **Assessing the Elderly: A Practical Guide to Measurement** by Kane and Kane, 1984. A recently developed assessment, the **Therapeutic Recreation Activity Assessment**, 1994, measures fine motor skills, gross motor skills, social behavior, expressive communication, receptive communication and cognitive skills for residents in long term care facilities.

# Resident Assessment Instrument

In the United States, the Health Care Financing Administration (HCFA) requires that the Resident Assessment Instrument (RAI) be used in addition to the individual professional assessment. This is a standardized assessment and must be used by all nursing facilities accepting Medicare and Medicaid funds.

The RAI is composed of two parts, the Minimum Data Set (MDS) and the Resident Assessment Protocols (RAPs). The MDS is a functionally based assessment and screening tool. The MDS will be updated as needed. At the time this book was written, facilities were using the MDS 2.0 and the MDS + versions. The RAPs are used for problem identification. Together they form the basis for developing a resident care plan.

## RAI = MDS + RAPs

The MDS has two purposes. First it has scoring instructions which indicate treatment needs. The team is responsible for scoring the entire MDS and then developing the treatment plan (or RAPs) from the needs "triggered" by the MDS. Additional treatment needs may have been identified in the professional's initial assessment. These needs may also be addressed through the treatment plan.

The second purpose of the MDS is the standardization of treatment. Because it is used throughout the United States, extensive data can be collected on the typical treatment goals and the length of time needed for care based on the original MDS score. This information helps the government fund health care needs more accurately.

The Federal regulations specify that a standardized assessment be conducted no later than 14 calendar days after admission, promptly after a significant change of condition and again within 365 days of the date of the last complete assessment. Assessments must be reviewed once every three months using the standardized MDS quarterly review form and revised as needed to assure the continued accuracy of the assessment.

Because the Minimum Data Set comprises the "minimum" information necessary for evaluation, your state regulations or facility policy may require you to use a more detailed assessment form in addition to the MDS 2.0 or the MDS +. The time requirements for completing these assessments may differ from the Federal requirements for completing the RAI. In any case, it is always permissible to document more than the requirements mandate.

## MDS

The MDS is a minimum of core assessment items. It is a functionally based assessment tool. The MDS form has specific instructions for completion. The Health Care Financing Administration (HCFA) has published an excellent guide for the RAI, which should be available for use in the facility. Portions have been included in the Appendix on the MDS 2.0 and RAPs for those sections specific to activities and social services. However, to complete the RAI correctly, the Activity or Social Service Professional should be familiar with the entire manual.

The Item by Item Guide to the MDS from the RAI manual[38] should be used alongside the MDS form, keeping the form in front of you. It gives the definitions and procedural instructions necessary for sound assessment. Completion of the MDS provides a picture of the resident at an instant in time. It provides a baseline by which the resident's progress and/or regression can be assessed at intervals during the resident's stay. Completion of the MDS also provides a preliminary assessment and screening of resident problems. Specific responses will "trigger" or "screen out" actual or potential problems. If the MDS can be thought of as a sieve, then the potential problems identified can be thought of as sifting through to the next screening process, the RAPs.

## RAPs

The RAP process can seem overwhelming. It helps to remember that the RAPs are the second screening process to determine whether or not a potential problem requires further follow-up. There are 18 RAPs developed to provide more clinical information, understanding of problem situations, their possible causes and their impact on the resident.

A review of the triggered RAPs is required for new admission, significant change and the annual MDS. Completion of RAPs is not required for the quarterly MDS.

The RAPs function as decision facilitators. They provide the basis for developing a problem list and formulating the resident's plan of care. After the MDS and the RAPs are completed, the interdisciplinary team will be able to decide if:
- The resident has a troubling condition that warrants intervention and addressing this problem is necessary condition for other functional problems to be successfully addressed.
- Improvement of the resident's functioning in one or more areas is possible.
- Improvement is not likely, but the present level of functioning should be preserved as long as possible, with rates of decline minimized over time.
- The resident is at risk of decline and efforts should emphasize slowing or minimizing decline and avoiding functional complications (e.g., contractures, pain).
- The central issues of care revolve around symptom relief and other palliative measures during the last months of life.

There are three steps to completing the RAP process. The appendix on the MDS 2.0 and RAPs shows the *Resident Assessment Protocol: Activities* and *Resident Assessment Protocol: Psychosocial Well-Being.* Refer to it in the steps that follow.

---

[38] Health Care Finance Administration, **RAI Training Manual**, Chapter 6 (also shown in the appendices to this book).

I. Review Section II, "Triggers," to determine if the trigger criteria are met. If the RAP meets the trigger criteria, determine why the RAP triggered. This is the most important step in the RAP evaluation process. The RAP cannot be completed correctly if the reason it triggered is not understood. Ask the question, How did I get here? Also remember that a RAP review must always be done if the trigger criteria are met. After the review you decide whether to proceed or not. As an example, the Activity Rap is triggered for several reasons:

A. The resident is involved in activities little or none of the time [N2 = 2,3]. Why is this a problem? The RAP identifies two types of residents with this question:
1. The first is the cognitively intact, distressed resident who may benefit from an enriched activity program.
2. The second is the cognitively intact, distressed resident whose activity levels should be evaluated.
In both cases, an evaluation and revision of the care plan may be required.

B. The resident prefers a change in daily routine [N5a = 1,2] [N5b = 1,2]. Why is this a problem? The RAP identifies residents that have additional activity choices that may not be met by the facility. An evaluation and revision of the care plan may be required.

C. The resident is awake all or most of the time in morning and involved in activities most of the time. [N1a = checked and N2 = 0]. Why is this a problem? The RAP identifies residents whose health may be in jeopardy because of their failure to "slow down," as in a diagnosis of Congestive Heart Failure. An evaluation and review of the care plan may be required to be sure the resident is not overstimulated or fatigued.

II. Review Section III — Guidelines of each RAP to:

A. Establish the nature of the condition. Ask yourself each of the questions in relation to the resident. Some may be relevant, some may not. It is not necessary to record all of the items referred to in the RAP guidelines, listing all factors that do and do not apply. Documentation should focus on the key questions that pertain to the resident.

1. Is the triggered condition actually a problem for the resident?
2. Does it place the resident at particular risk?
3. Should it be addressed in the plan of care?
4. Is the resident a good candidate for a rehabilitative intervention?

B. Evaluate methods to reverse or eliminate the condition. If the triggered condition is actually a problem or places the resident at risk, plan a program of services to ensure that the resident attains or maintains the highest practical physical, mental and psychosocial well-being.

1. What actions can staff take?
2. What activities are appropriate?
3. What corrective actions are possible for environmental factors?

III. Determine if the resident has a need for a revised activity plan. In other words, does a problem really exist or did the RAP review fail to identify a problem? Document your rationale for proceeding or not proceeding to the care plan. Identify the decision to proceed or not proceed with care planning on the RAP summary sheet and the location of the information. In this second screening process, the problem is evaluated in greater depth. Causal factors are identified, their impact on the resident is determined and a decision is made on how to proceed.

When the review process becomes familiar, the RAP key can be used to provide a quick review of the condition triggers (left column) and key items from the clinical Guidelines specified in Section III of the RAP (right column). How do you decide whether or not to proceed with care planning? The key is to know why the RAP triggered. The MDS preliminary screening will trigger many potential problems. In an attempt not to miss any potential problem, some items may trigger a check for a problem that does not actually exist. In other cases, the problem may exist but the physician, resident or family may not agree to pursue the interventions suggested by the RAP.

The method for documenting the RAP review will vary according to personal preference and facility policy. Some methods that are used include: a narrative progress note, a computerized printout, a standard RAP module form or a standard RAP review form. Two examples are given below of a narrative progress note. The case study gives a picture of the resident. Refer to the Activity RAP guidelines as each note is read to see which questions were addressed.

## RAP Example 1

Mr. Z is 86 years old with a diagnosis of endstage Alzheimer's. He is a retired accountant. He no longer recognizes his family or staff. He is on an antipsychotic medication for aggressive behavior. His main occupation is wandering around the facility clutching a newspaper (or any other paper object he can get his hands on ). He has very little interest in activity programs. He can't sit still for more than a few minutes before he wanders off. He seems content to amble around the facility and only becomes angry when he is made to participate in ADLs or is stopped from his wandering. He is marked as N2 = 3 on the MDS and triggers the Activity RAP.

Sample RAP note for Mr. Z

Triggered due to spending no time in activities. Mr. Z's main impediment to activity participation is his diagnosis of end stage Alzheimer's which precludes involvement in activities that would be of interest to him. There are no other diagnoses that contribute. He has had no other decline in functional status and remains ambulatory. He has retained some connection to "paperwork" and it seems at times as if he is "going to the office," but he has no ability to learn new skills or practice old skills. The antipsychotic medication has improved his tolerance of others around him and he is safer in his wandering behavior. He seems unaware of his environment, weather, etc. and doesn't particularly care whether he is inside or outside. He shows some awareness of holidays, especially Christmas, but only fleetingly. His wife and son visit 3-5 times a week but he shows no recognition of them. As lack of involvement is due to his severe Alzheimer's and there are no reversible impediments, a care plan revision is not required. Will not proceed. He is content and occupied in his routine. J. Jones, AC.

## RAP Example 2

Mrs. Y is a 72 year old woman with a recent CVA which has left her right side paralyzed. She is right hand dominant. She was very active prior to her CVA, participating in community events and maintaining a household for herself and her husband. She misses her dog and is worried it is not being taken care of. She is very depressed over her losses, feels she will never get better and is not participating fully in her rehab program. Her depression has caused a loss of appetite and she is losing weight and strength. Her speech is affected but she is cognitively unimpaired. The therapists and MD feel she has very good potential for recovery.

Sample RAP note for Mrs. Y

Mrs. Y's main impediment to involvement in activities is her severe lack of hope that she will ever get better. Her recent CVA has left her unable to participate in her prior activity patterns. Her lack of energy reserves contribute to her inability to participate in activities as her limited reserves are spent with therapy. She has retained the knowledge of how to perform her past interests but lacks the physical ability to perform. This contributes to her high level of

frustration and feeling of hopelessness. Her speech is very difficult to understand which also contributes to her frustration, but she makes it clear that she "hates this place." Her family and church group are frequent visitors and provide spiritual support that she responds to positively. The IDT has requested a psychologist evaluation and she and her husband have been introduced to the stroke support group. The main impediment to overcome is her feeling of hopelessness before she can proceed to recovery. Will proceed to careplan.
J. Jones, AC.

## Focus of RAPs

There are 18 RAPs. Each RAP has a particular focus. To document correctly and meet federal regulations, you need to understand the particular focus of each RAP and why it triggered.

Different types of triggers can change the focus of the RAP review. There are four types of triggers:
1. Potential Problems — factors may be present which suggest a problem may exist
2. Broad Screening Triggers — identify hard to diagnose problems. Because these are very broad, there are many "false positives." These RAPs overtrigger to prevent a problem from being overlooked. The Dehydration and Delirium RAPs have broad screening triggers.
3. Prevention of Problems — identify residents at risk for developing problems. An example is the resident with limited bed mobility. This triggers the Pressure Ulcer RAP.
4. Rehabilitation Potential — identify residents with rehabilitation potential. These trigger areas of resident strengths. In these cases, the care plan should focus on the areas with the highest potential for improvement.

To illustrate this point, review the Psychosocial RAP in the appendix. Notice in Section II, "Triggers," that *Establishes own goals [F1d = checked]* triggers the Psychosocial RAP and is identified as a strength.

In reviewing the RAP for this resident, the focus is to maintain and/or build on the strength of independent goal setting and to develop a plan to accommodate lifestyle issues. A resident who establishes his/her own goals may also be at risk for clashing with the staff or facility routine if lifestyle issues are not accommodated. There may be a need to develop a plan to avoid any resulting perceived behavior problems.

The following pages describe the eighteen RAPs, their focus and the suggested care planning goals from the RAP guidelines.

# RAP Descriptions

| RAP NAME | FOCUS OF RAP | CARE PLAN GOALS |
|---|---|---|
| Delirium | • detect signs and symptoms of delirium<br>• review the major causes of delirium and treat any found. | 1. prevent cycle of worsening symptoms (e.g. infection, fever, dehydration, confusion syndrome).<br>2. resolve delirium. |
| Cognitive Loss or Dementia | • enhance quality of life.<br>• sustain functional capacities, minimize decline and preserve dignity.<br>• identify potentially reversible causes for loss in cognitive status.<br>• identify and treat acute confusion. | 1. provide positive experiences for the resident.<br>2. define appropriate support roles for each staff member in the resident's care.<br>3. lay the foundation for reasonable staff and family expectations. |
| Visual Function | identify two types of residents:<br>1. those who have treatable conditions that place them at risk for permanent blindness.<br>2. those who have impaired vision whose quality of life could be improved through use of visual appliances. | 1. proper use of eye medications.<br>2. examination and follow-up by a vision consultant.<br>3. appropriate use of vision appliances.<br>4. modification of environment to meet individual's needs. |
| Communication | identify three types of residents:<br>1. those with serious communication deficits who have retained some decision making ability.<br>2. those with serious communication deficits in addition to no ability to make decisions but no underlying CVA or neurological problems.<br>3. those with hearing deficits and some ability to make decisions. | 1. restorative communication treatment program.<br>2. address behavioral, mood, environmental limitations that complicate communication.<br>3. restorative hearing program.<br>4. compensation strategies for communication loss (e.g. nonverbal communication skills). |
| ADL Functional Rehab Potential | • identify residents who either have the need and potential to improve or the need for services to prevent decline. | 1. restore function to maximum self-sufficiency.<br>2. replace hands-on assistance with a program of cueing and task segmentation.<br>3. restore abilities to a level that allow functioning with fewer supports.<br>4. shorten time required for providing assistance.<br>5. expand the amount of space in which self-sufficiency can be practiced.<br>6. avoid or delay additional loss of independence.<br>7. support the resident who is certain to decline to lessen the likelihood of complications (e.g. ulcers and contractures). |

# RAP Descriptions

| RAP NAME | FOCUS OF RAP | CARE PLAN GOALS |
|---|---|---|
| Urinary Incontinence and Indwelling Catheter | • improve incontinence either by bladder training or by detecting reversible causes of incontinence such as infections, medications, situationally induced stress incontinence.<br>• identify harmful conditions such as bladder tumors or spinal cord diseases.<br>• consider the appropriateness of catheter use. | 1. improve incontinence.<br>2. resolve incontinence.<br>3. discontinue use of indwelling catheter. |
| Psychosocial Well-Being | • identify distressing relationships and concern about loss of status.<br>• identify situational factors that may impede ability to interact with others.<br>• focus on areas where resident may lack the ability to enter freely into satisfying social relationships.<br>• identify lifestyle issues. | 1. develop treatment for mood/behavior problems.<br>2. develop staff interventions to change environmental and situational problems without "changing the resident." |
| Mood State | • determine if an altered care strategy is required (e.g. sad mood, feelings of emptiness, anxiety or unease, weight loss, tearfulness, agitation, aches and pains which persist with current care strategy). | 1. resolve mood problem. |
| Behavior Problems | • draw a distinction between serious behavior problems and others that can more easily be accommodated.<br>• identify potential reversible causes or factors involved in the manifestation of problem behaviors.<br>• develop a management plan to avoid the use of restraints. | 1. resolve causes and factors manifested by behavior problems.<br>2. adapt environmental and staff responses.<br>3. involve resident in psychological treatment plan.<br>4. limit use of restraints. |
| Activities | • focus on cases where the system has failed the resident or where the resident has distressing conditions that warrant a revised activity plan.<br>• identify factors that impede resident involvement in activities. | 1. help resident overcome distressing conditions.<br>2. remove factors that impede involvement in activities. |
| Falls | • identify and assess those who have fallen and those who are at risk for falls. | 1. identify and address risk factors.<br>2. manage risk factors and/or eliminate. |
| Nutritional Status | • focus on signs and symptoms that suggest that the resident may be at risk of becoming malnourished.<br>• early detection is the key. | 1. identify and address risk factors.<br>2. adjust feeding patterns.<br>3. compensate or correct food intake problems. |

# RAP Descriptions

| RAP NAME | FOCUS OF RAP | CARE PLAN GOALS |
|---|---|---|
| Feeding Tubes | • focus on reviewing the status of the resident using tubes.<br>• assess risks vs. benefits of tube use. | 1. remove tube.<br>2. prevent complications and serious negative consequences. |
| Dehydration and Fluid Maintenance | • identify any and all possible high risk cases.<br>• early intervention with hydration programs to prevent the condition from occurring. | 1. restore normal fluid volume.<br>2. identify and resolve risk factors for dehydration.<br>3. avoid consequences of dehydration. |
| Dental Care | • identify compounding problems which may prevent a resident from adequately removing oral debris.<br>• identify residents who may benefit from dental treatment. | 1. resolve compounding problems.<br>2. promote good oral health.<br>3. obtain appropriate dental services. |
| Pressure Ulcer | • ensure a treatment plan is in place to treat actual pressure ulcers.<br>• identify residents at risk for pressure ulcers. | 1. resolve ulcers following specified treatment plan.<br>2. prevent development of pressure ulcers. |
| Psychoactive Drug Use | • evaluate the need for the drug.<br>• start low, go slow.<br>• evaluate side effects and interaction with other medications.<br>• consider symptoms or decline in functional status as a potential side effect of medication. | 1. reduce or eliminate use of drug.<br>2. assess and prevent side effects of drug use.<br>3. assess and prevent decline in functional status. |
| Physical Restraints | • evaluate the need for the physical restraint.<br>• evaluate needs, problems, risk factors that if addressed could eliminate the need for the restraint.<br>• evaluate side effects of restraint use. | 1. reduce or eliminate use of physical restraint.<br>2. assess and prevent side effects of restraint use.<br>3. eliminate factors requiring restraint use. |

*Excerpted from the HCFA RAI Training Manual*

Although the Activity and Social Service Departments may only be responsible for completing a few of the RAPS, it is necessary for these disciplines to review the entire MDS and all triggered RAPs prior to completing the care plan. This is usually done in care conference; but if not, each discipline must take the responsibility to complete a thorough review of the RAI.

The MDS responses, especially in Cognition, ADL, Incontinence and Nutrition, will give more in-depth assessment information and possibly more current information than was gathered on admission. Many of the RAPS require or suggest interventions by the Activity and/or Social Service Professionals in conjunction with the other interdisciplinary team members.

The following charts list the RAPs and suggested interventions to be considered when developing the resident care plan.

# RAPs Requiring Activity Intervention

| | |
|---|---|
| Delirium | • Caused by recent relocation: Orientation program to provide calm, gentle approach with reminders and structure to help resident settle in.<br>• Caused by diagnosis: Activity program to help prevent further cognitive decline and improve quality of life while problem is being treated. |
| Cognitive Loss | • Provide positive experiences for the resident (e.g., enjoyable activities) that do not involve overly demanding tasks and stress.<br>• Design programs to enhance resident's quality of life.<br>• Provide opportunities for independent activity, participate more in decisions about daily life.<br>• Task segmentation.<br>• Small group programs.<br>• Special environmental stimuli (e.g., markers, special lighting). |
| Communication | • Provide opportunities to communicate, e.g., availability of partners.<br>• Provide tactile approaches to communication.<br>• Participate in restorative communication treatment program. |
| ADL | • Provide a program that supports rehabilitative goals for the resident. |
| Psychosocial Well-Being | • Provide social relationships.<br>• Alter environment to allow access to others or routine activities.<br>• Provide activities to address cognitive/communication deficits that may cause a lack of interest in activities or interactions with others.<br>• Focus on a daily schedule that resembles the resident's prior lifestyle. |
| Mood State | • Passive residents with distressed mood may be overlooked.<br>• Evaluate those with no involvement in activities (alone or with others) or little initiative. |
| Behavior Problems | • Participate in support programs that focus on managing behaviors.<br>• Participate in activities where coping skills, relaxation and anger management techniques are taught. |
| Activities | • Focus on: residents who have indicated a desire for additional activity choices; cognitively intact, distressed residents who may benefit from an enriched activity program; cognitively deficient, distressed residents whose activity levels should be evaluated; and highly involved residents whose health may be in jeopardy because of their failure to slow down. |

# RAPs Requiring Social Service Intervention

| | |
|---|---|
| Delirium | Assess and intervene if caused by:<br>• isolation,<br>• recent loss of family/friend,<br>• depression/sad anxious mood,<br>• recent relocation and/or<br>• sensory losses. |
| Cognitive Loss or Dementia | • Develop strategies to assist staff.<br>• Learn to live with behavioral manifestations of cognitive loss.<br>• Develop a behavior control program.<br>• Assess if problem could be remedied through improved staff education, referral to OT/RT for training or an innovative counseling program.<br>• Assess if emotional, social, excess disability and/or environmental factors play a role in cognitive decline. |
| Visual Function | • Referral to optometrist/ophthalmologist if necessary.<br>• Evaluate for appropriate use of visual appliances: glasses clean, labeled, reading glasses not used for walking.<br>• Evaluate for effect of sad or anxious mood on visual dysfunction.<br>• Evaluate for appropriate devices for level of vision: large print calendar, clock, high wattage light, large print signs.<br>• Refer to activities if necessary. |
| ADL | • Evaluate the effect of mood or behavior problems on ADL performance and motivation.<br>• Develop a behavior control program that could improve functioning. |
| Incontinence | • Evaluate the effect of incontinence on psychosocial well-being and social interactions and assist resident with coping with the dysfunction. |
| Psychosocial Well-Being | • Evaluate the effect of mood and behavior problems on feelings about self and social relationships.<br>• Develop treatment program to focus on mood and behavior problems.<br>• Develop corrective strategies to address distressing relationships and concern about loss of status. |
| Mood State | • Evaluate for need for new or altered care strategy when manifestations of mood state problem are present: sad mood; feelings of emptiness, anxiety or unease; loss of weight; tearfulness; agitation; aches and pains; bodily complaints and dysfunction. |
| Behavior Problem | • Develop alternate interventions and treatments to address behavior problems.<br>• Identify the various factors involved in the manifestation of problem to identify behaviors that could be resolved and eliminate the problem. |
| Psychoactive Drug Use | • Develop monitors and care plan to address possible decline or impairment of cognitive and behavior status. |
| Physical Restraints | • Evaluate conditions associated with problem behaviors and physical restraint use: delirium impaired, cognition impaired, communication unmet, psychosocial needs, sad or anxious mood, resistance to treatment, medication, nourishment, motor agitation, confusion, gait disturbance.<br>• Evaluate residents response to restraint use.<br>• Evaluate the philosophy, values, attitudes and wishes of the resident regarding restraint use.<br>• Develop monitors and care plan to address possible negative outcomes from restraint use. |

# Resident Care Plans

The assessment process is a comprehensive system of problem identification that provides the foundation for care planning. The care plan is the road map to resident care and treatment. It matches the individual resident's strengths, problems and needs with appropriate interventions and programs for care.

After the assessment is complete, the interdisciplinary team develops the initial plan of care for the resident. This is done by holding a care conference with members of the treatment team, the resident and the resident's family or guardian. In the past it was normal for each discipline to have its own set of goals. Now it is more common for many of the goals to require a coordinated effort from more than one discipline on the treatment team.

After the conference, the plan is formalized in a written document. New resident care plans are also required every time a new MDS is required, any time the resident's condition changes and at least once a year. Conferences to be sure that the plan of care is on track are held quarterly.

When you make a resident care plan, it is vital to remember that the resident is the consumer of our services and therefore has the absolute right to have input into the type of care and treatment objectives developed for him/her. Federal law (Tags F155 and F156) also mandates that we extend the resident and/or family the right to participate in this process and the right to make the final decision in any plan of care.

It is important to be aware of a resident's *capacity* to make decisions for themselves. This information can be determined by the physician and/or the courts, based on input from the entire treatment team. Determination of capacity will appear either on the physician's order sheet or in the advanced directives section of the chart. If a resident has the capacity to make decisions, you must ask his/her permission to contact the family for involvement in the care conference and for obtaining additional personal information. If the resident does not have the capacity to make these decisions, then the staff must request involvement from the responsible party or family member.

Involvement can take one of two forms: 1. actual participation in the care conference or 2. discussions between the resident and/or family and a designated staff member (usually a Social Service Professional or someone from nursing). Either method is acceptable as the intent of the law is for involvement in the care plan process, but not specifically at resident care conferences.

To program success into the care conferences, send invitations to the responsible party or conservator well in advance. Allow at least ten minutes per resident/family, more for the initial care plan or if you know there will be significant concerns that need to be covered in a team situation. Explain clearly that this is a time to see what the resident's problems are and to assess whether or not the concerns still exist and are being addressed.

At the resident care conference, listen carefully to each perspective. Nursing will speak to disabilities and health problems; dietary to nutritional needs and expectations; activities to sociability, lifestyle and interests; therapies to functional potential. Cognitive ability and orientation are important for all to be aware of. Usually the Activity and Social Service Professionals are the ones who formally assess these areas. The Social Service Professional can help identify the resident's mental status. For example, can we expect him/her to know the difference between fantasy, paranoia and reality?

Resident and family are then given the opportunity to discuss particular worries with the attending staff. Should grievances surface which will take longer than the scheduled time, the team should make an appointment for further discussion with the appropriate members of the team (often social services).

Many residents and families do not respond well in the group situation. In that case, the individual conference is especially worthy of merit. It is generally less anxiety-provoking and, we have found, more comfortable for many. It is also an opportunity to work more closely with residents and families to resolve ongoing concerns by addressing them at a comfortable pace and with undivided attention.

Use this opportunity four times a year to review Residents' Rights with the residents. Don't assume that because you have done this once that it is done! It is also a good time to review Advanced Directives to be sure that the wishes of the resident still remain as stated in the record.

# Resident Care Plan Documentation

The purpose of the care plan is to aid the resident in attaining or maintaining their highest practicable physical, mental and psychosocial well-being.

To achieve this the interdisciplinary team uses the information identified in the RAPs to address the needs, strengths and preferences of the resident. The care plan is required to be oriented toward preventing avoidable declines in functioning, managing risk factors and building on strengths.

The resident care plan is functionally oriented, rather than medically oriented. This means that, rather than planning care for the medical diagnoses, the care plan addresses the losses that the resident has sustained from the condition and how they affect the resident's functioning. For example, a care plan for a resident with Congestive Heart Failure could include dealing with the issues of mobility limitations, diet restrictions, loss of energy and the need to "slow down." Diagnoses are assessed as contributory factors, but usually only short term, acute diagnoses (e.g., urinary tract infections) are included in the plan.

Writing entries on the resident care plan requires experience. It is frightening to think of committing your ideas to paper when you first face this process, but over time you will learn to use your MDS, RAPS and assessment tools to help you do your work. As a history emerges, so will the material for your resident care plan entry.

Before you make your entry, read carefully what the other disciplines have discovered about the resident. Review all of the triggered RAPs for the resident and using the RAP chart shown in the assessment section of this chapter, consider what interventions your department can use to help address the problem or need. The ideal is to be working on the issues with other departments in an interdisciplinary fashion. It may be possible to "tie on" to existing entries in the care plan. Your care plan entry will address the issue and contributing factors. The teamwork will be reflected in the approach column. Refer to the care plan example for Mrs. Y for an idea of how to merge RAPs and disciplines.

The resident care plan is an interdisciplinary form. Although it is not required that every goal have an interdisciplinary approach, it is rare that a professional in one discipline will make an entry pertaining to that discipline alone. The care plan should "merge" disciplines and RAPs into holistic programs that represent the resident's strengths and needs.

All care plan entries are reviewed quarterly. If there is a change of condition, this entry will be reviewed before the quarter is up and revisions will be made, if necessary. If the resident's condition has been stable, the entry will be reviewed and updated with the next quarterly review. If you find that a goal is met and the problem no longer needs to be addressed, it will be changed at the time of update. Remember, a change to the care plan always requires an explanatory progress note.

# Care Plan Components

Care plans may follow many different formats, may be computerized or preprinted, may use different terminology, but they all contain a specific set of information shown in the table below. The three key elements (problem, need or strength statement; objective; and a plan of action) are discussed in more detail following the chart.

## Components of a Care Plan Entry

| Date | Today's date: day, month and year |
|---|---|
| Initials | Your initials to identify the person writing the care plan |
| Discipline | Discipline responsible for carrying out the care plan — Activity or Social Service Department |
| Problem, Need or Strength | "Resident needs ..." |
| Objective | "Resident will ..." |
| Plan of Action | Team actions that will help the resident achieve the goal. Number these and be very specific as to who, what, where and when. These approaches will be reflected in attendance records. |
| Review Date | Three months from entry date unless there is a change of condition |
| Resolve Date | Date the problem/need was resolved or discontinued |

## Problem, Need, Strength Statement

A problem is a condition or behavior that you feel should be changed to improve the quality of life for the resident. A need is a requirement of something essential or desirable that is lacking. A strength is an inherent capacity to act upon or affect something. How to write each type of statement is shown below.

    1. Problem:
        A. What is the problem?
        B. Where is the problem?
        C. When is there a problem?
        Example:        A. Can't hear
                            B. Right ear
                            C. Hearing aid lost
        Statement:      Can't hear from R ear due to lost hearing aid.
    2. Need:
        A.       What is the need?
        B.       Why is there a need?
        Example:      A. needs to be fed
                              B. paralysis of upper extremities
        Statement:      Needs to be fed due to paralysis of upper extremities.
    3. Strength:
        A. What are the strengths?
        B. What is to be acted on?
        Example:      A. desires to go home
                              B. when mobility regained
        Statement:      Desires to go home when mobility regained.

## Objective

An objective is something for the resident to try to achieve. An objective needs each of the characteristics shown below.
        What — the actions that are to be done and by whom
        Measurable — how far, how often, how many times, how much
        Observable — experienced with the senses: see, feel, smell, hear, taste
        Time — limited date to achieve desired result

Example:
What: resident will walk to maintain function
Measurable: walk 100 feet, 2x day, 5 days a week
Observable: staff observe walk
Time limit: 4-3-96 to 6-4-96

Objective: Resident will walk a minimum of 100 feet (distance from room to activity room) two times a day, five days a week to maintain skill — 3-4-96 through 6-4-96.

## Action Plan

The action plan lists the actions to be taken by each discipline to solve the problem, meet the need or improve the strength and achieve the objective. The action plan has the following information:

Who — Specific to each discipline
What — instructions for resident care
When — time frames
How — realistic to staffing and equipment

Example:
Who:    Social Service
What:   take resident for walk
When:   after lunch Mon., Wed., Fri.
How:    with front wheeled walker

Statement: Social Service will take resident for walk after lunch Mon., Wed., Fri. using front wheeled walker.

## Care Plan Examples

Mrs. Y has triggered the Mood, Psychosocial, ADL, Activities and Nutritional RAPs. The Interdisciplinary team has decided that her most acute need is to resolve her mood problem as this is causing most of her other problems and impeding her rehabilitation goals. The team care plans merging all of the above RAPs are shown below.

| Problem, Need, Strength | Objective | Interventions | Dsc |
|---|---|---|---|
| 5/15/96<br>Alteration in Mood as evidenced by:<br>• expresses sadness over lost status<br>• anger at nursing home placement<br>• spends little time in activities<br>• leaves 25% > uneaten | will eat 80% of breakfast & lunch QD by 5/20/96 | 1. Hipro with each meal<br>2. DSS to provide substitutes for food refused<br>3. Encourage husband and friends to bring in favorite foods | D<br>D<br><br>All |
| • lacks interest in rehab<br>• frustration over lack of speech<br><br>Contributory factors:<br>• Recent CVA with dysphasia<br>• Recent decline in ADLs<br>• Recent nursing home placement | will verbalize acceptance of disability and need to participate in rehab by 5/25/96 | 1. Introduce to stroke support group<br>2. Visit with facility dog<br>3. Discuss Discharge Plan in positive terms<br>4. Ask yes/no questions<br>5. Allow time to express thoughts<br>6. Psych visit 1x wk<br>7. PT to describe interim goals to be met to achieve discharge | SS<br><br>AC<br>DC<br><br>All<br>All<br>Psy<br>PT |
| Strengths:<br>• Close family and church group support<br>• Good rehabilitation potential | | 1. Space to be arranged for daily visits from friends | AC |

# Sample Activity Care Plan Entries

The **Activity Care Planning Cookbook** by Hall and Nolte[39] contains problem/need statements, goals and over 300 care plan approaches and interventions. A sample care plan on anxiety in shown below. Choose the entries that are appropriate for the resident and integrate them into the care plan. Tie on to existing problems/needs if possible.

Category:       Emotional Issues
Subtopic:       Anxiety

| Problem Description, Concern, Need or Strength | Goal/ Objective | Approach/ Interventions |
|---|---|---|
| Refer to MDS Section E<br><br>• Resident often appears to become anxious during activity programs evidenced by wringing hands, jumping at every sound, rigid posture, frequently yelling for help, _____.<br><br>• Resident often states, "I'm not sure I should be here. I have lots of things to do in my room."<br><br>• Resident needs one-on-one attention to promote participation during activity programs secondary to displaying anxious behaviors. | • Resident will not exhibit anxious behavior of _____, for \_\_\_\_ minutes, at _____ group activities, \_\_\_\_ times per week.<br><br>• Residents will participate in _____ activity programs by following the groups general directions, \_\_\_\_ times per week. | • Invite, assist Resident to group activities of interest (i.e. _____ _____).<br><br>• Explain the activity program's format to Resident prior to the start of program.<br><br>• Allow Resident to choose seating placement at program.<br><br>• Introduce to other alert peers. Identify similarities between Residents to promote conversation/friendships.<br><br>• Ask the Resident direct questions to promote participation.<br><br>• Refocus the Resident's attention to the specific activity task of _____ if anxious behavior is exhibited.<br><br>• Compliment the Resident for following the activity program's directions. |

---

[39] Hall, Beth A., CTRS and Michele M. Nolte, CTRS, ACC, 1996, **The Activity Care Planning Cookbook 2.0**, p. 5-3, Recreation Therapy Consultants, San Diego, CA.

The chart below shows more possible entries in a resident care plan specific to activities. These could be combined with existing problems/needs on the care plan.

| Problem/Need | Goal | Approach |
|---|---|---|
| Poor pathfinding skills — needs to go between room and dining room | Resident will be able to go between room and dining room without assistance within 3 months. | 1. Visual cue on door.<br>2. Walk with Resident to and from dining room.<br>3. All staff to praise efforts of Resident. |
| Sensory deprivation — needs tactile stimulation | Resident will receive a minimum of 20 minutes of tactile stimulation a day. | 1. Pet visits 2x weekly.<br>2. Massage hands with lotion 3x weekly.<br>3. 1:1 with sensory stimulation kits 2x weekly |
| Personal appearance sloppy, beard stubble, uncombed hair, body odor — needs to improve grooming | Resident will shave at least every two days, comb hair daily and bathe daily. | 1. AC to visit with grooming items 2x weekly.<br>2. Grooming group 2x weekly.<br>3. CNAs to assist with AM care. |
| Hearing impairment — needs to be seated next to group leader | Resident will learn to sit next to leader where s/he can hear and respond to reminiscing questions. | 1. Seat Resident next to leader in Current Events 1x weekly.<br>2. Reinforce advantages of sitting where s/he can hear.<br>3. Use visual cues. |
| Blindness and deafness — needs increased social contact | Resident will have at least 20 minutes of structured social contact 7x weekly. | 1. AC to assist weaving hand over hand 4x weekly.<br>2. Resident will roll yarn ball for project.<br>3. Include in cooking, gardening and out door events for social interactions 5x weekly. |
| Self-stimulation — needs to keep hands busy due to dementia | Resident will fold napkins for social events by 3 months. | 1. AC to set up folding station for Resident 1x daily.<br>2. AC/volunteer to visit Resident with tactile 2x weekly. |

## Other Resident Care Plan Considerations

If your facility uses hand-written resident care plans, you can leave a few lines between your entry and the ones above and below. As the residents needs change and interventions are revised, there is room to add new entries.

Be realistic, both in your identification of a problem and the approach. Do not enter "will visit 4x weekly" on the care plan, if you realistically cannot visit more than 2 times weekly.

Be specific in your interventions. For example, do not enter "Group activities 1 x wk," but rather "Go to sing-along 1x week."

Be sure that the goal which is stated on the care plan is the same as the one discussed in the quarterly note. You must be sure that all parts of the care plan come from observations in the assessments and that every observation of problems or needs in the assessments — especially triggers in the MDS if the team decides to proceed — are addressed in the care plan. The team may choose not to proceed with a triggered RAP, but they must document why they made that decision.

There are some terms to avoid in identifying a problem on the care plan. The following chart offers some alternatives which are more descriptive and offer clearer connections between the problem and the treatment.

| Don't say this | Say this to be more descriptive |
|---|---|
| social isolation<br>or<br>loneliness | needs to be aware of people around him/her<br>or<br>needs to feel useful to others |
| non-responsive | fear of answering inappropriately in a group setting. |
| confusion | needs to improve problem solving skills |
| short attention span | needs to follow one directive in exercise class<br>or<br>needs to stay on task with project for 5 minutes |
| disorientation | needs to locate room |
| too tired | needs energy conservation techniques due to COPD |
| boredom | needs to develop one new leisure interest |
| lack of awareness | needs to stimulate short term memory retention |
| anxious | cries easily due to CVA or has anxiety due to CVA |
| need for diversional activities | needs diversion to decrease agitation |
| needs sensory stimulation | needs to respond to _____ stimulation as seen by (blinking eyes, holding object etc.)<br>Be specific as to what type of stimulation — tactile, visual, auditory, etc. |
| refuses to attend | This is the resident choice and is not a problem for the resident. Your problem is to devise activities that the resident will participate in. |
| needs transportation to activities | no alternative, this is your problem, not the resident's |

# Monitoring the Care Plan

Assessing the resident and writing the care plan are not the end of the process of resident care. There must be an ongoing process to monitor the status of each resident. You must make notes in the resident's chart whenever there is any change of condition that affects the residents functioning or ability to participate in programming. Every quarter the care team must meet to perform a quarterly review of each resident's care plan which includes determining if the most recent assessment of the resident's condition is still correct.

As we will discuss in the nest section. *Updating the Care Plan*, significant changes in the resident's condition indicate the need for a new care plan. (OBRA requires a new RAI, too, under certain circumstances.)

# Monitoring Documentation — Activities

There are several ways to make sure that your treatment plan is still appropriate for the resident. The methods include:
- Thirty-day Re-evaluation Note (optional)
- Daily Activity Attendance (Participation ) Records
- Bedside Log Notes for one-on-one visits
- Progress Notes

### Thirty-Day Re-evaluation Note (Optional)

Thirty days after admission, the Activity Professional should review the initial assessment, the MDS and the RAPs to determine whether there has been any change of condition or if there is a need for a change of plan. S/he should document the results of the re-evaluation in the care plan including the date of the review and a signature.

This note is not required by federal law, but we feel that significant changes in the resident or in your perception of the resident occur often enough in the first thirty days to justify this as a recommended standard of practice. If everything stays the same, you can initial and date the original form to document this review.

If there has been a change or there is additional information which you feel is important to document, use the activity progress note page and title it "30 day re-eval note." An example of what this note might say:

> 4/22/96      30 day re-eval note
> Resident has adjusted to the environment and schedule of the facility. She is still very involved with rehab therapies with the goal of returning home. She is spending time with AC reinforcing PT goals through short walks outdoors 2 x weekly. This is the same goal but we have added onto the frequency per week as her level of endurance seems to be improving.
> E. Best CTRS, ACC

### Participation Records

Records must be kept on each resident's participation in activities and treatment programs. The records must be kept seven days a week. The following pages show a set of forms you can use to keep a record of participation. We recommend that the Activity Professional use two different kinds of forms for documentation of participation:
1.   Activity Participation Record
2.   Special Programming/Bedside Log

The first form, the Activity Participation Sheet, shows a way to keep track of resident participation in group activities. You don't have to use this exact form, but it includes the set of information that you do need to keep. (You, of course, need to have the activities from your facility listed). The important components to include are resident name, type of activity, date and length of time. You may also want to use a code which shows the level of participation (active or passive). When a resident refuses an invitation to an activity or room visit, be sure to mark R for refuse. This will document that you attempted to include her/him and that it is her/his right to refuse.

For residents who are restricted to their beds or who do not attend activities 2–3 times per week you need to keep additional documentation to show their involvement in activities. One way to do this is with a bedside log shown in the second form. Whatever type of log you decide to use, it must describe the type of visit (what you did), length of the visit, date and the resident's response.

In 1996 the Health Care Financing Administration released a report showing Tag F248 as the tenth most cited deficiency across the nation. One of the causes for this Tag to be found out of compliance is that the activity staff recorded only attendance. The activity staff are expected to show the degree of independence demonstrated by each resident for each activity. We recommend activity staff use the FIM Scale (or modified FIM Scale) when documenting participation. The complete FIM Scale can be found in the *Glossary (Appendix A)*.

**Modified FIM Scale**

| Symbol | Term | Description |
|---|---|---|
| I<br>(7-6) | Independent | The resident doesn't require the assistance of another person to engage in the activity. The resident is able to engage in the activity at a reasonable pace, with or without the use of adaptive equipment and does not present undo safety concerns. |
| S<br>(5-3) | Semi-independent | The resident requires assistance in set-up, and/or standby assistance, and/or cueing/coaxing, and/or touching assistance while still completing at least 50% of the activity himself/herself. |
| D<br>(2-1) | Dependent | The resident requires physical assistance to engage in activity. Resident completes less than 50% of the activity with his/her own effort. |

# ACTIVITY PARTICIPATION SHEET

**Resident Name** _____

**Month** _____

**Room #** _____

Independent = I
Dependent = D
Refused = R

Semi-independent = S
Observed = O
Non-cooperative = N

| | 1 | 2 | 3 | 4 | 5 | 6 | 7 | 8 | 9 | 10 | 11 | 12 | 13 | 14 | 15 | 16 | 17 | 18 | 19 | 20 | 21 | 22 | 23 | 24 | 25 | 26 | 27 | 28 | 29 | 30 | 31 |
|---|---|---|---|---|---|---|---|---|---|---|---|---|---|---|---|---|---|---|---|---|---|---|---|---|---|---|---|---|---|---|---|
| | | | | | | | | | | | | | | | | | | | | | | | | | | | | | | | |
| | | | | | | | | | | | | | | | | | | | | | | | | | | | | | | | |
| | | | | | | | | | | | | | | | | | | | | | | | | | | | | | | | |
| | | | | | | | | | | | | | | | | | | | | | | | | | | | | | | | |
| | | | | | | | | | | | | | | | | | | | | | | | | | | | | | | | |
| | | | | | | | | | | | | | | | | | | | | | | | | | | | | | | | |
| | | | | | | | | | | | | | | | | | | | | | | | | | | | | | | | |
| | | | | | | | | | | | | | | | | | | | | | | | | | | | | | | | |
| | | | | | | | | | | | | | | | | | | | | | | | | | | | | | | | |
| | | | | | | | | | | | | | | | | | | | | | | | | | | | | | | | |

# Special Programming Bedside Log

## How to Use the Form

The Activity Professional must provide specialized and individualized programs for residents unable and/or uninterested in attending group activities at least 2–3 times per week.

Each resident who needs in-room activities will have a Bedside Log Form. The form is used and kept by the month and the year.

*Activity Code:*    These are the types of activities that you may be providing. They need to be the same as on the care plan "approaches." Numbers 16 and 17 are there in case you wish to add any activity not listed on the form.

After the visit, which should be at least fifteen minutes in duration and two to three times per week in frequency, you record onto the log.

*Example:*

| Date | Length of Visit | Code | Resident Response |
|---|---|---|---|
| 4/16/96 | 20 minutes | 2 & 4 | Resident held and petted the kitten and afterwards we wrote a letter to her son. She expressed thanks and enjoyment for the visit. |
| OR | | | |
| 4/18/96 | 15 minutes | 15 a, c | Resident opened his eyes when I turned on relaxation tape. He visually followed my movement around his bed and seemed to be intent on listening to the sound of my voice while I was talking to him. |

These records can be kept either behind the residents' attendance participation records or in a separate binder. If the bedside logs are not in the attendance participation records, you need to note in the participation records where the bedside logs can be found.

# Special Programming: Bedside Log

Resident Name _____

Month _____

**Activity Code:**

1. Reality orientation
   - a: oral
   - b: written
   - c: picture book/board
2. Pet visits
3. Art projects
4. Creative expression
5. Exercise

6. Music
7. Religion
8. Games
9. Reading material
10. Grooming
11. Resident volunteer
12. Community involvement
13. Work type activities/project oriented

14. Discussion, conversation
15. Sensory stimulation
    - a: scent
    - b: tactile
    - c: sound
    - d: visual
16.
17.

| Date | Length of Visit | Activity Code | Initials | Resident Response |
|------|-----------------|---------------|----------|-------------------|
|      |                 |               |          |                   |
|      |                 |               |          |                   |
|      |                 |               |          |                   |
|      |                 |               |          |                   |
|      |                 |               |          |                   |
|      |                 |               |          |                   |
|      |                 |               |          |                   |
|      |                 |               |          |                   |
|      |                 |               |          |                   |
|      |                 |               |          |                   |
|      |                 |               |          |                   |
|      |                 |               |          |                   |
|      |                 |               |          |                   |
|      |                 |               |          |                   |
|      |                 |               |          |                   |
|      |                 |               |          |                   |

## Activity Involvement Reference Sheet

The Activity Involvement Reference Sheet is a communication tool between the Activity and Nursing Departments. This form can be posted in a conspicuous place in the resident's room. The back of the closet door is a usually good place.

The Activity Professional should write all of the activity groups that are listed in the resident care plan. In addition, the Activity Professional should list the one-on-one activities that the resident enjoys or responds to well.

Each morning the CNA should refer to this sheet, review the calendar for time and location and transport the resident to the appropriate activity.

For residents who stay in their rooms, the one-on-one supplies should be available for resident, staff and family use.

# Activity Involvement Reference Sheet

_____     _____
**Resident Name**                                                        **Date**

## Nursing Staff:

Please be aware of this resident's activity treatment plan as shown below:

| Group Activities<br>(* = transport to location) | One-on-One Activities |
|---|---|
|  |  |
|  |  |
|  |  |
|  |  |
|  |  |
|  |  |
|  |  |
|  |  |
|  |  |
|  |  |
|  |  |
|  |  |
|  |  |

Please request sensory supplies for your residents' needs from the activity department.

Thank you,


Activity Coordinator

**Progress Notes**

Progress notes are written to document a significant event in the life of the resident. They can be written in a narrative format, telling the story of the resident's progress or in a problem-oriented format, a structured note specific to the resident's problems. (This is also called a SOAP note.)

An example of a narrative note:

> 3/11/96    Progress Note
> Resident has been active with the living history project as well as the sewing club. She attends coffee group every morning, helping pass out napkins & silverware. She states satisfaction with the activities offered. Functional status remains the same. Will continue with program as it meets needs at this time.
> J. Jones, AD.

The SOAP note (from Subjective, Objective, Assessment, Plan) has the following format:
S: Subjective — What the resident states, information from family, caregiver or chart.
O: Objective — What you see, hear, touch. Measurable information.
A: Assessment — What you assess to be the problem or need.
P: Plan — What you will do to address the problem, need or concern.

An example of a SOAP note:

> 3/11/96    Progress Note
> S: "I like everything here." Family states she seems much happier at this facility.
> O: Attends history 1x wk, sewing club 2x wk, coffee club daily. Fills time with visiting & reading.
> A: MDS shows no change in functional status. Current program effective in meeting needs.
> P: Continue care plan with no changes.
> J. Jones, AD.

All progress notes regardless of format should include the date, content and signature (first initial, full last name and title). The exact time should also be included on all change of condition notes.

# Monitoring Documentation — Social Service

Keeping up with residents' needs (psychosocial and concrete) and changing conditions (health and behavior) is an ongoing challenge. It is only partly done if you know what the need/concern/problem is. To complete the cycle you must reflect your knowledge and your plan in writing in the resident's medical record.

Although this is not a regulation and will not even appear in any of the surveyors' guidelines, it is a good social service practice to make an entry in the resident's chart every week for at least the first two months. You can start it with each new resident and use it as a form of tracking his/her adjustment to the facility. Chart each week on some significant clue to the adjustment (or lack thereof) by indicating such things as knowledge of the facility: locations of his/her own room, recognition of faces, if not names, of staff and roommates and familiarity with the approximate routine within the facility.

This charting will help you track the resident's moods, find behavior patterns which might escalate into problems or begin to work toward appropriate discharge planning. Very importantly, you can determine if your current entry on the resident care plan is still a reflection of the resident's need. Use a standard social service progress note form. A narrative style of documentation seems to work best for most social service entries.

If you find that weekly charting is not necessary because the resident's overall independence and adjustment or, at the other extreme, very poor orientation and inability to respond to standard reality orientation, you can record this observation in the chart by making a note to that effect and change the frequency of the tracking.

Another way to document social service interventions is to keep a Social Service Log for each resident. This log is a record documenting services and counseling provided to the resident by the Social Service Professional. The form could be a narrative or it might be similar to the Bedside Log used by the Activity Professional. Be sure to identify date, nature of service, resident's response and the follow-through that is required.

# Quarterly Care Conferences

Care conferences are held quarterly for each resident to discuss his/her current status and care plan. This is usually a relatively informal meeting designed to give the entire care team a chance to meet together and discuss each resident's care plan. The team needs to be sure that the information about the resident's condition is up to date and that the care plan reflects the resident's current condition.

Each member of the team should submit a written report summarizing his or her interactions with the resident during the last three months. Your responsibilities are to write a quarterly progress note and then carefully read the notes for the other disciplines before you attend the care plan meeting. (Activity Professionals are required to write quarterly notes. Social Service Professionals are only required to write annual notes, but we strongly recommend that they write quarterly notes, too.)

## Quarterly Progress Notes

When you write your quarterly progress notes, realize that you are reflecting on three months of a resident's life. It is essential, therefore, that you take the time to do a comprehensive review of all of the most recent entries in the medical chart: from the doctor's progress notes to nursing summaries, to dietary and therapy entries and your own interventions. Also check the resident care plan for any changes, the medication book for new drugs or discontinued ones and, when indicated, behavioral monitors that reflect a resident's mood or behavior. Review your last quarterly note to ensure that you have addressed unfinished issues from the last quarter.

The quarterly note for an Activity Professional should include:
1.  resident's participation record for the last quarter
2.  resident's response to the activity program
3.  whether the goals set last quarter have been met
4.  whether there are any necessary changes in the program to either achieve the goals or maintain status
5.  assessment of the effect of any changes in functioning (as per the MDS) in the resident's activity level
6.  any necessary changes in the program to address declines or improvements in functioning as seen by the MDS
7.  a statement of plans with goals for the next quarter *(Remember that changes require resident approval.)*
8.  behavior issues
9.  psychoactive medications
10. potential for falls
11. effectiveness of restraint minimization program, if applicable

On the next page you will find a checklist for a comprehensive activity quarterly progress note. Follow these guidelines for a note that identifies all important areas of an individual. If there are areas not needing attention such as special diets, skip them in the note.

# Checklist for a Comprehensive Activity Progress Note

**Directions:** When writing your quarterly note, review the necessary areas of information on this checklist form. Include as many of these areas as possible in order to document in a *comprehensive* manner.

## Content Areas

| | |
|---|---|
| | Cognitive Status |
| | Communication Deficits and Needs |
| | Behavioral Issues and Interventions |
| | Family Involvement |
| | Relationship with Roommate and Staff |
| | Previous Leisure and Lifestyle Interests |
| | Specific Involvement in Activity Program |
| | Level of Responsiveness in Group Activities |
| | Strengths and Abilities |
| | Necessary Info About Vision, Hearing and Speech |
| | Psychoactive Medications |
| | Restraint Use |
| | Special Notes About Diet |
| | Therapy |
| | All Areas on Care Plan, with Activity Approaches |
| | Activity Treatment Plan & Quarterly Goal |

The Social Service Professional looks at different parts of the resident's life. View your note as a summary of events; recap important occurrences in the quarter and note any changes. Consider the following:

1.  Is the resident alert? oriented? Has there been a change in his/her cognitive status?
2.  What is the resident's involvement with family or other residents?
3.  What is the resident's daily pattern: where does s/he spend most of his/her time (in his/her room; in activities)?
4.  Have there been any changes in the types of activities that the resident has chosen to participate in?
5.  Have there been any changes in the level of participation?
6.  Does s/he socialize with other residents or does s/he seek out staff?
7.  Does s/he have visitors? Who? How often? Has this changed since your last quarterly note (e.g., a family death or illness)?
8.  Who tends to his/her concrete needs (family, Social Service Professional)?
9.  In general, what has changed over the last 3 months: has s/he become agitated? calmer? why?
10. What comments do you have about personality, characteristics and special individual traits of this resident's individuality and previous lifestyle?
11. Has any special consultation been received (psych, etc.)?
12. Have there been any changes related to dentures, glasses, hearing aids, funding, durable equipment?

Let us reinforce the components of these elements of a resident's record:
*   review all physician's notes for the quarter
*   check to see if there have been any medication changes (especially regarding psychoactives)
*   assess the behavior monitors in the medication/treatment book. Are there any patterns emerging that can be analyzed?
*   assess restraint use and whether it has had any effect on psychosocial functioning
*   check for any consults and results during the quarter (e.g., psych or dental)
*   check for changes in function (see nursing notes)
*   reread your own interventions to refresh your memory

After you have finished thinking about the resident during the last quarter, you can begin to write. Again, using the narrative form keeps your notes interesting and allows you to present the true personality of the resident.

Both Activity and Social Service Professionals should end the note with a goal for the quarter. This goal will be the same as on the care plan.

## Resident Care Plan

Now it is time to reflect on your resident care plan entry.
*   How accurate has the problem/need/concern been during the quarter?
*   How close is the resident to the goal you established for him/her?
*   Have the planned approaches been successful/adequate?
*   Does the problem, need or concern still reflect your assessment of the resident?
*   Have things changed enough so that you need to start again or add to the care plan?

Your quarterly entry is the place to answer these questions. It is okay to change; in fact, it is essential to change any part or even all of the resident care plan entry if it is no longer a reflection of the resident. If the goal will never be accomplished, change it; then alter the approaches to support the goal. Remember that all changes in the care plan require input from the resident and/or guardian.

When you have done this, support your changes in the progress note. If you have been honest in your updated assessment of the resident, you will know whether the care plan needs changing. Remember — the resident care plan goal must be reflected in your progress notes. If your entry does not help to paint an accurate picture of the resident, it needs to be changed.

A few sample quarterly progress notes for Activity and Social Service Professionals are shown below:

# Activity Quarterly Progress Notes

6/8/96 Activity Quarterly Progress Note

Mary is alert and aware of people and things around her. She has occasional periods of confusion which seem to occur in the late afternoon. When in a group setting, she is hesitant to speak up due to an embarrassment about her word retrieval skills.

She spends most of her day in her room, feeding birds on the patio and waiting for her daughter to visit.

During one-on-one visits 2x weekly, she converses and expresses interest in our conversation.

Mary has a wonderful sense of humor and a strong sense of curiosity. She is receiving speech therapy 1x weekly for language deficits 2° to a mild left CVA. The speech therapy goals for her will be reinforced in one-on-one conversation and word/memory games. She will also be encouraged to join in the small morning discussion group for social interaction and communication building skills.

E. Best CTRS, ACC

9/8/96 Activity Quarterly Progress Note

Mary is alert with periods of confusion reported about 1x per day, usually in the early afternoon. Some progress is being made in conjunction with the speech therapist to solve problems pronouncing words, but she still has significant difficulty being understood at times.

Most of the day, she can be seen looking out of her window, waiting for her daughter or feeding the birds out on the patio. Her daughter visits weekly and she receives mail monthly from a distant relative in Iowa.

She seems to enjoy our visits 2x weekly and has enjoyed participating in the small morning discussion group. She has contributed a lot of insight to our discussions and is much appreciated. I have had to interpret what she said to the other members about 20% of the time (down from almost 50% when she first joined the group), but this has not been a problem for the group. We have worked with the speech therapist on the continuing areas of difficulty.

One thing that I have continued to appreciate is Mary's strong sense of curiosity and a wonderful sense of humor.

GOALS:

Res. will continue to practice communication techniques (see speech therapy goal for revised plan) during the small discussion group 2x per week for the next three months. Activity Professional will assist resident to practice new communication skills learned in speech therapy during the small discussion group.

Check more carefully to try to pinpoint time of confusion. Nursing is considering the possibility that it may be related to medication.

E. Best CTRS, ACC

## Social Service Quarterly Progress Note

3/8/96 SS    Quarterly Progress Note

Lydia has been here for three months now and has worked very hard to make an adjustment to this environment. She came here from a loving home environment which could no longer support her, given the escalation in her personal care needs related to a compression fracture in her spine which compounds the existing circumstance related to a CVA she suffered in 1994. She very appropriately mourned the loss of her life as she had known it and SSD spent at least an hour a week with her reminiscing, dissecting the pros and cons of her present situation and gradually looking to a future (something she had verbalized to me after about six weeks into her admission that she had no sense of).

Lydia has rejected the idea of an antidepressant (which her physician had asked her to consider) feeling instead that she would rather "feel her emotions and deal with the issues now — not prolong the pain of separation." There have been no observed indications of depression; Lydia has maintained as excellent appetite (gaining eight pounds over the quarter), sleeps well at night and says she has "nice dreams," all counter indications of the usual signs and symptoms of depression. Her weight gain of 8 pounds keeps her well within range of her normal body weight. (For further clarification, see dietary note.)

Lydia's family, husband and one of two daughters who lives nearby, visit several times a week and have made her room homey, reflecting Lydia's love of clowns and flowers.

Lydia remains oriented, interested in her care and gradually has entered into an activity of her choosing.

SSD goal of visiting at least once a week to allow her to verbalize her feelings related to adjustment, with the additional intention of establishing a trusting relationship with at least one staff member, has been met thus far. Because she is becoming more independent, emotionally and physically, within the facility, this goal will be revised to biweekly visitation for the next quarter.

M. A. Weeks, SSD

## Social Service Quarterly Progress Note

3/8/96 SS    Quarterly Progress Note

John is a very stable resident of three months duration in the facility. He has a diagnosis of Alzheimer's Disease (probable). His signs and symptoms are consistent with that as he is no longer able to identify himself, find his room or ask for what he needs. He is alert, however and seems interested in his surroundings; he is a passive observer in most activities, responds to his name by making eye contact and appears to recognize his wife when she visits (daily at lunch) because he will smile and reach for her.

John had been receiving Ativan for agitation and anxiety BID [two times a day]. He had been placed on this medication at home because of his behavior and the physician chose not to discontinue it upon admission, choosing instead to monitor and assess his behavior on the drug in this new setting.

At first John would become very restless, moving himself in his chair, reaching out to passersby and pulling at his clothes. This was noted especially in the evening, beginning at about 7 pm. After several weeks of a trial with the medication, the staff was not noticing a major change in his behavior pattern (per MAR) and it was decided to attempt behavioral interventions to address John's anxiety. The goal of reducing his episodes of nightly anxiety was addressed by removing John from the main activity room and putting him in the room where there was quiet music being played and there were never more than 5 other residents in attendance. Staff would speak very calmly and softly and if John began to show any signs of motor restlessness, he would be calmed with a gentle and reassuring touch to his hand. These approaches have been successful to the extent that the physician discontinued the Ativan at his last monthly visit.

SSD goal has been revised; John is visited at least monthly and during those visits, the goal is for him to respond in conversation by making eye contact when his name is used; he is also assessed for any personal care or clothing needs. If there are any, contact is made with his wife.

M. A. Weeks, SSD

The best advice we can give you on actually getting these done is to stay organized and try not to let progress notes pile up. Doing them each week before the resident care conference is the regulation. It is easy to put such a routine obligation on the "back burner," but you will be ignoring your responsibility if you do so and also depriving other members of the interdisciplinary team of your unique perspective as they, too, comply with quarterly entry requirements.

# Updating the Care Plan

There are two times when the resident care plan must be updated. Whenever there is a significant change in the resident's status, a new MDS and an updated care plan are required. The care plan must also be updated annually, even if there is no change of condition.

## Change of Condition

Sometimes there will be a significant change in a resident's behavior. You must document the change you see and create a new set of goals that reflect the change of condition. Significant changes in condition cannot wait until the next quarterly review. The following shows a sample change of condition note.

1/12/96     Change of Condition Note
Resident has been experiencing quite a change in terms of her daily routine and cognitive awareness. She appears more confused and disoriented when left on her own. As of late, she has been found lost in the hall coming back from the patio. She had been coming to the morning discussion group per last quarterly goal on a weekly basis. During the group she was alert, focused and witty. I feel that she needs this small structured group for reality awareness and orientation and also to be reminded of her many strengths.
GOAL: Resident will share one memory with the reminiscing/discussion group or
GOAL: Resident will respond to direct orientation discussion as seen by repeating the date from the board.
E. Best CTRS, ACC

A "significant change" is a major change in the resident's status that is not self-limiting, impacts on more than one area of the resident's clinical status and requires interdisciplinary review and/or revision of the care plan. A significant change reassessment is required if decline or improvement is consistently noted in 2 or more areas of decline or 2 or more areas of improvement. *Note that conditions not in this list may also require a reassessment.*

Decline:

- any decline in ADL physical functioning where a resident is newly coded as 3, 4 or 8.
- increase in the number of areas where Behavioral Symptoms are coded as "not easily altered"
- resident's decision making changes from 0 or 1, to 2 or 3.
- resident's incontinence pattern changes from 0 or 1 to 2, 3 or 4, or placement of an indwelling catheter
- emergence of sad or anxious mood as a problem that is not easily altered
- emergence of an unplanned weight loss problem, 5% in 30 days, 10% in 180 days
- begin to use trunk restraint or a chair that prevents rising for a resident when it was not used before
- emergence of a condition/disease in which a resident is judged to be unstable
- emergence of a pressure ulcer at stage II or higher, when no ulcers were previously present at stage II or higher
- overall deterioration of resident's condition and resident received more support

Improvement:

- any improvement in ADL physical functioning where a resident is newly coded as 0, 1 or 2 when previously scored as a 3, 4 or 8
- decrease in the number of areas where Behavioral Symptoms or Sad or Anxious mood are coded as "not easily altered"
- resident's decision making changes from 2 or 3, to 0 or 1
- resident's incontinence pattern changes from 2, 3 or 4 to 0 or 1, or catheter is removed
- overall improvement of resident's condition, resident receives fewer supports.

### Updates in the Progress Notes for a New RAI

Not only must you comment on the reason for the new RAI, but you must also reflect on any impact that this may have had on the psychosocial well-being of the resident. For example, if the resident has had a stroke, s/he may have lost some of his/her ability to socialize. Clearly this can have an effect on his/her ongoing orientation and a new plan must be developed to address this.

Remember, because the MDS starts the clock anew, this update note will in essence be a quarterly progress note. If it has been a while since you have written a comprehensive note, now is the time to write one.

# Annual Review

Once a year you will participate in an annual review of each resident. The purpose of the annual review, unlike the quarterly review, is to completely reassess the resident. The team does a new MDS and any RAPs that are triggered. New, rather than revised, care plans are written.

This is not to say that you should ignore everything that you know about the resident from working with him/her. The intention is to take a fresh look at the resident with the hope that this will allow the team to correct any misinterpretations about the resident's condition and about what the care plan should be.

Your participation is the same as it was in the initial assessment of the resident: supplying information for your section of the MDS, assisting with RAPs, reading through information from all the other disciplines and participating in the care plan conference.

The Social Service Professional is also responsible for an annual update in the progress notes. This note is an overall summary which reflects change over the entire year. A statement should be made in both the discharge planning section and the section you use for progress notes. The annual date is determined by the date of the previous, full, validated MDS.

Sample annual Social Service progress notes are shown below:

# Social Service Annual Progress Note

9/6/96 Social Service Annual Progress Note

Lydia has continued to make progress with an adjustment which started out with difficulties related to her mourning her previous life at home. She has been consistently verbal and able to express her feelings and has maintained an ongoing relationship with me which has included at least biweekly "check-in" visits after the first quarter of weekly visits.

Her health has remained stable with no further fractures or indications of new problems related to her original CVA. Her mood is optimistic and she has reached out to other alert residents and they have formed a dining group which meets every day at lunch. This group is also the nucleus of the Resident Council and Lydia seems delighted to use her organizational skills as the elected secretary.

Her daughters offer love and support to her; her husband has himself suffered some major health problems during the year and his pattern of visiting four times per week has been reduced to two times per week. Lydia has been able to accept this new pattern without evidence of a setback in her mood, probably, she says, because she realizes that her husband, after so many years of focusing on her, must allow others to tend him now. She misses him but is always so happy to see him when he does visit that they spend their time catching up on events in their separate lives.

There have been no new medications needed; the MD's progress notes regularly reflect Lydia's stability and good humor.

SSD goal of biweekly visits has been revised to quarterly visits which is a reflection of a well integrated resident.

M. A. Weeks, SSD

# Social Service Annual Progress Note

9/8/96 Social Service Annual Progress Note

John has had an expected decline due to his diagnosis of probable Alzheimer's Disease. He is no longer alert as evidenced by his keeping his eyes closed much of the time and he does not seem to respond to his wife any longer, not even opening his eyes when she speaks to him. He spends much of the day out of his room with the possibility that he will receive some form of stimulation. John seems calm with no restlessness or aimless body movements noted. He is nonverbal and all of his needs must now be anticipated. Additionally, John has had a weight loss over the year representing about 10% of his body weight. He remains well within range of his ideal body weight but with his diagnosis a gradual weight loss is not inconsistent, even though he is fed all of his meals, consumes 75–90% of each and receives protein drinks between each meal and at bedtime.

John signed a Durable Power of Attorney for Health Care when he was well and his wife is able to make decisions regarding his care. She has asked that all possible comfort measures be provided, including relief of pain if necessary; he will remain with us, even if he develops further health care problems. She does not wish him transferred out to the acute care hospital.

John's physician has noted the obvious decline during the past 5 monthly visits to him; there is no medication indicated.

The SSD goal has been revised to reflect these changes: during monthly visits with John, his concrete needs are assessed, he is monitored for any obvious change which should then be discussed with his wife.

M. A. Weeks, SSD

## Scheduling Updates

As important as documenting your service, is the design of a documentation update system. This is a means of having your own documentation audit system.

An easy system is a 3x5 card file. Each resident has a 3x5 card with his/her name, date of care plan entry and quarterly progress note date. You may find it helpful to include specific information related to interests, likes, dislikes, care plan problem and need, therapy goals, etc. The box is organized with monthly dividers from January to December.

If a resident has his/her first care plan entry on AUGUST 8, 1996, his/her card will be filed behind NOVEMBER. This will be the month that the review is due. Many facilities have due dates set up according to the resident care conference schedule. If this is the case in your facility, you will keep in sync with their calendar.

When the first quarterly update is due, be sure that this review date is the same date as for the care plan review. If both dates are the same, you will always have these two items due on the same day — a good time management technique.

Sample card:

```
MYRTLE SMITH
8-8-96
loves music, dislikes large groups. Responds well to pets
Speech therapy for improving communication by pronouncing words




```

# Discharge

Sadly, many residents and families regard admission to the long term care facility as the final move. What they do not realize, however, is that many residents are able to return to a lesser level of care, either as a result of rehabilitative service or a change of condition toward — not away from — wellness.

Although most residents are naturally hopeful about once again being in their own homes, for some this is just not a possibility due to the constraints of care needs or lack of support. Sometimes there simply are no close family or friends to manage the home care. However, other options do exist in most communities and you can explore the choices with the resident while s/he recuperates in the facility.

When home is the best answer, enlist the assistance of the occupational therapist for a home visit to assess the safety and accessibility of the home. S/he can make valuable recommendations about removing hazardous rugs and suggest ramps and safety bar placement (especially in bathrooms). The responsible party should be able to follow up on these suggestions using parts which can be found in most hardware stores to improve the safety of the home.

Once the environment has been made safe, follow up care can be arranged. Home care agencies, some hospital based, some private, are a rich source of assistance. They can provide physical therapists, occupational therapists, recreational therapists, skilled nurses and home health aides. The Social Service Professional makes the initial contact after receiving the doctor's order. The agency will then review the case, frequently meeting with the resident and/or the responsible party before the discharge to make the transition as easy as possible.

If there is a Meals on Wheels program in the community which can bring at least one hot meal a day, check to see if the resident would like to have the service. We like to recommend it for the first two weeks at home. It must be ordered by the doctor.

For the actual discharge, you may have to arrange transportation if the family is not able to do it. Check with your local resources to determine what will work best. Usually a private car or van service will suffice.

If the resident wants a homelike setting, but does not want all of the responsibilities that entails, you can look into assisted living complexes in the community.

There are several variations on this theme. Some include well care, supervised care and skilled nursing. Some have only the first two options. Some are only for those who are independent. Research the possibilities to find the best match for the resident.

The usual situation will allow the resident to have all the possible amenities in his/her apartment, including his/her own furnishings and kitchen facilities. S/he will be able to use congregate dining facilities and planned activities within the complex, too. This is often a good transitional environment from total independence to the beginnings of supervised care. It is an excellent option if the resident is still able to be independent and manage his/her own personal and health care needs.

The next step toward supervised care is a board and care facility. Most board and care facilities pride themselves on being homey but the sizes vary considerably and it is important to visit them to find the one that will best suit the resident's needs. Look for the availability of supervised care: medication administration and personal needs such as bathing and dressing. Then assess the match between the facility and the personal style of the resident:
- Do they prefer social settings or quiet and privacy?
- Are there grounds for strolling (and does the resident care)?
- Are there animals?

If there is family to help with this, they can usually be relied upon to provide accurate assessments. If there is not, perhaps you can take the resident for a visit. If this is not a possibility, ask the board and care facility operator to meet the resident and bring photographs of the facility.

Board and care facilities will allow the resident to bring personal possessions such as a favorite chair. This will help the move seem more like a return home rather than like being a guest in someone else's home.

For both assisted living and board and care facilities, home care agencies will follow residents who have a doctor's order for follow up. Take advantage of these resources since they provide an excellent bridge between long term care facility dependence and the next level of independence.

The process of planning for discharge begins at the time of admission. At the time of admission, the treatment team, including the Activity and the Social Service Professionals, will use the medical data base and the resident/family goals to begin the process of discharge planning. This includes an assessment of the change in medical status which has necessitated admission, an assessment of the home situation (from resident/family interview) and discussion with the rehabilitation staff concerning the possibility of improvement.

Then progress itself must be monitored. To do so, it is essential to attend weekly rehab meetings; in fact, in terms of any successful determination of discharge potential, this may be the most important meeting of the week. At this session, you will have available to you all of the resources which are acting in either a rehabilitative or a supportive role with the resident. You will be able to examine his/her daily pattern from every aspect: dietary to therapy to activity level to nursing. From this comprehensive overview, you will be able to note progress (if any) and to inform the resident and the family of the consensus opinion so that: 1. neither becomes unnecessarily discouraged or encouraged and 2. they can begin to plan and prepare the home environment if this seems feasible.

Meanwhile, the Social Service Professional uses the interdisciplinary team's assessments to continue to evaluate the resident for home care needs. With this information, s/he will make referrals, under the doctor's orders, for follow-up home care to be initiated at the time of discharge.

As exciting as the prospect of a discharge might seem to the health care workers, do not forget that the time leading up to the long term care facility placement may have been extremely traumatic for the resident and the family and they may be reluctant to accept a discharge plan, seeing it as another opportunity for failure. In fairness to everyone, the Social Service Professional should make every effort to give weekly progress reports to all concerned parties, assuring them always that a support system (usually home care) will be built into any discharge plan and that they, as the major components of the plan, must be honest and forthcoming with their input and their anxieties. Involving them at all levels of planning and organizing the discharge will give the discharge the best chance of success.

Sometimes, even with your best effort, you will not be able to convince the resident or their family that the planned discharge is appropriate. In those cases OBRA regulation require that someone in the facility initiate a **Right to Appeal** document with the resident. The **Right to Appeal** says that when a long term care facility decides to discharge or transfer a resident, it needs to give the resident reasonable notice of the change. If the resident does not feel that the change is appropriate, there is a formal process, outlined in OBRA, which describes the rights and responsibilities for both parties and the process for the appeal. (The specific requirements for notice and the right to appeal are given in the *Management* chapter.)

Often this task is done by the Social Service Professional. Inform the resident that s/he can contest the discharge plan and can speak to a resident advocate (such as an ombudsman) or may contact the Department of Health Services directly. By federal law, these phone numbers must be posted where staff, residents, family and/or guardians can see them. If there is no expressed interest in contesting the discharge, ask the resident and the responsible party to sign the discharge document and place it in the resident's medical record.

In anticipation of the discharge, an interdisciplinary discharge summary must be completed by the interdisciplinary team. (See the glossary entry **Discharge Summary** for a description of how to write a discharge summary.) In this way, resident and family will be given some of the tools needed to insure that successful return "home."

All of those involved in a discharge, from the resident to the CNA, wish for a successful homecoming, one that will "stick." Communication among all members of the health care team, especially at rehabilitation meetings and ongoing communication with the resident and the family, are the key factors for a successful discharge from the long term care facility.

In the **discharge plan**, you might write something like one of these:

> 9/6/96      Annual Note
> Lydia has remained stable in her care needs over the last year but she continues to require assistance with all of her personal care. She transfers and ambulates only with two person assistance. She is not able to be cared for at a lesser level of care.
> M. A. Weeks, SSD

> 9/6/96      Annual Note
> At this time discharge is not the preferred option for John. John is incontinent, unable to ambulate, even with assistance and requires total assistance with all of his personal care needs. His wife has voiced her desire to have him remain at this long term care facility instead of being placed in acute care. He continues to be appropriate in long term care placement.
> M. A. Weeks, SSD

> 9/6/96      Annual Note
> Mary continues to make progress with communication. If the periods of confusion could be eliminated, the daughter says placement in her home is a distinct possibility. (The daughter works and would not be available to help her mother if she had problems during the afternoon.) AC will prepare a set of activity information and community leisure resources if discharge becomes possible.
> E. Best CTRS, ACC

# Letting Go: The Way We Die

We wonder what act we perform in our whole lives that is more personal, more private, more self-centered than death! What a privilege it is to be allowed to share this experience with someone.

It is unnecessary for us to repeat what others have written so eloquently about the stages leading up to death. If you are not informed about preparing for death, you should read one or more of these books.[40]

Death is inevitable and we know that it causes the least negative impact on the survivors when the person who is dying has reached an "acceptance" of his/her death. Please don't misunderstand that this also means "dependent" or "morose." Instead, it means that the person understands the inevitability of death and feels prepared to die. We are often fortunate to have a chance to help our residents prepare for death and to be a witness to the hopefulness of impending death.

Let's draw a context here. Imagine having lived a full life; having created positive associations and memories; imagine further having lost close family, then friends, then function and, finally, a physical environment which was supportive of one's illness and disabilities. Having dealt with loss and change,

---

[40] If you are interested, see the books:
Kübler-Ross, Elizabeth, **On Death and Dying**. Collier Books, 1969.
Lewis, C. S., **A Grief Observed**. Bantam Books, 1961.
Manning, Doug, **Comforting Those Who Grieve: A Guide for Helping Others**. Harper and Row, 1985.
Harris Lord, Janice, **Beyond Sympathy: What to Say and Do for Someone Suffering an Injury, Illness or Loss**. Pathfinder Publishing, 1988.
Lightner, Candy and Nancy Hathaway, **Giving Sorrow Words: How to Cope with Grief and Get on With Your Life**. Warner Books, 1990.
Staudacher, Carol, **Men and Grief.** New Harbinger, 1992.
Caplan, Sandi, **Grief's Courageous Journey: A Workbook**. New Harbinger, 1995.

step by step, problem by problem, people will usually arrive at the point of acceptance with a degree of relief. Ongoing love, support and counseling will allow them to find peace in that emotional setting and, instead of mourning what life has been, there is pleasure in one's memories and hope for a peaceful end.

One does not have to have lived a life of comfort and joy to be able to arrive at such a state. In fact, one can still produce a positive face for the future, even without the pleasant memories that we would hope would accompany each of us. It is no secret that, as with placement in a long term care facility, it is the resident who frequently accepts the inevitable before the family does. We sense that it relates to the comfort of letting go of all the unnecessary trappings in our lives, of already having made the hard choices and now being stripped to that part of self that is most vulnerable, most human. Without the distractions of the world, there is peace in having our needs met; peace in the assurance that we will be made comfortable to the end of our lives.

This does not mean that the need to control is not still in evidence. In fact, that need is so ingrained in us that many people orchestrate their own dying. It is with pleasure that they cause families to rally round, to feel the power of being responded to, of being capable of living by choice until the end.

This is not true, of course, for everyone; but, among us, we often discuss — and believe — that people die the way they wish to. Some wish to die with family nearby; others prefer to be alone (to save family the possible pain of witnessing this final separation?). All wish to die pain free which is often our only viable goal as caregivers — comfort for the dying resident.

Frequently there is useful and wonderfully productive time to be lived as people proceed toward death. This can be a more open time, more emotional, more honest, with communication among family members at its best. Reminiscing is appropriate, especially if family members have never taken the time to explore the past with each other. (Amazingly, we find this is often true, as when we ask a resident for a social history and become aware that the family members are hearing life details for the first time, too. "Oh that's how your parents chose your name, Mom.") Sharing memories and stories revives lives led and provides the material for future reminiscing and for creating family legends and folklore.

The care givers need to pay special attention to changes in health status that may be leading to the terminal state. At such times, it is imperative that you be even more available to resident and family in order to address any terminal care needs:
- Do they wish clergy to be phoned?
- Do they wish a private meal with friends and family?
- Are there special arrangements that need to be made (an autopsy)?

Sometimes your presence, sitting with the resident and being with the family, is the best you can do. If appropriate, participate in the reminiscence. Help the family interact with the dying resident by modeling: speak to the resident, assure him/her that s/he is not alone and that his/her family is with him/her. Ask if the family wishes to be alone or if they are more comfortable having others in the room. The family may wish you to interpret physical changes; encourage them to speak with nursing as they observe alteration in color and breathing patterns and body temperature.

Finally, determine if anyone in the family wishes to view the resident after death and before the body is removed to the mortuary. Some people draw great comfort in this final good-bye, this private time. Most facilities are able to make accommodation for this.

When there is a death, be certain that the residents most involved with the deceased have the opportunity to verbalize feelings of lose or fear. Include them in the dying process. If it seems feasible, allow them to sit with the dying person. Predictably, there is seldom any anxiety displayed by other residents after a death. There is sadness and a sense of lose and of missing a companion, but the pervasive feeling is of peace with the inevitable. We witness the ability of people to carry on when the natural has occurred.

It often seems to us that when we lose a resident, we lose twice, especially if the person had an active and interested family. The staff misses the spirit and energy of the resident but also the socializing and the communication with the family.

In order to allow all of us to have our final good-byes, to the deceased and to the family and the routine that have become a part of us, we strongly recommend having a memorial service. We are not proposing that you conduct one after each death, but having one monthly or quarterly can be very much of an emotional release. Be sure to invite the families and special friends of all the residents who have died.

The service is simple with perhaps a prayer or a Psalm reading led by a clergyman; this brings the appropriate solemnity to the occasion. These formalities are followed by spontaneous reminiscences, with staff and other residents also making their contributions. When the formal service is concluded, there is time for refreshments and informal exchanges. For some, this is the only memorial service they will have had. For others, it is their second, more private one. For everyone, it provides the opportunity for closure.

It never ceases to amaze us how truly uplifting it is to be with someone who is dying. We will qualify this by saying that this is especially true if the death is accepted, anticipated with joy as the natural ending to a life that has been well spent and is essentially pain free at the end. The emotional release is cathartic for all involved and opens our hearts to emotions that keep us most human: compassion, sympathy and, in some cases, empathy.

It is always a privilege for caretakers who witness and ease the way to death; and no matter how one chooses to let go, it is always personal and private and special.

# 9. Councils

## Resident Council

According to OBRA every long term care facility is required to have a Resident Council. The Activity Professional is usually the chairperson for the council and is responsible for assuring that this very important meeting occurs each month and that minutes are kept and issues resolved.

### What is the Resident Council?

The Resident Council is the political voice of the individuals who reside in a long term care setting. Many of the residents are *unable* to voice their opinions and/or concerns and need to rely on those residents who are capable and interested in the facility events to speak for them.

A president, vice president and secretary/treasurer should be elected from the group. Because the Resident Council is so important, during the annual survey process, the surveyor team will ask to meet the president and or vice president of this council.

The meeting consists of all interested residents, representatives from the Ombudsman program, any guests that the residents invite and/or request to speak and the chairperson. The resident council members need to approve any staff member or visitor to these meetings. They can also request to have time alone without any staff present in order to discuss issues confidentially.

Many residents will be hesitant to take on the responsibility and leadership of a council position as it may be a new and intimidating experience. Because of this, be sure to explain how the meetings work, what the responsibilities are and encourage members to share a position if they are interested. The president is the spokesperson for the council. This resident sits at the head of the group along with the chairperson and other officers. Each council has its own personality. Create the positions to meet the needs of the current group along with the stated responsibilities of the council.

The Resident Council is required to take place *one time per month*. In large facilities, there may be additional meetings called as the need occurs. The minutes of these meetings are kept by the chairperson.

A copy of the meetings minutes always goes to the administrator for review so that s/he is always current on issues, concerns and resolutions.

# How should a meeting be organized?

Each meeting should begin with attendance and recognition of each member. The chairperson usually opens the meeting unless the president wishes to open. Because this is an official meeting, there should be an agenda to follow. An example of an agenda would be:

- Attendance.
- Review of last month's minutes including resolutions to each issue addressed.
- Department heads speak on any issues that may have come up. Residents need to know that when an issue is addressed, the responsible discipline follows through with the concern and speaks to the group in regards to policy, changes and educational information.
- Review of one or two specific resident's rights.
- Reminder of the right to review the past year's survey results and where they are located. These should be both available and accessible for review.
- Discussion of activity planning so that the residents have a voice in future events and evaluation of the program.
- Voting issues should always be mentioned so that all members know that they can register to vote, can request assistance with absentee forms and change of address forms. A current list should always be kept of residents who are registered to vote.
- Open forum for any and all residents in the council to voice an opinion and add additional information and recommendations for group projects.

As with any group, if complaints and concerns are the only agenda, members will become disinterested in attending. Find worthwhile projects for the council to become involved in. Some examples could be: welcome cards and visits to new residents, Employee of the Month award voted by council members, inservice training, invitations to outside speakers, congratulation letters to community groups and individuals recognized for special efforts, recognition projects for staff and other residents in the facility, a council newsletter, inspirational announcements each morning and the list goes on and on.

# What if only a few residents attend the meetings?

In relationship to the census in a facility, the number of council members is always on the low end. Some very alert and independent individuals may be found in their rooms because they are not interested in attending these meetings. Others may not attend because the effort required is too great. Sometimes it is appropriate to bring the meeting to them. After the official meeting is adjourned, go individually to the rooms of residents so they can review issues and address concerns with you on a one-on-one basis. Keep a record of these council room visits attached to the council minutes. If there are issues addressed, be sure to document these and have the responsible department head write up the resolutions. These should be signed and dated also.

# How do you document tough issues in the minutes?

As the legally responsible chairperson, your duty is to document the facts and issues verbalized by the council members. There must be an atmosphere of trust and responsibility in these meetings. If a resident requests to remain anonymous, this is his/her right and you must respect this right. If there are individuals who are "chronic complainers" even when the issue has been resolved, discuss the resolution during the meeting and add this to the minutes. This documentation will substantiate both the resolution and the fact that this resident needs to vent each meeting regardless of past resolutions. Be sure that this resident does not have the opportunity to take over the meeting. The chairperson may have to designate a five minute period near the end of the meeting for this member's voice to be heard.

When documenting tough issues in the minutes, be specific but not narrative. The minutes are not the place to write the story, but to record the information so that the responsible department head can address and help find resolution to the issues and concerns.

## What exactly are the chairperson's responsibilities?

The chairperson is responsible for scheduling the monthly meeting, announcing the meeting and posting an invitation to family members, creating the agenda, facilitating the meeting, recording the minutes and typing them up and, most importantly, taking the issues and concerns to the responsible department head for review and resolution. This is not *your* meeting. This is a legal requirement of the facility and you are the designated chairperson.

All grievances and concerns need to be resolved by identified departments. You must get these staff members to write a plan of action, date it and sign it on the council forms. These minutes are kept on file and are always to be made available for surveyor review, corporate review, administrative review and ombudsman review. They are never thrown away as they are legal documents for the facility.

## Use of the Resident Council Forms

The Resident Council form on the next page has an area for attendance, old business, review of resident rights, activity review and new issues. The new issues area is very important. Write the issue and then have the responsible discipline write the plan of action and date and sign it. Your signature is on the bottom of the form along with the date. More lines could be added to the back of the form. The one-on-one form needs to be completed by the chairperson also. Any issues that come from the one-on-one form should be addressed the same way as issues from the Resident Council meeting.

# Resident Council Meeting Minutes

**Attendance:** _____  _____  _____  _____

**Business:**

1. **Review of Past Month's Issues/Resolutions:**

   _____
   _____

2. **Review of Resident Rights : Review at least two specific rights per meeting**

   _____
   _____

3. **Activities: Review of Calendar/Input by Residents:**

   _____
   _____

4. **New Issues**

| ISSUE | PLAN OF ACTION (Completed by Responsible Department) | RESPONSIBLE DISCIPLINE (Signed and dated by dept. member) |
|---|---|---|
| _____ | _____ | _____ |
| _____ | _____ | _____ |
| _____ | _____ | _____ |
| _____ | _____ | _____ |
| _____ | _____ | _____ |

Resident Council Chair _____     Date _____

# Resident Council Meeting
## In-Room Form

| Resident Name | Comments/Concerns |
|---|---|
| | |
| | |
| | |
| | |
| | |
| | |
| | |
| | |
| | |
| | |
| | |
| | |
| | |
| | |
| | |
| | |
| | |
| | |
| | |
| | |
| | |
| | |
| | |
| | |
| | |
| | |
| | |

_____

Resident Council Chair                    Date

# Family Council

Organizationally, the Family Council is wide open and its success is dependent upon the available family population and the associated energy level and interest. Theoretically, it is a self-governing body which serves in an advisory capacity to the administration. Underlying its motivations is the support which can only be given and received by people sharing situations in common. Because each council sets its own standards and determines its own needs, each is unique.

Family Council provides a wonderful opportunity for personal support within the group and also forms a ready and willing audience for giving information about the facility, the staff and the long term care system in general. The ideas generated by those most directly affected by facility policies can make a difference in the overall atmosphere. When the group is part of the decision making process (from remodeling to laundry problems), everyone — residents, families, staff — benefits.

The presence of staff should be occasional and limited to 1 to 2 people who have been invited or have a direct purpose for being in attendance (e.g., explanation of a program or policy). The Social Service Professional is the appropriate resource person and his/her presence will be monitored by those in charge of the Family Council.

It can be very difficult to convene an entirely autonomous Family Council. For some, any leadership commitment is an additional drain on an already taxed spirit and some feel the transitory nature of their involvement in the facility. The size of the group doesn't matter. Whether it is five or fifteen members, regard the council as the body which speaks for all of the families. As the members begin to become involved in the facility through the family council, they will be the best advertisement for new members.

Family Councils are not mandatory but facilities must allow such organizations to exist. The support required by the long term care facility is space for meetings, privacy and, by invitation only, staff. The other obligation is to follow-up on grievances and recommendations which are directly related to the resident and his/her quality of life.

The meeting can be announced by direct mail, newsletter and/or posters within the facility. Vary the time, the day and the topics in order to appeal to the schedules and interests of a number of family members. Coming together for a meal will frequently create the informal, relaxed atmosphere desired in the early stages of a Family Council. Speak with your dietary manager, plan a meal or a snack, choose a program (the ombudsman, Medicare, your rehabilitation program, etc.), announce the meeting and see what happens.

Once convened, families will soon realize what a relief it is to share with others. Long-lasting friendships are often made through these meetings because most find that their concerns, complaints, recommendations and emotional highs and lows are remarkably similar. Proceed from this point of sharing, encourage varying agendas, projects (e.g., a facility garden), a newsletter or legislative activity. Be creative.

Even if no one agrees to take on the leadership roles, you do not need to abandon the Family Council concept. You must simply assume more responsibility yourself, at least temporarily, especially if it appears that there are very interested families and very real concerns. Be mindful always of not imposing on the families' right to privacy.

The Family Council may be one of your most frustrating ventures as a Social Service Professional; not because it isn't worthwhile, but because of the turnover of families and the frequent lack of interest in being in charge. We find that families really enjoy coming together and they like receiving new information. When the time is right and someone feels that s/he would like to do more, step aside. Until then, continue to provide a welcoming environment yourself.

Someone once told us to expect it to take 18 months for a Family Council to get organized. We think that's an underestimate, but keep at it and it will get done.

The form on the next page can be used to record the minutes of a Family Council meeting.

# Family Council Meeting

Meeting Date: _____

Attendance: _____  _____  _____

_____  _____  _____

_____  _____  _____

_____  _____  _____

_____  _____  _____

_____  _____  _____

Agenda: _____

_____

_____

_____

Minutes: _____

_____

_____

_____

## Action Items:

Concern: _____

Department: _____

Response (including Plan of Correction): _____

_____

Concern: _____

Department: _____

Response (including Plan of Correction): _____

_____

## Recommendations:

_____

_____

_____

# 10. Volunteers

*Volunteers* is the first word that you will hear from the administrator after you accept the position of an Activity or Social Service Professional. Not only do you need volunteers as part of your departmental team, the residents need a variety and collection of personalities and talents to enhance the quality of their interactions. It is important however to inject a word of caution. Do not begin recruiting volunteers until there is a structure to your program. In terms of priorities, the department needs to be well organized and structured and you need to know both the resident needs and the volunteer needs. If you encourage volunteers without a vision for how the experience will benefit them and the residents, it will be disappointing to all involved. And most importantly, the volunteer will not stay long.

Both federal and state regulations identify the need for volunteers and address this as a function of the Activity Department. Social Service also has a need for volunteers working more on a one-on-one basis. LITA, which is a good example of a one-on-one volunteer program, is discussed at the end of this chapter.

## Activity Department Volunteers

There are many excellent resources on designing and developing a volunteer program. Contact the local volunteer center in your community and request brochures and job descriptions. Arrange to go to training sessions that they offer. Go to facilities and organizations that have a strong and successful program in place. Although the settings and needs are different, the basic development of a volunteer program is similar.

**Priority Steps in developing a volunteer program:**

- Identify what needs the department has for volunteers.
- Write volunteer policies and procedures.
- Design a job description with specific responsibilities, qualifications and time needed.
- Have a choice of possible work and responsibilities for volunteers to choose from.
- Identify volunteer skills, talents and strengths for the growth of both volunteer and program.
- Create forms for applications, orientation to facility, work, attendance records, evaluation.

- Recruit and select volunteers. This process should be as structured as it was for you to be interviewed and selected.
- Train and orient all volunteers well. The more information that a volunteer has, the better able they are to meet the demands of the work, residents and setting.
- Supervise. By working with a volunteer on site you continue their training and assure follow through with the responsibilities of the work.
- Evaluate. It's easiest to evaluate volunteers according to the duties and outline of the specific work. Everyone needs feedback on how they are doing and this is one of your responsibilities as the volunteer coordinator. Evaluation should be on a regularly scheduled basis.
- Recognize. Individuals who volunteer are doing so for personal reasons. There is a personal goal that they have identified as being important in their lives. For most it is the opportunity to help others in need or to build up on their work skills that can be transferred to employment. There are other volunteers who are completing hours either for school or to work off minor violations through a community service program. These volunteers also need feedback and recognition for their work. The ways to recognize volunteers are many. What is more important than "prizes" is recognition and individual honors. Volunteers need to know that they are making a difference to the organization and lives of the residents in long term care settings. Having residents involved in this recognition is very meaningful.

If you have ever volunteered, you know how important it is to manage this time into your already busy schedule. Be clear on how much time is needed per day or week or month. If a volunteer feels that there is not enough organization or direction, s/he will seek out another agency that is better prepared.

Another important area to consider is how you identify needs to determine what volunteer jobs should be created. Think beyond the needs of group activity and individual visits. These both are very important and demand assistance from volunteers. However, there are many other ways that individuals and groups can be involved. Some ideas are

- writing and typing the newsletter,
- decorating the facility,
- shopping,
- letter writing,
- sewing and mending,
- caring for facility pets,
- sharing talents in performances,
- creating visual aids and cards for residents who are sensory impaired,
- making the new month's calendar of activities,
- monitoring residents who are confused and disoriented in structured parallel sensory activities,
- filing and organizing the office,
- reaching out to the community with presentations and flyers,
- developing an intergenerational exchange program with a local school or agency, and
- having a business or agency adopt your facility one time monthly.

The list is endless so the best way to begin is with a wish list. Volunteers help create a quality activity program! It takes work to recruit and supervise a good set of volunteers, but the benefits are felt by all staff, residents and families.

*"Sometimes our light goes out, but is blown again into flame by an encounter with another human being. Each of us owes the deepest thanks to those who have rekindled this inner light." — Albert Schweitzer*

# Social Service Volunteers

The social service volunteer differs significantly in function from the volunteer in the activity program mainly because emphasis is on one-on-one contact as opposed to group involvement. This means that a volunteer who wishes to interact directly with a resident must maintain contact with the Social Service Professional to stay abreast of changes in the emotional or physical status of the resident.

In our experience, however, it can be difficult to recruit and train the true social service volunteer — the person who is not threatened or intimidated by the ongoing contact with one person at a potentially intimate/emotional level. There is a high turnover rate with one-on-one volunteers as they begin to feel that they are not qualified or are not prepared to interact with a resident so intensely. Often a volunteer will come to the facility with some time to share but with no idea of how emotional this experience can be. Also, some volunteers begin to relate too personally in this setting because they themselves are elderly or have an aging relative. These factors also contribute to the high turnover rate among volunteers.

When we are fortunate enough to find individuals who are willing and able to take on the role of social service volunteers, they act as a direct adjunct to the social service program and extend the contact that the Social Service Professional is able to have with the resident.

The social service volunteer may be a Friendly Visitor (some begin in this rather casual role and stay for years), a support to someone in the adjustment crisis, a source of support for someone in the terminal state or one of several variations on these themes. The key to success in terms of residents' needs is a solid mix of warmth, compassion, consistency and a true interest in the residents.

The Social Service Professional has the responsibility of providing ongoing support for the volunteer, beginning with a well-rounded orientation to the facility and a definition of role expectations. An introduction to Resident Rights, especially confidentiality, is essential. After that, a weekly check-in is vital. The volunteer can offer "untrained" insights and ask questions which will assist in a better overall psychosocial plan for the resident; the Social Service Professional can share information from a professional perspective and elicit feelings and concerns from the volunteer.

Your support may be what makes the difference in keeping a volunteer in your facility — for the benefit of all concerned.

# LITA — Love is the Answer

## A volunteer program that every facility needs.

One of the most important gifts that you can give to a resident is the gift of ageless friendship. A volunteer not only adds to the services provided by activity and social service departments, s/he also adds to the quality of life of individual residents. The losses associated with living in a care setting are profound and depression is prevalent in every facility. One way to lessen the loneliness is to bring in volunteers of all ages to visit on a one-on-one basis and match them with a resident who has no family or visitors close by.

Such a volunteer program exists under the name of **LITA,** *Love is the Answer.* The mission statement of this non-profit organization is to lessen loneliness in long term care settings by providing one-on-one friends for isolated residents. The concept is a simple one, to be a friend. The commitment for the volunteer is a weekly visit of at least 15–30 minutes with their matched resident friend. Matches are made with only one resident at a time as developing relationships takes time and attention.

The uniqueness of this program is that it is provided *to* a long term care facility by the organization LITA. The volunteers are recruited and trained by the LITA organization and each facility has a LITA coordinator who works with either the Activity or Social Service Professional. Together, they identify residents in need and work on making a match to meet the needs of both resident and volunteer.

In order to start up a LITA program in your community, contact the National LITA Association for information on getting started. To begin with you will need to identify community members who are interested in getting a LITA program established and going through the process of applying to be a non-profit organization. This will entail the development of a board of directors. The local newly formed LITA organization will work with all the facilities in the geographic area to meet the needs of lonely residents.

The National LITA Association has a start up kit and all other information necessary for the establishment of this important agency in your community. Contact their office for more information.

The National LITA Association
714 "C" Street #207
San Rafael, California 94901
(415) 453-6130

# 11. Quality Assurance, Safety and Risk Management

This chapter covers three important aspects of working in any health care setting: quality assurance, resident safety and risk management. *Quality assurance* looks at the ability to provide the highest quality services and treatment, *safety* is concerned with the ability to modify the environment so that, in most situations, everyone is safe and *risk management* discusses the ongoing process of making the environment safer.

Providing the resident with quality services — meeting his/her needs — does not happen by accident. It takes knowledge, thoughtfulness and some old fashioned self-evaluation to do good work. And, it does not matter how good your services are or how successful your treatment is if you cannot guarantee the resident a basic level of safety while s/he is in your facility. Each resident has the absolute right to be free from bodily harm or psychological damage while receiving care. It is up to each staff person to act in a manner that ensures that each resident is safe. A solid quality assurance program, knowledge of the basic principles of safety (as well as the regulations concerning safety) and a solid understanding of risk management are required to ensure a good program. These issues are discussed in this chapter.

## Quality Assurance

Quality assurance is a process of continually self-evaluating the services you provide and then improving the service based on problems you have identified and corrected. In order to continually evaluate your department, you must have a Quality Assurance Program in place.

Quality Assurance is not a new term but is much more frequently used in nursing homes now that OBRA regulations (Tags F520 & F521) have mandated that each nursing facility have a quality assurance program. A quality assurance program must include policies and procedures for quality assurance and a committee which meets at least quarterly to review current studies and issues.

A facility must maintain an ongoing assessment of the quality of services provided and have a quality assurance committee to monitor the overall effectiveness of the facility's quality assurance program. The quality assurance committee consists of:

1.   the director of nursing services,
2.   a physician designated by the facility and
3.   at least three other members of the facility staff.

The quality assurance committee must meet at least quarterly to identify areas which could and should be improved and then to develop and implement appropriate plans to correct identified quality deficiencies.

*What is Quality Assurance?*

Quality assurance is the process of internally monitoring your own work. It is an on-going program that looks at the quality of the services provided as well as the cost effectiveness of those services. It is not enough to find out at survey time that there are problems. We should always know, during the entire year, what our weak areas are. And we should always be working on improving our services by taking a systematic approach to problem solving. Just as we have written out care plans identifying ways to meet resident needs (with measurable objectives) we have a written out quality assurance program which identifies ways to meet our quality improvement needs.

*How can a facility assure that the QA process will be successful?*

The best way to begin the process is by educating all staff on the importance of monitoring their performance. Stress that they are not only a part of the process but also accountable for the end results.

Quality assurance has been a part of the long term care setting for many years but it became all the more important when OBRA added it to the regulations. The Final Rule (OBRA 1995) included quality assurance as a part of the survey process and plan of corrections guidelines.

*How do I start a Quality Assurance Program or study?*

Your facility already has a quality assurance program, policy and procedure manual and quality assurance committee. If you are not a member of the committee, ask to sit in on these meetings to better understand the process. Activity and Social Service Professionals should be a strong element of this committee because of their involvement in the area of *Quality of Life, Resident Behavior and Practices* and *Quality of Care.*

The quality assurance process is, by definition, an interdisciplinary process. When the committee has identified an area needing attention, all departments will work on to solve the problem. But in addition to working on identified problems, each department should be on the lookout for potential problems and issues specific to their service.

*What type of studies would Activity or Social Service Departments address?*

There are many areas to study. Some of these might include:
*   Does the current program meet the needs of the current resident population?
*   Are some residents having difficulty getting to activity groups of interest? If the resident is not getting to the activity, this is an issue to address in QA.
*   Is the role of Activity or Social Service Professionals in the behavior management programs to decrease the use of psychoactive medications clearly defined?
*   Is the role of Activity or Social Service Professionals in the physical restraint reduction programs for use in groups or one-on-one activities clearly defined?
*   Are residents satisfied with their rooms, food, opportunities, interactions with staff or any other Quality of Life issues?

- Is the space where activities are held large enough? Is the lighting at the proper level for residents who have visual impairments?
- Are all levels of cognitive and functional needs being met in group or individual settings?
- According to the percentage of men or younger residents in the facility, are there appropriate and available leisure activities for their interests?

There are specific steps involved in the design of a quality assurance study. The chart on the following page shows the five steps you need to take for a successful quality assurance program. For more information about quality assurance programs see Cunninghis and Best Martini's book, **Quality Assurance for Activity Programs, Second Edition** (1996) from Idyll Arbor, Inc.

The following forms can be used as quality assurance review forms for survey preparedness. The first two forms (one for activities and one for social services) provide a review of what you should be doing that will help you prepare for survey. The next two department checklist forms can be used to review your activities. They can be used as time management tools and for orienting new employees to their duties. The last form can be used to make sure that you meet all of the requirements for admitting a new resident.

# Steps of Quality Assurance Programs[41]

| Step 1 | *Identifying Issues and Selecting Study Topics* | Obviously it is essential to begin with a determination of what service needs to be improved to provide quality service. This first step has you look closely at the problem to specifically identify what is not right. Unfortunately, many quality assurance programs concern themselves with issues that are not important or with procedural items that can be easily remedied, rather than those that justify being part of long-range planning. |
| --- | --- | --- |
| Step 2a | *Establishing Indicators* | Identifying elements that can be monitored to measure changes made. The elements or characteristics of the service you select to measure should be a general statement about what the service would look like if there was not a problem. |
| Step 2b | *Developing Criteria* | Developing criteria for each indicator. Writing a plan that spells out exactly what should be found and ideally in what quantity and in what time frame. |
| Step 3a | *Determining Methodology* | Establishing the exact method to be used to collect information: from which sources, by whom, how often, how long and how the results are going to be used. |
| Step 3b | *Collecting Data* | Implementing the chosen methods of data collection. |
| Step 4a | *Understanding the Problem* | Reviewing and assessing collected data to see what, where and how serious the problems are. Deciding which problem areas should be the focus of further study. |
| Step 4b | *Setting Standards* | Standards are set to describe the desired outcomes in a measurable way. |
| Step 4c | *Finding Solutions* | Searching for possible ways to reach the standards set. |
| Step 4d | *Writing an Action Plan* | The methodology for implementing a change is determined along with decisions about who is to have the responsibility and what the time frames will be. |
| Step 4e | *Implementing the Plan* | Putting into action the strategies that have been developed. |
| Step 5a | *Assessing the Outcomes* | Did the plan work? Do the problems still remain? Has there been some improvement? This procedure often entails a repeat of steps 3 and 4: going back and re-collecting the data and then analyzing the results to see if the standards have been reached. |
| Step 5b | *Identifying New Issues or Continuing to Work on the Old* | If the problems are not solved, new strategies must be planned. If, however, the process has been successful, a new plan should be developed for the next area of focus. As stated earlier, quality assurance is an ongoing process and does not stop once a particular problem is corrected. It is also necessary to periodically go back and monitor earlier plans and see if the goals are continuing to be met. Two or three past issues may be chosen at random for an on-going audit in addition to the main topic of study. These could be changed periodically on a rotating basis to assure that new problems have not arisen in any of these areas. |

[41] Cunninghis, R. N. and E. Best Martini, 1996, **Quality Assurance for Activity Programs, Second Edition**, pp. 18-19, Idyll Arbor, Inc., Ravensdale, WA.

# Quality Assurance Checklist for Activities

Reviewed by: _____ Date: _____

Review this list to determine the level of compliance for your department.

**Staff:**                                                                    Yes/No
1.   proof of training/qualifications ......................................................................... _____
2.   consultation reports & qualifications ................................................................ _____
3.   job descriptions ............................................................................................... _____
4.   weekend coverage ........................................................................................... _____
5.   evening coverage............................................................................................. _____
6.   professional involvement................................................................................. _____
7.   inservice training............................................................................................. _____

**Documentation:**
1.   initial activity assessment form........................................................................ _____
2.   MDS form, activity portion .............................................................................. _____
3.   input to RAP summary sheet............................................................................. _____
4.   resident care plan entry ................................................................................... _____
5.   30 day re-eval .................................................................................................. _____
6.   daily attendance (7 days per week) ................................................................. _____
         Did you include level of participation and refusals?................................... _____
7.   bedside log....................................................................................................... _____
         Did you include type, frequency and response to visit? .............................. _____
8.   resident included in assessment and care plan process ................................... _____
9.   quarterly activity progress note ....................................................................... _____
         Did it end with a goal? ................................................................................ _____
         Is this the same as on the care plan?........................................................... _____
10.  change of condition note.................................................................................. _____
11.  physicians orders for activities, outings, work related activities ................... _____

**Physical Environment**
1.   large calendar posted and legible to visually impaired ................................... _____
2.   individual calendars in each room.................................................................... _____

**Program Evaluation**
1.   Activity Analysis Form completed for all activities offered............................ _____
2.   Activity Program Review completed................................................................ _____
3.   programs offered that meet the diversity of resident needs and abilities ........ _____

**Resident Rights**
1.   Resident Council minutes ................................................................................ _____
         proof of resolution to issues........................................................................ _____
         posted invitation to monthly meetings. ....................................................... _____
2.   review of resident's rights................................................................................ _____
3.   review of last survey results ............................................................................ _____
4.   accessibility of survey results to interested residents ..................................... _____
5.   opportunity to register to vote......................................................................... _____

# Quality Assurance Checklist for Social Service

Reviewed by: _____ Date: _____

Review this list to determine the level of compliance for your department.

**Staff:**                                                                              Yes/No
1. proof of qualifications ........................................................ _____
2. job description.................................................................... _____
3. consultant reports & qualifications ......................................... _____
4. professional improvement.................................................... _____
5. inservice training ............................................................... _____

**Documentation**
1. social history..................................................................... _____
2. initial psychosocial assessment............................................. _____
3. initial discharge plan........................................................... _____
4. MDS form, psychosocial aspects ........................................... _____
5. RAP summary sheet input .................................................... _____
6. resident care plan entry....................................................... _____
7. quarterly social service progress note .................................... _____
8. annual social service progress note ....................................... _____
9. annual discharge plan update ............................................... _____
10. MDS update (change of condition)......................................... _____
11. resident care conference attendance sign in............................ _____
12. durable power of attorney for health care, living will directive to physicians and/or conservatorship papers ....................... _____
13. advance directives signed (such as no CPR)............................ _____
14. surrogate decision maker listed............................................. _____
15. room change notification; introductions made.......................... _____

**Optional Recommendations:**
1. community resource file ...................................................... _____
2. family council minutes......................................................... _____
3. theft and loss log................................................................ _____
4. social service groups .......................................................... _____
5. social service newsletter ...................................................... _____
6. social service log................................................................ _____
7. social service volunteers ...................................................... _____
8. grievance log..................................................................... _____
9. log for marked dentures, glasses, hearing aids.......................... _____
10. client follow up after discharge ............................................. _____
Notes:

# Activity Department Checklist

Starting Date _____

Activity Professional _____

| **Daily** — Areas to be completed | Mon | Tue | Wed | Thu | Fri | Sat | Sun |
|---|---|---|---|---|---|---|---|
| Attendance | | | | | | | |
| MDS — RAP Summary | | | | | | | |
| Care Conference | | | | | | | |
| Initial Interviews & Assessments Completed | | | | | | | |
| Schedule Changes and Revisions | | | | | | | |
| Shopping & Inventory | | | | | | | |
| Community Contacts | | | | | | | |
| Completion of Special Planning | | | | | | | |
| Quarterly Progress Notes | | | | | | | |
| Volunteer Sign-in & Supervision | | | | | | | |
| Resident Council Minutes | | | | | | | |
| Interdepartmental Meetings | | | | | | | |
| Room Visits/Bedside Log | | | | | | | |
| Calendars/Decorations/Newsletter | | | | | | | |
| Department Head Meetings | | | | | | | |
| In-service Training | | | | | | | |
| Office/Department Ready For Next Day | | | | | | | |
| Other | | | | | | | |

**Notes:**

# Social Service Department Checklist

Starting Date _____

Social Service Professional _____

| **Daily** — Areas to be completed | Mon | Tue | Wed | Thu | Fri | Sat | Sun |
|---|---|---|---|---|---|---|---|
| Department Head Meetings | | | | | | | |
| Complete New Resident Assessments | | | | | | | |
| Complete Multidisciplinary Discharge Summary | | | | | | | |
| Paperwork Related to Room Changes | | | | | | | |
| Introduce Residents to New Roommates | | | | | | | |
| Fix Up Room Changes with Visit About Move | | | | | | | |
| Chart Room Changes and Adjustments | | | | | | | |
| Document Significant Behavior Changes | | | | | | | |
| Document Significant Changes in Condition | | | | | | | |
| Record Lost Dentures, Glasses and Hearing Aids | | | | | | | |
| Clothing and Personal Care Needs | | | | | | | |
| Transportation Needs | | | | | | | |
| Family and Resident Counseling | | | | | | | |
| Deaths | | | | | | | |
| Other | | | | | | | |
| **Weekly** | | | | | | | √ |
| Quarterly, Annual Progress Note Updates (Including MDS) | | | | | | | |
| Attend Resident Care Conferences | | | | | | | |
| Attend Rehabilitation Meetings | | | | | | | |
| Organize Rehabilitation Meetings with Resident and Family | | | | | | | |
| New Resident Adjustment Issues | | | | | | | |
| In-Service Training | | | | | | | |
| Staff Meetings | | | | | | | |
| **Monthly** | | | | | | | √ |
| Send Out Notices for Next Month's Resident Care Conferences | | | | | | | |

**Notes:**

# New Resident Checklist
## For Activity and Social Service Departments

Name of Resident _____

Date of Admission _____

Date Assessments to be Completed _____

Date MDS to be Completed _____

Social Service Professional _____

Activity Professional _____

| | |
|---|---|
| Social history | |
| Capacity statement completed by physician and in chart | |
| Psychosocial assessment, activity assessment | |
| Discharge plan | |
| MDS and RAPS | |
| Resident care plan entry | |
| Letter inviting resident or responsible person to resident care conference | |
| Review resident care plan with resident and/or responsible person if not in attendance at resident care conference | |
| Add resident name to voting status form, birthday list, alcohol list, outing list | |
| Mark glasses, dentures and hearing aid(s) | |
| Weekly charting by social service for the first two months | |

**Notes:**

# Standards of Practice

One of the best ways to determine if your department or facility is providing quality services is to compare your services to your professional organization's standards of practice. Standards of practice are written statements which outline the minimum level and scope of services that a professionally trained individual will perform. While each professional organization has its own set of standards, common threads weave through each. Below are the National Association for Activity Professionals Standards of Practice.[42]

# National Association of Activity Professionals

## Standards of Practice

### STANDARD 1: ACTIVITY ASSESSMENT

1.1     Information about the client/resident is recorded systematically and continuously. It is coordinated with information from other professionals involved with the care of the client/resident. Information is communicated to the care team when appropriate and accessible to staff, within the bounds of client/resident confidentiality.

1.2     The client/resident is the primary source of information. Other sources may include, but are not limited to:

- Family, friends, significant others
- Records and reports
- Other professionals directly involved in the care of the client/resident

Information is obtained through interviews, observation and reading of reports and records.

1.3     Information to be gathered should include, but not be limited to:

- family history
- ethnic and cultural background
- educational background
- social habits
- lifestyle choices
- vocational background
- recreational interests/hobbies
- talents
- membership in clubs/organizations
- volunteer activities
- political involvement
- spiritual activities
- past profile of a typical day/week
- future profile
- life goals, aspirations, dreams
- physical/mental/emotional conditions which may impact on client/resident's ability to participate in an activities program

1.4     The Activity Assessment shall be completed in a timely manner in a format acceptable to facility practice.

---

## STANDARD 2. ACTIVITY ASSESSMENT ANALYSIS

2.1    Assessment information is analyzed to provide a baseline of strengths and needs which can be emphasized and met through the activity program.

2.2    This baseline is recorded in the client/resident record and determines the structure of the client/resident's individualized activity program.

2.3    This analysis contains, but is not limited to, an identification of the client/resident's present and past health status; capabilities and limitations; and need for adaptation, both in equipment and environment.

## STANDARD 3. ACTIVITY PLAN OF CARE

3.1    The activity plan of care is based on the analysis and is designed to enable each resident to achieve and/or maintain the highest practicable level of physical, spiritual, social, intellectual and emotional well-being.

3.2    The client/resident is involved in determining the plan of care to the maximum extent possible.

3.3    The activity plan of care contains goals which are measurable, objective, timely and realistic.

## STANDARD 4. ACTIVITY PROGRAM

4.1    The activity program reflects the assessed individual and community needs of the clients/residents served.

4.2    The activity program can be categorized in three ways:

1.    Supportive

Supportive activities promote a comfortable environment while providing stimulation or solace to clients/residents who cannot benefit from either maintenance or empowerment activities. These activities are generally provided to clients/residents who may be severely impaired and/or unable to tolerate the stimulation of a group program.

2.    Maintenance

The primary function of maintenance activities is to provide the client/resident with a schedule of events which promotes the achievement and continuation of the highest practicable level of physical, emotional, cognitive, psychosocial and spiritual well being.

3.    Empowerment

Empowerment activities emphasize the promotion of self-respect by providing opportunities for self-expression, choice and social and personal responsibility. They differ from maintenance activities in that they assist clients/residents directly in redeveloping a sense of purpose in their lives. *(Supportive, Maintenance and Empowerment, Perschbacher, 1986)*

4.3    Activities shall be conducted in such a way as to allow for both passive and active participation by the client/resident.

4.4     The activity program is consistent with the facility's Mission Statement.

4.5     The activity program is flexible enough to accommodate changes in client/resident.

4.6     The client/resident is involved in the planning and implementation of the activity program to the extent possible.

4.7     The activity program is implemented, evaluated and monitored to ensure the safety of the client/resident and of the environment.

4.8     The activity program is implemented in such a way that it does not conflict with the civil, legal or human rights of the client/resident.

## STANDARD 5. EVALUATION

5.1     The activity program and the client/resident's participation in the program shall be evaluated on an on-going, regular basis.

5.2     Program evaluation shall be utilized in the continuous re-development of the activity program,

5.3     Evaluation of client/resident shall include, but not be limited to:

- Progress toward goal
- Appropriateness of activity plan
- Resources used
- Level of functioning in activity program
- Development of new goals based on current information
- Any changes in the information initially gathered

5.4     Client/Resident evaluation shall be included in his/her record, in acceptable facility format, in a timely manner consistent with facility practice.

## STANDARD 6. LEGAL RESPONSIBILITIES

6.1     The Activity Professional shall adhere to all applicable Federal, State and Local laws regarding the provision of activity services.

# Ethical Aspects of Practice

An "ethic" is a belief that is shared by members of an occupational group. Ethics statements let us know which behaviors are considered appropriate and which behaviors are considered unacceptable. They are formalized and approved by professional organizations. Ethical statements are developed by the organizations through past experiences with behaviors on the part of individual professionals. These behaviors either made the profession proud or disturbed the profession as a group. In essence, these standards for professional behaviors are developed along with, and because of, information about practice that came to light because of quality assurance programs and the developing body of knowledge.

The code of ethics statement below is from the National Association for Activity Professionals.[43]

---

[43] ©1996, National Association of Activity Professionals, *Code of Ethics* adopted April 1996. Used with permission.

# National Association of Activity Professionals

## Code of Ethics

Preamble:

The National Association of Activity Professionals and its members are dedicated to providing activity services and programs which meet the unique needs and interests of the individuals we serve.

Principles:

| | | |
|---|---|---|
| I. | Conduct | The Activity Professional shall maintain high standards of personal conduct and professional integrity on the job site at all times. The Activity Professional shall treat colleagues with professional courtesy and ensure that credit is given to others for use of their ideas, materials and programs. |
| II. | Dignity/Rights | The Activity Professional shall treat the client/resident with a regard towards personal dignity at all times. The Activity Professional shall respect and protect the rights, civil, legal and human, of the residents at all times. The Activity Professional shall report abuse, exploitation and work through appropriate channels to protect the rights of clients/residents. |
| III. | Confidentiality | The Activity Professional shall treat as confidential any information about the client/resident. Information which must be shared in the course of care to other staff and volunteers shall be exchanged in a professional manner. |
| IV. | Empowerment | The Activity Professional shall enable clients/residents to participate in the planning and implementation of their care, as well as to make independent medical, legal and financial decisions. |
| V. | Participation | The Activity Professional shall enable clients/residents to maximize their potential in activity participation through adaptation, cues/prompts, protection from undue interruption and assistance in the rescheduling of other events which may interfere with the client/resident's ability to participate in activities of their choice. |
| VI. | Record Keeping | The Activity Professional shall maintain client/records in an accurate, confidential and timely manner. The Activity Professional shall follow facility policies and procedures in the formatting of such records. In the absence of facility policy, the appropriate state and/or federal guidelines shall be followed. |
| VII. | Professional | The Activity Professional shall participate in continuing education opportunities, strive for professional competence, ensure accurate resumes and differentiate between personal comments/actions and official NAAP positions. |
| VIII. | Supervisory | The Activity Professional shall treat persons supervised with dignity and respect, protect their rights and provide accurate and fair evaluations. |

IX.    Communication        The Activity Professional shall strive to maintain open channels
                            of communication with other departments, with administration
                            and with families and clients/residents.

X.     Provision of Services The Activity Professional shall provide programs, regardless of
                            race, religion or absence thereof, ethnic origin, social or marital
                            status, sex or sexual orientation, age, health status or payment
                            source, which assist the client/resident in achieving and
                            maintaining the highest practicable level of physical, intellectual,
                            psychosocial, emotional and spiritual well-being.

XI.    Legal                The Activity Professional shall comply with all applicable
                            Federal, State and Local laws regarding the provision of
                            services.

# Safety

Providing residents with a safe living situation implies that the environment within the facility has been modified so that, in most situations, everyone is safe, free from physical or mental harm. For the Activity or Social Service Professional that means awareness of infection control principles, pressure sores and safe transfer techniques. This section will provide the professional with an overview of all three.

# Infection Control

The spread of infection requires three elements: 1. a source of the infectious material, 2. a resident who is susceptible to the infectious material and 3. a means of transmitting that infectious material to the susceptible resident. Just by the nature of health care facilities it is not possible to exclude infectious material (residents come in sick), nor is it possible to exclude residents who might be susceptible to infection. The only way to truly control the spread of infection in facilities is to control the transmission.

There are four main routes of spreading infections:

1.  Contact transmission
    a.  Direct Contact (staff to resident or resident to resident)
    b.  Indirect Contact (germs transmitted by touching an object, e.g. a tape recorder passed from one resident to another)
    c.  Droplet Contact (transmission of germs from a person sneezing, coughing or talking within a distance of three feet)
2.  Vehicle Route Transmission Through Contaminated Items (food, water, drugs, blood)
3.  Airborne Transmission (infectious materials which adhere to moisture or dust in the air and are suspended for long periods of time)
4.  Vectorborne Transmission (infection spread through an insect or animal as in mosquito-transmitted malaria)

Handwashing is the best way to control the spread of infections. Staff will need to wash their hands after coming into physical contact with any resident, using the restroom or coming into contact with activity supplies which may have contaminated surfaces. It would not be unusual for Activity Professionals to wash their hands over 30 times a day — Activity Assistants even more.

Using good handwashing technique is important. First, get the hands wet. Place soap in the hands and lather up the soap. Once the soap is lathered, scrub all parts of the hands while slowly counting to ten. The hands should be rinsed under running water while continually rubbing the hands, again counting to ten slowly. Dry the hand using disposable towels or air dry them. Turn off the water using the paper towels, not the newly cleaned hands, to turn the handles.

# Cleaning Activity Supplies

Many of the supplies used by Activity Professionals are considered to be "reusable equipment" versus "disposable equipment." Nursing and other health care professionals have turned to using disposable equipment to help significantly reduce the spread of microorganisms but this would prove too costly for activity departments. It is therefore important that the Activity Professional learn the basics of good disinfecting techniques.

When cleaning items that can tolerate getting wet, use the following technique:
- The staff or volunteer doing the cleaning should wear waterproof gloves while cleaning all items.
- When using equipment which has moving parts or which comes apart to be cleaned and which has body secretions on it, take apart the item immediately after it is used by the resident. This allows cleaning to take place later without the pieces becoming stuck together after the secretions dry.
- When rinsing the item to be washed, always use cold water first. Body secretions are more likely to coagulate (to thicken and become glue-like) when placed in hot water versus cold water.
- Soap and sudsy water work well for loosening up dirt. Let items soak if possible.
- When doing the actual cleaning, use water as hot as your hands will tolerate. Hot water and soap help break the dirt into tiny particles, making them easier to rinse off.
- Use a cloth or sponge if you need to clean using friction (scrubbing). This friction, combined with hot water and soap, breaks down the dirt and microorganisms into even smaller pieces, allowing for easy rinsing.
- Use a stiff bristled brush to remove dirt and microorganisms from groves in the equipment, being careful not to allow any of the dirt to fly up into your face. Wear a face shield or a mask and goggles for extra precautions.
- Use abrasive cleaners to remove stains that soaking doesn't remove. Use alcohol or ether to remove oily stains that don't come out with just soap and water. Remember to rinse items cleaned this way thoroughly.
- Rinse all items under hot, running water to detach any remaining dirt and microorganisms.
- Thoroughly dry all supplies prior to putting them away.
- Clean all of your cleaning supplies and then wash your hands, even though you wore gloves.

For items which cannot be washed using water and soap, follow your agency's disinfecting or sterilization techniques for these items. When using disposable equipment, dispose of the equipment immediately after use to reduce the change of further contamination of other equipment.

# Isolation Techniques

There are seven different types of isolation precautions used in the United States. Each one is designed to reduce the transmission of infection. All staff should be familiar with the reasons each precaution is required, the procedures used with each one to reduce the transmission of infectious material and the color of the precaution notice. (Each type of isolation precaution has been assigned a color for the notice sign. This color is the same for that isolation type no matter where you are in the country.) The seven types of isolation precautions are listed below.

1. **AFB Isolation** An isolation procedure for residents with current pulmonary TB who have a positive sputum smear or a chest X-ray appearance that strongly suggests current (active) TB. The isolation procedure includes: 1. masks are indicated only when resident is coughing and does not reliably cover mouth, 2. gowns are indicated only if needed to prevent gross contamination of clothing, 3. gloves are not indicated, 4. hands must be washed after touching the resident or potentially contaminated

articles and before taking care of another resident, 5. articles should be discarded, cleaned or sent for decontamination and reprocessing. The sign for AFB Isolation is always gray.

2. **Blood/Body Fluids Precautions** (Also known as "Universal Precautions".) An isolation procedure for residents who have AIDS; Arthropod borne viral fevers; Hepatitis B, non-A and non-B; malaria, rat-bite fever, syphilis and other selected diseases. The isolation procedures include: 1. masks are not indicated, 2. gowns are indicated if soiling with blood or body fluids is likely, 3. gloves are indicated for touching blood or body fluids, 4. hands must be washed after touching the resident or potentially contaminated articles and before taking care of another resident, 5. articles contaminated with infective material should be discarded or bagged and labeled before being sent for decontamination and reprocessing, 6. care should be taken to avoid needle-stick injuries, used needles should not be recapped or bent; they should be placed in a prominently labeled, puncture-resistance container designated specifically for such disposal and 7. blood spills should be cleaned up promptly with a solution of 5.25% sodium hyprocholorite diluted 1:10 with water. The sign for Blood/Body Fluids Precautions is always pink.

3. **Contact Isolation** A specific type of isolation precaution used when residents have acute respiratory infections: conjunctivitis; influenza; multiply-resistant bacteria, infection or colonization of specific bacteria; pneumonia (viral); rubella; scabies; and skin, wound or burn infection. The specific isolation procedures are: 1. masks are indicated for those who come close to resident, 2. gowns are indicated if soiling is likely, 3. gloves are indicated for touching infective material, 4. hands must be washed after touching the resident or potentially contaminated articles and before taking care of another resident and 5. articles contaminated with infective material should be discarded or bagged and labeled before being sent for decontamination and reprocessing. This sign for Contact Isolation is always orange.

4. **Drainage/Secretion Precautions Isolation** An isolation procedure for residents with infectious diseases which are producing an infective purulent material, drainage or secretions. The isolation procedure includes: 1. masks are not indicated, 2. gowns are indicated if soiling is likely, 3. gloves are indicated for touching infective material, 4. hands must be washed after touching the resident or potentially contaminated articles and before taking care of another resident and 5. articles contaminated with infective material should be discarded or bagged and labeled before being sent for decontamination and reprocessing. The sign for Drainage/Secretion Precautions is always green.

5. **Enteric Precautions** An isolation procedure for residents with amebic dysentery, cholera, diarrhea, gastroenteritis, hepatitis (viral, type A) and other specifically listed diseases. The isolation procedures include: 1. masks are not indicated, 2. gowns are indicated if soiling is likely, 3. gloves are indicated for touching infective material, 4. hands must be washed after touching the resident or potentially contaminated articles and before taking care of another resident and 5. articles contaminated with infective material should be discarded or bagged and labeled before being sent for decontamination and reprocessing. The sign for Enteric Precautions is always brown.

6. **Respiratory Isolation** An isolation procedure for residents with epiglottitis, measles, meningitis, meningococcal pneumonia, meningococcemia, mumps, pertussis (whooping cough) and some types of pneumonia. The isolation procedure includes: 1. masks are indicated for those who come close to resident, 2. gowns are not indicated, 3. gloves are not indicated, 4. hands must be washed after touching the resident or potentially contaminated articles and before taking care of another resident and 5. articles contaminated with infective material should be discarded or bagged and labeled before being sent for decontamination and reprocessing. The signs for Respiratory Isolation are always blue.

7. **Strict Isolation** An isolation procedure used with residents with diphtheria, lassa fever and other viral hemorrhagic fevers, plague, smallpox, varicella (chicken pox) and zoster. The procedure for strict isolation is: 1. masks are indicated for all persons entering room, 2. gowns are indicated for all persons entering room, 3. gloves are indicated for all persons entering the room, 4. hands must be washed after touching the resident or potentially contaminated articles and before taking care of

another resident and 5. articles contaminated with infective material should be discarded or bagged and labeled before being sent for decontamination and reprocessing. The sign for Strict Isolation is always yellow.

Nosocomial infections are infections which a resident develops after being in the facility for 72 hours. These infections have usually been spread to the resident after his/her admission to the facility and indicate that the staff may need to review their infection control techniques.

# Pressure Sores

When a resident develops pressure sores, the Activity and Social Service Departments should be notified by nursing department. The Social Service Professional should determine if the resident is refusing care, e.g., turning and repositioning, food or fluids that could contribute to the development of the pressure sores. The Activity Professional should, in consultation with the nursing department, determine if a revised activity schedule is required.

The activity programming can address the resident confined to his/her bed, assist in encouraging turning and repositioning and additional food and fluid intake.

Prevention of pressure sores can also be addressed through exercise programs, health education programs, programs that encourage nutritional intake and programs that develop self-esteem, interest in life and encouraging residents to remain out of bed.

# Transfers[44]

Many of the residents require assistance to move from one location to another. If a resident is in bed and wants to attend an activity, the activity staff should be able to transfer the resident correctly and safely from the bed into a wheelchair if that is part of their job description. In some facilities the Activity Professional is expected to help with transfers and has received formal training. If the Activity Professional works in a facility which allows him/her to transfer residents and if s/he has been trained to do so, the Activity Professional must ensure that s/he knows what s/he is doing.

There are six main types of transfers as described on the following two pages. Use the descriptions of the transfers as a basic overview. Each staff person should receive an inservice in the facility prior to attempting to transfer residents.

Remember that you are assisting the resident so that s/he may be more independent and involved in his/her community. Always work with the resident as much as possible, asking him/her to direct as much of the transfer as possible. Your mind and your conversation should be on the resident and what s/he is doing, not talking with other staff at the time of the transfer.

There are a few points a professional should know about transfers:
- Transfers are inherently safer for both the staff person and the resident when the resident is transferred between two objects which are the same height.
- When ever possible, transfer **toward** the resident's stronger side of his/her body.
- Do not allow the resident to place his/her arms around your neck while you are executing a transfer. Encourage the resident to hold on to your upper arms.
- To protect your back, always transfer a resident with your back straight, knees bent, stomach muscles tight and feet shoulder width apart.
- When transferring a resident, hold his/her body close to yours for increased stability and to protect your back.

[44] By joan burlingame, used with permission from Idyll Arbor, Inc. *Quick Reference Series.*

**Transfers**

| Transfer Type | Functional Ability Required of Resident | Transfer Sequence |
|---|---|---|
| Stand Pivot | Ability to support weight through legs with standby assistance or with physical assistance. Ability to cooperate with staff. | 1. Ask if resident is ready to transfer.<br>2. Have resident don gait belt.<br>3. Place wheelchair at an angle to the resident's intended seat (bed).<br>4. Lock any applicable wheel brakes.<br>5. Remove arm and foot rests, drop side rail of bed.<br>6. Have resident scoot to edge of seat as independently as possible.<br>7. Have resident check to ensure that his/her feet are flat on the floor.<br>8. Place and hold the resident's knees between yours.<br>9. Staff person takes hold of the gait belt.<br>10. Instruct the resident to lean toward you.<br>11. Instruct the resident to push out of the sitting position to a full stand, then to pivot and then to sit.<br>12. Insure that resident has stable balance in new seat.<br>13. Remove gait belt. |
| Sit Pivot | Ability to partially bear weight with legs. Ability to lean and to scoot forward in chair with standby assist. Ability to cooperate with staff person. Skin not prone to tearing with moderate sheer. | 1. Ask if resident is ready to transfer.<br>2. Have resident don gait belt.<br>3. Place wheelchair at an angle to the resident's intended seat (bed).<br>4. Lock any applicable wheel brakes.<br>5. Remove arm and foot rests, drop side rail of bed.<br>6. Have resident scoot to edge of seat as independently as possible.<br>7. Have resident check to ensure that his/her feet are flat on the floor.<br>8. Place and hold the resident's knees between yours.<br>9. Staff person takes hold of the gait belt.<br>10. Instruct the resident to lean and scoot forward, the momentum for the transfer will come from the staff person.<br>11. Staff pulls the resident forward and guides a pivoting move into the new seat.<br>12. Insure that resident has stable balance in new seat.<br>12. Remove gait belt. |
| Two-Person Sit Pivot | Ability to bear part of the weight with legs. Requires physical assistance to lean body forward, to scoot to edge of chair. May be able to lean & scoot, but body weight is in excess of staff person's strength to bear safely. | 1. Ask if resident is ready to transfer.<br>2. Have resident don gait belt.<br>3. Place wheelchair at an angle to the resident's intended seat (bed).<br>4. Lock any applicable wheel brakes.<br>5. Remove arm and foot rests, drop side rail of bed.<br>6. Have resident check to ensure that his/her feet are flat on the floor.<br>7. With one staff person in front of resident and one behind, assist the resident in scooting forward to the edge of the seat.<br>8. The staff person in front will place and hold the resident's knees between his/her knees.<br>9. The staff person in front of the resident will be in charge of timing of the transfer and will count "one, two, three". On "three" both staff will provide physical assistance for the transfer.<br>10. Insure that resident has stable balance in new seat.<br>11. Remove gait belt.<br>12. Have resident apply lap belt if appropriate. |

**Transfers**

| Transfer Type | Functional Ability Required of Resident | Transfer Sequence |
|---|---|---|
| Sliding Board Transfer | Inability to support weight through legs but has adequate sitting balance. Can scoot sideways along board with standby to full assistance. Ability to cooperate with staff person. | 1. Ask if resident is ready to transfer.<br>2. Have resident don gait belt.<br>3. Place wheelchair at an angle to the resident's intended seat (bed).<br>4. Lock any applicable wheel brakes.<br>5. Remove arm and foot rests, drop side rail of bed.<br>6. Gently place one edge of the sliding board at least 3" under resident's thigh and the other edge at least 3" onto the resident's next seat.(If the next seat is a bed or any soft surface, allow more than 3" to rest on the surface.) Ensure that the placement of the board does not compromise the resident's skin integrity.<br>7. Have resident scoot to edge of seat as independently as possible.<br>8. Have resident check to ensure that his/her feet are flat on the floor.<br>9. While providing standby assistance, encourage the resident to scoot to the other end of the board.<br>10. Have resident scoot onto the new surface. If resident is not able to scoot onto new surface independently, do a pivot transfer.<br>11. Remove sliding board.<br>12. Insure that resident has stable balance in new seat.<br>14. Remove gait belt. |
| Two Person Lift | Ability to tolerate a sitting position. Ability to cooperate with staff person. | 1. Ask if resident is ready to transfer.<br>2. Have resident don gait belt.<br>3. Place wheelchair at an angle to the resident's intended seat (bed).<br>4. Lock any applicable wheel brakes.<br>5. Remove arm and foot rests, drop side rail of bed<br>6. The physically strongest staff person should place himself/herself behind the sitting resident, place his/her arms around the resident's torso and hold on to either the resident's wrists or to the gait belt.<br>7. The second staff person should stand to the side of the resident and place his/her arms under the resident's thighs and calves.<br>8. The staff person holding the resident's torso will count "one, two, three" and on "three" both staff persons will lift the resident out of the chair and onto the desired surface.<br>9. Insure that resident is stable on the new surface.<br>10. Remove gait belt. |
| Prone Cart or Stretcher Transfers | No specific functional ability required. | 1. Ask if resident is ready to transfer.<br>2. Lock all applicable wheel brakes.<br>3. Line up cart/stretcher so that it is parallel to the bed/mat.<br>4. Place draw sheet under the resident if the resident is not able to roll onto the cart/stretcher himself/herself.<br>5. For residents unable to assist with the transfer, use four staff to slide the resident to the edge of the bed/mat using the draw sheet.<br>6. Either remove the draw sheet or tuck the ends in under the cart/stretcher mattress.<br>7. Secure resident to cart/stretcher with a seat belt. |

# Risk Management

Risk management is the act of identifying situations in the workplace that may harm the resident, the staff or the facility. Most facilities will have many policies and procedures related to making the workplace safe. This section will talk about how the staff controls for risks.

Controlling risk is like placing a safety net under the resident. It requires around-the-clock management by each staff person — on duty as well as off duty. Krames Communications, in the booklet "Risk Management: Your Role in Providing Quality Care" (1989) lists the eight areas of around-the-clock management. Specific questions for the Activity and Social Service Professionals have been added to Krames Communications" categories.

### Around-the-Clock Risk Management

**On the Job**

**Safe Environment**

- Are the activities supplies appropriate for the residents' abilities?
- Are all the fire exits unblocked?
- Is the water temperature below 110°F?

**Ongoing Monitoring**

- Do resident assessments represent the resident's actual abilities and needs?
- Are staff diligent in changing the resident's care plan as the resident's abilities change?
- Are staff continuing to be careful about resident safety and infection control?

**Clear Communication**

- Do staff communicate important information to each other concerning resident status and workplace concerns?
- Do staff communicate with the residents and their families in a timely and appropriate manner?

**Handling Incidents**

- Do all staff know the facility's policies and procedures well enough to implement them all of the time?
- Have staff had the proper training to be able to carry out the administration's intent for handling the different types of incidents?

**Off the Job**

**Continuing Education**

- Have you kept your knowledge and skills up-to-date by continually seeking out new information?
- Are you seeking continuing education in the areas where you have the weakest knowledge and skill, not just the areas that are convenient or interesting to you?

**Journals**

- Do you regularly (e.g., at least monthly) spend an hour or more reading up on new information and developments in your professional journals?
- Do you support the body of knowledge by writing up important information or developments and submitting them for publication?

**Professional Groups**

- Are you an active member in at least one national and state/local organization?
- Do you find time to discuss issues with other professionals outside of your facility, especially if you are a one person department?

**Healthy Lifestyle**

- Are you responsible enough to make sure that you get enough sleep prior to going to work to reduce the chance of mistakes being made?
- Do you eat food that is good for your physical health and exercise on a regular basis to be able to perform your job well?
- Do you balance your work life with your play life to be able to be refreshed?

How do you ensure that each resident is safe while they are in your environment and receiving your services? One of the most successful ways of ensuring that the resident is receiving quality care and services is to make sure that your department is adhering to professional standards of practice. Standards of practice usually outline minimum standards for management of the service, minimum standards for delivery of the service and minimum qualifications for staff. However, even when you seem to be following standards of practice completely, you may still run into problems. Risk management and quality assurance are similar — only on different ends of the continuum. Quality assurance is the process of improving good services to make them better. Risk management is the process of reducing or eliminating harmful or dangerous situations.

The ability to identify and control harmful or dangerous situations in the environment and in the delivery of service is called Risk Management. Risk Management has six steps:
1.  To recognize that there is a problem.
2.  To be able to identify what in the system is causing the problem.
3.  To be able to identify who is impacted by the problem.
4.  To be able to identify if the problem is changeable (or if other systems need to be changed to accommodate for what cannot be changed — a long term care facility cannot decide to exclude all residents who are HIV positive — they need to change their systems of infection control to accommodate those residents).
5.  To develop a method of correcting the problem.
6.  To develop a means to measure if the problem was corrected.

joan burlingame studied the worst breakdowns in resident safety in her 1992 study. (A summary of her study may be found later in this chapter.) She was able to identify ten basic principles of reducing risks to resident safety. By being aware of these risks, the Activity Professional can help manage harmful or dangerous situations within his/her own facility. These basic principle are:
1.  Water temperature at the taps should never be over 110 degrees Fahrenheit.
2.  Fire doors and fire routes must always be free of clutter. Fire safety standards must always be followed.
3.  Floors should be free of objects which may cause the resident to slip or to trip.
4.  Walkways (including hallways) must be free of protruding objects — many residents have poor vision and may walk into a protruding object and injure themselves. (Protruding objects may stick out only 4 inches from the wall between the height of 27" to 80" from the floor. Exceptions are made for drinking fountains or telephones which are mounted on posts. They may stick out 12 inches.)
5.  The building must be maintained in a manner that ensures it is always structurally safe.
6.  Staff must always talk to and treat each resident respectfully.
7.  Only life threatening events should get in the way of any staff helping a resident move/turn who is at risk for pressure sores and is in need of movement/turning.
8.  Good infection control principles should always be practiced by all staff.
9.  Staff should always ensure the physical safety of each resident — including protecting him/her from self-inflected injuries.
10. Food and fluid should always be treated as if they were a prescription item — never given to a resident unless in a manner which follows the medical orders.

The most important thing for staff to remember is — if something does not seem right, it probably isn't. Even if your supervisor assures you that the manner that a resident is being treated is all right because the treatment team agreed to the treatment, if you feel that it may be abusive or neglectful treatment, *act!* Approach your facility administrator. If that doesn't work, each state has a law that says a staff person must report a potential case of resident abuse or neglect (usually in 24 hours or less). It is not up to that staff person to obtain proof that the treatment is abusive or neglectful. If the staff person suspects abuse or neglect, s/he is to leave it up to the state investigators. When you call, you do not need to give your name. Remember, you may be the best advocate that the resident has!

# Immediate Jeopardy[45]

When a survey is conducted, the surveyors determine whether or not a facility meets the Conditions of Participation (the federal regulations) for receiving Medicare and Medicaid funding by assessing whether the facility meets all of the requirements in the federal regulations. Usually, a deficiency means that the provider must submit a plan of correction to be acted upon within 30 days.

However, sometimes the surveyors discover situations which are so severe that stronger sanctions are required. In these cases, the guidelines for determining "immediate jeopardy" (also known as "fast track") are applied. The provider must correct a condition of "immediate jeopardy" immediately or "immediate termination action" will be taken; i.e., the residents will be removed and the facility closed.

To assist surveyors in determining when circumstances pose an "immediate jeopardy" to resident health and safety, a set of criteria has been developed. This guide is intended to provide greater consistency among surveyors when reviewing specific situations and assessing provider failures.

The standards for the funding for health care services (and therefore, the standards of health care practice) in the United States depends heavily on the actions of the Congress of the United States. For administration purposes, health care is divided into two separate entities, the Health Care Financing Administration and the Public Health Service. Almost every Activity or Social Service Professional who works in a clinical setting is under the auspices of the Health Care Financing Administration or HCFA. (In the Fiscal Year 1991 HCFA was responsible for oversight on 54,586 facilities.)

Specific minimum standards are set for each type of facility, e.g., hospitals, home health care, long term care (nursing homes), etc. All changes and new health care laws are released on October 1st of each year in the government publication called the **Code of Federal Regulations** or **CFR**. While most regulations are facility-type specific, there are two federal health care regulations that apply to all health care under the jurisdiction of HCFA. The first regulation is the Civil Rights Act (Title Six). The second regulation, the most stringent, is called **Immediate Jeopardy**, also known as Appendix "Q". (Prior to October 1, 1992 it was called "Immediate and Serious Threat.")

With just a few exceptions, every facility that is surveyed by either the Joint Commission or by CARF fall under the jurisdiction of HCFA. The loss of HCFA certification is actually more severe than the loss of accreditation by either the Joint Commission or by CARF. A facility may maintain its business license without Joint Commission or CARF Accreditation. Without HCFA certification, it is not likely that a facility can maintain its business license. In such a case, it often requires legislation on the state level to maintain the facility.

## Definitions from Appendix Q and Appendix J

**Immediate and Serious Threat**  An immediate and serious threat is defined as having a high probability that serious harm or injury to residents could occur at any time or already has occurred and may well occur again if residents are not protected effectively from the harm or the threat is not removed.

**Patients**  Includes all persons receiving treatment, care or services from the provider.

**Physical Abuse**  Refers to any physical motion or action (e.g., hitting, slapping, punching, kicking, pinching, etc.) by which bodily harm or trauma occurs. It includes use of corporal punishment as well as the use of any restrictive, intrusive procedure to control inappropriate behavior for purpose of punishment.

---

[45] This section is by joan burlingame, CTRS. Used with permission.

**Provider/Facility** Means all Medicare providers and suppliers and Medicaid only facilities (intermediate care facilities for the mentally retarded — ICF-MR).

**Psychological Abuse** Includes, but is not limited to, humiliation, harassment and threats of punishment or deprivation, sexual coercion, intimidation, whereby individuals suffer psychological harm or trauma.

**Verbal Abuse** Refers to any use of oral, written or gestured language by which abuse occurs. This includes pejorative and derogatory terms to describe persons with disabilities.

**Guiding Principles** (taken directly from Appendix Q)

1. An immediate and serious threat need not result in **actual** harm to the resident. The threat of probable harm is perceived as being as serious or significant.
2. The threat could be perceived as something which will result in potentially severe temporary or permanent injury, disability or death and must be perceived as something which is likely to occur in the very near future.
3. Mental abuse can be as damaging as physical abuse and may constitute an immediate and serious threat.
4. Only one resident needs to be jeopardized; the entire or large percentage of resident population **does not have** to be threatened or injured.
5. The absence of adequate staff training does not, in and of itself, pose the threat. However, if the staff lacks the skill or knowledge necessary to properly care for the residents, this may present the same serious problems as when there are insufficient numbers of staff and will make it more difficult for the provider to correct or eliminate the problems.
6. The situation is severe enough that it outweighs potential concerns of resident transfer to another facility.
7. The situation may or may not be a threat considering such factors as season of the year and geographic location.
8. The deficiency cannot be corrected quickly to prevent a resident from being severely harmed.
9. Immediate and serious threat termination is the only response to the problem.

(Immediate Jeopardy may be "called" without having to close a facility. By citing an Immediate Jeopardy the survey team is stating that there exists an unacceptable threat to a resident which must be corrected within hours or days or else termination action will begin. Termination action usually does not officially occur (with public notification) until the fifth day after Immediate Jeopardy has been called.)

# Immediate Jeopardy

**Note:** Idyll Arbor, Inc. has analyzed the actual Immediate Jeopardy citations across all ten HCFA regions for the calendar years 1990 and 1991. The actual citations listed in this paper come from HCFA Regions II, VIII and X (the only regions analyzed at the time this paper was prepared). These three regions account for 12,134 of the 54,586 facilities (or 22% of the facilities) around the United States.

While only a few Immediate Jeopardy citations in this sample directly applied to recreation and/or activities, many of the citations may have been avoided if the activity staff had been professionally trained and certified. The author found only one Certified Therapeutic Recreation Specialist involved with any of the citations listed in this paper. All the other staff appeared not to be certified as a CTRS. (It is unknown how many, if any, held other credentials.)

The three most common Immediate Jeopardy violations cited which involved therapy and activities in this sampling are:
1. Lack of appropriate intervention with SIB (Self-Injurious Behavior) and PICA behaviors.
2. Water temperature in excess of 110 degrees F.
3. Lack of safe egress due to locked or blocked fire exits.

# Immediate Jeopardy — Actual Citations

In this section the information in Arial type are direct quotes from survey documents.

## I. Core Statement: Failure to Protect Residents from Disease and Infection

### I.1. Failure to protect from nosocomial infections and/or communicable diseases.

> (Nosocomial infections are infections that a resident catches after being admitted to the nursing home.)
>
> One nursing home in the Midwest had an unusually high rate of a nosocomial infection. The surveyor observed the activity coordinator use a game with one resident who had pussy eyes and who constantly touched her eyes and then the game pieces. Without washing her hands or the game, the activity coordinator then took the game to the next patient!

## II. Core Statement: Failure to Provide Care or Services Essential to Maintaining or Improving Resident Health

> An Immediate Jeopardy call is frequently made because of an overall pattern of poor care and not just one single event. Citation after citation noted that the residents' right to receive quality care was lacking. In many of the surveys reviewed, the dehumanization of the individual was so pervasive that I doubt that the nursing homes met even the minimal standards for prisoners of war.
>
> On July 16, 1991 during the group interview, only one of the ten residents responded that s/he received an absentee ballot. The administrator acknowledged that the staff does not assist the residents to exercise their right to vote.
>
> The facility failed to provide access to the private use of a telephone. The phone was in the dining/recreation room, where the television was in use. The phone was not adapted for the hearing impaired. The lack of access to a private telephone was confirmed during the interview process.
>
> One facility was undergoing renovations. To help empty out one unit to put down a new floor, the residents were sent to "activities" for the day:
>
> Renovations and construction was in progress on the fourth floor. On April 26, 1991, all 57 residents on the fourth floor were evacuated to a small activity room on the first floor. The following problems were identified: 1. These residents were seated in this room for over a ten hour period with no provisions for fresh water or exercise. There was no area provided to lie down to rest., 2. Several residents were observed asleep with their faces lying directly on a table in front of them., 3. One male resident restrained in a wheelchair fell asleep with his right arm extending over the back of the chair. His arm was a mottled purple color due to lack of circulation., 4. At approximately 9 p.m. when residents were returned to their rooms, alert residents constantly asked for water to drink; staff did not respond.

### II. 1. Failure to protect from bodily harm

> One facility in Indiana had a 189 page survey document outlining physical harm to residents, primarily in the form of pressure sores. After a description of each resident's pressure sore the surveyor indicated the lack of documented time spent in activities by that resident (usually only one or two times documented for each resident over a 3 month period).

The following citation is one that directly implicates the Activity Professional as one member of the treatment who failed to follow a very specific physician's order. The consequences for the resident was severe, requiring invasive procedures (surgery).

Resident A1290 with a physician's order for Activities, "Out of Bed Q.I.D. x 30 minutes" and "Don't keep out of bed more than 30 minutes at a time" was not addressed on nursing care plan, nor were these instructions conveyed to care givers on nurse's aide instruction for resident care. Activity documented a problem: "In bed most a.m. and p.m. Gotten up only for noon meal. By observation this resident was out of bed in excess of 1 hour on 11/2/90."

Another facility had an excessive percentage of residents with pressure sores. One of the citations as a result was the lack of documented activities.

There were no planned activities and no activities were observed during any of the days of this survey for residents who were bed-bound or room-bound. Due to the lack of staffing, many residents were not assisted out of bed during the days of the survey to attend activities. For examples [in a survey done 3/15/91]: 1. resident #73 an elderly bed-bound resident had documentation of having one in-room activity in January 1991 and none during February 1991. 2. resident #72 had no activity assessment or progress notes. Since admission 1-14-91 there was no documentation of any activities offered. 3. Resident #3 had only three activities offered in January 1991 according to documentation and none in February 1991. 5. Resident #69 had no activity assessment and only two activities offered in January 1991. No activities were recorded for this resident for February 1991.

## II. 2. Failure to ensure that residents received medications as prescribed.

The Activity Professional should not be giving medications. However, when the Activity Professional finds the resident's medications in medicine cups still on the resident's bedside table, action should be taken. In one situation dated 12/06/91 the staff person had found numerous medicine cups by a resident's bed (with the medications still inside). She took these pills to the administrator to express concern. The administrator did not follow through, however, the surveyor noted in the citation that the staff had tried to alert the appropriate staff to the problem. The nursing home was cited with an Immediate Jeopardy for multiple situations similar to this one that were not being resolved.

## II. 8. Failure of provider to furnish supervision or monitoring consistent with resident needs

## II. 11. Failure to monitor resident status to identify conditions or changes in conditions which potentially could lead to resident harm and/or deterioration

The Activity Professional, as a member of the professional health care team, must have an assessment that is specific enough for him/her to know the resident's actual ability in many areas. The types of treatment objectives that the Activity Professional has listed **must come directly from the activity assessment**. The activity assessment must be specific enough to be able to determine honestly if the resident's ability has changed at all.

The care plan lacked quantifiable objectives for the highest level of functioning the resident may be expected to attain, based on the comprehensive assessment: failed to reflect intermediate steps for each outcome objective; failed to reflect resident's assessment; lacked orientation towards preventing declines in functioning and/or functional levels.

The two most prevalent citations for Immediate Jeopardy found for nursing homes were lack of quality control for dietary needs and lack of prevention of pressure sores. While the Activity

Professional does not provide nursing care for pressure sores, s/he must take responsibility to ensuring that appropriate positioning and pressure releases are done and that all new (or worsened) pressure sores are immediately noted. If the Activity Professional is not trained to modify a resident's positioning himself/herself, s/he should notify nursing for them to change the resident's position.

There are 42 bed or chair bound residents in the facility. Seventeen residents (41%) have pressure sores. Eleven residents (65%) of the 17 either formed them in the facility or the status of the pressure sores declined or worsened in the facility. During the survey, the surveyors identified 10 previously unidentified pressure sores; nine were stage II's and one was a stage I.

**III. Core Statement: Failure to Maintain Equipment and Supplies at an Acceptable Level to Ensure Health and Safety**

**IV. Core Statement: Failure to Prevent Situations/Conditions in Environment or Physical Plant Which Prevent a Hazard and Would Jeopardize Resident Health and Safety**

**IV. 2. Failure to ensure that equipment, furnishing or supplies do not present hazards to residents**

At 7:10 p.m. one wheelchair was observed to have a torn back, a portable commode chair had torn pads and a chair in the living room had tears on the vinyl back, rendering these items uncleanable.

Observation and inspection of wheelchairs revealed 2 of 5 had faulty brakes. For example, observed on 6/26/91 at 11 am of resident #6 being transferred from bed to w/c revealed the chair rolled backwards despite the staff having set the brakes. This startled the resident who attempted to brace himself against falling.

The enclosed back lawns of the facility were not safe for residents. High weed and tall grass presented a tripping hazard for residents who would like to walk outdoor in these areas. Thickets were overgrowing on the interior side of the back perimeter fence.

**IV. 10. Failure to store, prepare, maintain and serve food to ensure against the growth/transmission of pathogens**

Note: Hot foods must be held at not less than 140 degrees Fahrenheit and served promptly (within 15 minutes of being removed from temperature control devices). Cold foods must be held and served at 45 degrees Fahrenheit or cooler.

This citation is one that is directly attributable to the activity department:

Observation of the walk-in freezer on 6/29/91 at 11 am revealed a large plastic garbage bag filled with unprocessed, unskinned muskrats open to the air. Interview with staff disclosed that the muskrats were to be used at a skinning contest. Traditional game foods which are unprocessed, uncleaned and with animal hair provide avenues for contamination and disease.

**IV. 11. Failure to control temperature of hot water used by residents**

Water temperature may not exceed 110 F.

**IV. 15. Failure to maintain physical plant in safe condition**

The Activity Professional should be familiar enough with physical plant maintenance that s/he can identify when an activity room is unsafe for occupation or at least know when to call for a maintenance person.

There were numerous examples cited of water damage resulting from a leaking roof. Both the fire safety and health surveyor provide information that indicates water has entered electrified systems which now have malfunctioning conditions. In addition, there is information that water or other elements have damaged the building's structural components. The most pronounced indicator of this is a sagging support beam in the resident's activity room which is being temporarily supported by a 4x4 post. This arrangement would present the most risk during earthquake or if additional weight were added to the roof as snow or ice.

**V. Core Statement: Failure to Uphold Resident Rights Whereby Violations Can Result in Harm or Injury**

**V. 1. Inappropriate Restraints: Failure to ensure that restraints in the form of devices, drugs or procedures that in some way restrict a resident's physical and/or mental independence/autonomy are appropriately used and monitored.**

As a member of the team, the Activity Professional is partially responsible to ensuring that reasonable care is taken when restraints are used. I was so appalled at this next citation that I called the Region X office to see if this wasn't also a case of resident abuse. This situation qualified as resident abuse and should have been called in and reported by any of the staff who observed this situation. The federal surveyor I talked with said that this situation could have actually been a criminal violation and could have ended up with jail time for the staff involved.

Resident #1 resides behind a "Dutch Door" that is secured in a locked position with three (3) slide bolt locks, that are positioned at the base of the door. The resident is currently diagnosed with Alzheimer's. The resident is incontinent of urine and feces, the room reeks with the foul odor of urine which permeates the entire room and hallway. On one occasion the resident was observed eating the excrement of her roommate, another occasion the resident was found to have feces smeared on her mouth. The facility did not assert, protect or facilitate the rights of this resident. Review of this resident's clinical record and comprehensive care plan revealed that a trial of less restrictive measures had not been implemented. The locked Dutch Doors were used for the convenience of the staff to control the resident's behaviors and wandering. No documentation per the resident's care plan and/or clinical record indicated what measures the facility's staff would initiate to promote the highest practicable physical, mental and psychosocial well being of the resident.

One additional question I had about the situation above (but did not see it cited in the survey document) is: How would the staff be able to evacuate all of the residents in time during a fire if every door had 3 bolts!

Often the nursing staff (as well as the activity staff themselves) do not look upon the Activity Professional as a key professional member of the treatment team. However, the law considers the Activity Professional to be a key member and **expects** him/her to act accordingly. This expectation includes the use of standardized assessments and procedures to determine the type of restraint the resident may need during activities and determining the type of interventions needed to reduce the need for a restraint. The following citation indicates that the entire treatment team was in grave error.

Sixteen of sixteen residents reviewed for restraint use did not have documentation that reflected:

1. Multidisciplinary evaluations prior to restraint use for: a) restraint need,
b) consideration or trials of less restrictive approaches.

2. Discussion of: a) the reasons necessitating the use of a restraint, b) the potential risk/benefits of the restraint to be used with the resident and/or appropriate responsible persons, c) permission for the use of the restraint by the resident and/or responsible persons.

3. The plan of care did not include: a) when the restraint was to be used, b) a periodic planned activity/exercise program during the restraint release times.

Observations of residents in physical restraints revealed that they were not monitored and/or released from their restraints on a regular basis.

Resident #38098 had an order for wrist restraints to prevent him/her from pulling at a colostomy. During two days of the survey the wrist restraints and a waist restraint were observed on continuously, both in bed and in a wheelchair. The ties connected to the wheelchair were released from the chair during a group activity, however, the restraints were not removed from the wrist for a period of exercise and/or activity. It was also noted that while the restraints were tied to the wheelchair the resident was able to easily reach the colostomy. She was not observed to pull at the colostomy nor was there documentation since 4/13/91 (60 days) of any attempts. This resident was also observed in the Station I dining area on 6/13/91 from 10:40 a.m. until 4:00 p.m. with the waist restraint not released.

**V.2. Inappropriate Psychiatric Seclusion: Failure to ensure that the removal of residents from their normal environment to an area from which their egress is prevented, is done appropriately and/or failure to ensure that there is adequate and appropriate monitoring of residents while in seclusion.**

**V.3. Neglect: Failure to provide necessary physical or psychological care, attention or treatment, resulting in gross neglect.**

The activity staff are responsible for helping the rest of the team identify those residents who are not receiving adequate care. This resident was seen by the activity staff occasionally and yet the condition continued to exist.

During the interview, the resident emitted a body odor and his nails were long and had an accumulation of dark debris. He stated that he did not get care on a regular basis and when he asked staff for assistance he was made to feel like he was imposing on their time. He stated he did not like to eat his food with "filthy" hands, but he had no choice.

**V.4. Mental Abuse: Failure to prevent mental abuse whereby residents suffer psychological harm or trauma.**

**V.5. Physical Abuse: Failure to protect residents from bodily harm or trauma.**

**Other Citations that Helped Lead to a Facility's Receiving an Immediate Jeopardy Call**

At times the lack of activities or activity room space is cited as one of the factors that caused a nursing home to receive an Immediate Jeopardy call. Below are some examples that were contained in survey documents associated with Immediate Jeopardy.

Although the dining room usually used for activities was not large enough to hold even one half of the residents, there had been no alternative plans to provide similar activities to the residents who would appropriately benefit from the same activity but who were unable to attend due to space constraints.

There were no organized activities on Sundays other than religious programs. The Activity Cart which was indicated on the monthly calendar consisted of only a cart with various games and activities for residents who were able to make those selections for personal use. There were few activities for the residents who were confused or confined to their rooms and these activities were inappropriate for their individual needs. For instance, one activity observed for a resident who was unable to leave her room, consisted of gently touching her hand with a feather dusters, Consideration had not been made of the decreased tactile sense of the elderly when planning this activity.

**The Activity Professional should not use the term "participate"** when s/he is writing the care plan objectives!! Not only is it unprofessional to base wellness on where one's body is, it is also a violation of the resident's right to refuse treatment. Instead use terms like "maintain fine motor manipulation skills through activity" or "decrease visual neglect through cueing and practice during activity."

For residents #10, #21, #5, #37,...(etc.) care plans had goals which were not stated in specific individualized, measurable terms. For instance, "decrease episodes of sadness, provide opportunity for individual activities within three months, increase physical and social activities at least three times a week, increase tolerance of others"

One facility had multiple citations because of the poor quality of activity objectives. This citation is part of that survey document:

The requirement is that the activities program must be directed by a qualified professional. This requirement is not met because the Activity Coordinator has not attended an approved school in activities. Per interview of staff the activity coordinator will not attend a course until February [four months later].

(The facility solved this problem by firing the Activity Professional and hiring someone else who was qualified.)

The resident's rights as a human being must be respected.

On June 5, 1991, at 9:30 am, the surveyor observed an activity assistant taking resident #131 from her room in her wheelchair to bible study. The resident was not asked by the assistant if she wanted to go to this activity or informed where she was going until the surveyor intervened. When the assistant asked the resident if she wanted to go to bible study, the resident declined because she was in pain. The assistant did not give the resident the choice of attending the bible study nor inform her where she was going.

This study done by Idyll Arbor, Inc. is looking at all of the citations across the United States for the years 1990 and 1991 in long term care settings. It seems apparent that the surveyors did not hold Activity Professionals to the same stringent standards for quality of work as they did other Activity Professionals in other settings (Intermediate Care Facilities for the Mentally Retarded, General Hospitals, Psychiatric Hospitals, etc.). This may be in part because the surveyors for nursing homes do not understand the importance of activity for residents and/or because the surveyors do not really consider the Activity Professional as a separate professional entity from nursing. With the citation from Indiana being the only exception, the surveyors did not consistently identify the partial responsibility the Activity Professional has to help reduce pressure sores in each and every resident.

The typical activity staff to resident ratio is about 1/70; a ratio that makes it impossible for the Activity Professional to have any serious impact on the health and well being of the residents. It may be time to change the role of the Activity Professional. The Activity Professional would be much more effective if s/he spent more time working with the nurses' aides to teach them how to carry out sensory stimulation, range of motion and other vital activities. Ten short sessions (five or ten minutes at the most) of sensory stimulation or range of motion activities is more beneficial then one or two longer periods a day. The nurses' aides could help with these activities during normal care.

A few citations were not noted in this paper but were cited time and again. The most common violations stated after pressure sores and dietary issues — not just those relating to activities — were blocked fire exits. The Activity Professional may also want to have the water temperature in his/her activity room measured from time to time to make sure that it is **never** over 110 degrees.

# Summary

While it is important for the professional to have the knowledge and skills required to provide services and treatment, other areas of knowledge and skill are also required. Three of these areas are quality assurance, safety and risk management. The three areas are not really separate entities, but part of a continuum for providing the types of services that residents need.

# 12. Management

This chapter discusses some of the important management issues not covered in the rest of the book. The issues include resident rights, restraints, behavior management, time management, budgets, writing policies and procedures, OBRA regulations, surveys and medications for the elderly.

## Resident's Rights

Residents in nursing facilities have specific rights outlined in federal and state laws. This section discusses some of the most important rights. The primary right of a resident is to make decisions. This right is never taken away, just modified. If the resident is no longer competent to make decisions, another individual is named to represent the resident's wishes. Other resident rights include the right to informed consent, the right to participate in his/her care plan and the right to be free of unreasonable restraint.

### Determining Competency

If the resident is unable to make decisions for himself/herself, these rights are granted to his/her legal representative. Many states have provisions for representation of the resident who has no legal representative or who may not have any interested family member and is not capable of making decisions. The capacity of the resident may be established in several ways. A court may determine that the resident is unable to make his/her own health care decisions and formally declare him/her incompetent. In this case a *conservator of person* will be appointed. If an individual is not available to act as conservator, a public guardian may be appointed. It is important when reviewing conservatorship papers to determine whether the conservatorship is for *person* or *property* or both. Only a conservator of person can make health care decisions for the resident.

In the absence of a court order, the physician may make the determination of capacity. This will be documented in the health record. The physician, with the help of the facility, will designate a surrogate decision maker or interested family member to make health care decisions. If the resident has executed a Durable Power of Attorney for Health Care, the surrogate decision maker will be specified on the form. In interviewing a resident and in developing a care plan, it is important to be aware of who the legal decision maker is. At times we mistakenly defer to the family member when the resident is the one who must make the decisions.

# Informed Consent

Informed consent is a legal term which means that the resident has the right to understand both the positive reasons for making a decision and also the possible negative consequences of any decision made. To meet the legal test of informed consent, the resident must have been presented five types of information. The first type of information is a clear description of the problem presented in a language and manner that the resident can understand. The second is a description of the suggested solution presented in a language and manner that the resident can understand. The third is an explanation of the possible negative consequences (or possible side effects) of going along with the proposed solution. The fourth piece of information is the possible negative consequences of not going along with the proposed solution. The fifth type of information is other, possible treatment options. When the resident is given these five different types of information, s/he should be able to make a decision about the proposed solution.

Agreement or consent, by itself, is not enough. The resident must: be capable (or represented by a legally recognized representative), receive all of the information that is necessary to make an intelligent decision and not be coerced.

# Right to Participate in Care Planning

An important right the resident has is the right to participate in the plan of care *including the right to refuse a treatment or a service* (Tags F154, F155, F157 and F280). In other words, the resident must give consent before any treatment or service is initiated. In some cases, informed consent is required (e.g. for a restraint program). The regulations specify that even if the resident's ability to make decisions is impaired or the resident is formally declared incompetent by a court, the resident should still be informed of changes in his/her plan of care and consulted about preferences. OBRA requires that a resident be fully informed in advance about care and treatment and of any changes in that care or treatment that may affect the his/her well-being (483.10 (d) (2)). The resident must receive information necessary to make health care decisions, including those involving activity and social service. When planning an activity program for a resident or when developing social service interventions, be sure to include the resident or the surrogate decision maker in the planning.

Residents (or their legal representative) have the right to refuse any and all treatments or services. When a resident refuses medication, treatments, food, fluids, socialization or activities, the Social Service Professional must assess the cause of the refusal and discuss with the resident or surrogate decision maker the risks and consequences of refusal. The counseling of the resident must be clearly documented. The refusal must be shown to be consistent and persistent. Alternative treatments must be offered and all attempted interventions should be documented in the progress notes and on the care plan. Every effort should be made to safeguard the resident's health and safety while also respecting his/her right to refuse treatment.

# Right to be Restraint Free

The resident has the right to be free from any physical or chemical restraint not used to treat medical symptoms (Tags F221 and F222). In fact, the resident is guaranteed the right to make an informed choice about the use of restraints. Except in a few situations (e.g., medical crisis), informed consent must be obtained before restraints can be used. Posy vests and lap belts are easily recognized restraints, but bed rails, geri-chairs and seizure medications may also be used to modify a resident's behavior. Any piece of equipment, furniture or medication which is used to control any aspect of the resident's behavior is considered to be a restraint and requires specific consent.

Before using restraints, the facility must show that reasonable attempts were made to determine the cause of the problem and that non-restraint interventions were exhausted. It must be determined if the resident's behavior is due to a lack of a meaningful activity program or the need to manipulate his/her environment. Is the resident's behavior is due to environmental factors — i.e., too hot, too cold, too noisy, too crowded — or if it may be related to a recent loss, such as the loss of a family member or a roommate? Perhaps individual needs are not met or customary routines are not being followed. The Activity Professional and Social Service Professional, because of their expertise in these areas, should participate in these assessments and interventions. See the section on restraints in this chapter for more information on when and how restraints can be used.

# Visitation Rights

The resident must be given immediate access to his/her immediate family or relative, his/her physician, the State Ombudsman or other individuals of his/her choosing. *Visiting hours are not legal!*

# Transfer and Right to Appeal

Each resident has the right to remain in the facility and not be transferred or discharged unless one of the following is true. Even if one of the following is true, the resident has the *Right to Appeal* the decision.
1.  The resident's needs cannot be adequately met with the current placement — this must be documented in the resident's clinical record and signed by the resident's physician.
2.  The resident's health has improved to the point that s/he no longer needs the services provided in a long term care facility — this must be documented in the resident's clinical record and signed by the resident's physician.
3.  The resident's presence significantly endangers the safety of other individuals in the facility — this must be documented in the resident's clinical record and signed by the resident's physician for those who are receiving Medicare; needs only to be documented in the resident's clinical record and does not require the signature of the physician for a resident receiving Medicaid.
4.  The resident's presence significantly endangers the health of other individuals in the facility — must be documented in the resident's clinical record and signed by the resident's physician.
5.  The resident has failed to pay (or to have Medicare or Medicaid Pay) for stay at the facility — this must be documented in the resident's clinical record.
6.  The facility is ceasing to operate.

**Prior to transferring and/or discharging any resident the facility must:**
1.  notify the resident (and family member or the resident's legal representative) of the intent to discharge/transfer and the reasons why,
2.  record the reasons for the discharge/transfer in the resident's clinical record, including a copy of the notice sent to the resident/family/legal representative,
3.  notify the resident of his/her *Right to Appeal Under Established Appeal Process*,
4.  provide the resident/family/legal representative with the name, mailing address and telephone number of the State's Long Term Care Ombudsman and
5.  provide the additional necessary notifications for those who are receiving Medicaid.

**When less then 30 days notice of discharge/transfer is given to the resident, the following must be done:**
1.  the notice must be given at least 30 days prior to discharge/transfer unless one of the following situations has occurred: a. the safety or health of others in the facility is endangered, b. the immediate transfer or discharge is due to the resident's significantly improved health or significantly deteriorated health (and the need for urgent care) or c. the resident has been in the facility for less then 30 days,
2.  the maximum available notice must be given to the resident as practicable,
3.  the facility has furnished sufficient preparation and orientation to the resident to ensure that s/he has a safe and orderly transfer/discharge and

4. additional notices and actions must be completed for the resident whose stay is being funded through Medicaid.

# Protection of Resident Funds

The long term care facility may not require that the resident deposit his/her personal funds with the facility.

If the resident does choose to deposit his/her funds with the facility, there are strict guidelines for the handling of the resident's funds. If the resident's funds are in excess of $50, they must be deposited in a separate account and the resident must receive all interest earned on the deposited money. If a resident's deposited funds stay under $50 at all times, they may be deposited in a non-interest bearing account or in a petty cash fund as long as full accounting is kept.

The facility has five legal responsibilities for the funds deposited:
1. to assure a full and complete separate accounting of each resident's personal funds,
2. to maintain a written record of all financial transactions involving each resident's personal funds deposited with the facility,
3. to provide the resident or his/her legal representative with reasonable access to the record of deposits, withdrawals and interest,
4. to convey promptly the resident's personal funds and final accounting record to the administrator of the resident's estate upon the resident's death or transfer and
5. to purchase a surety bond to provide assurance that the resident's funds are protected from staff theft.

# Theft/Loss: An Issue of Identity

Theft and loss occur in long term care facilities. The way to handle situations of theft and loss are part of both federal and state law. It serves a facility well to explain its philosophy about theft and loss very early in the admission process to prepare residents and families for the reality of the situation. It also behooves all of us in the facility to take very seriously any claims concerning missing items and to use the quality assurance process to reduce the number of incidents of theft and loss by eliminating situations that allow theft and loss to occur.

The prevailing philosophy is that everything, from a misplaced robe to a lost radio, is assumed stolen until it is found again. It is our experience, however, that episodes of theft are less frequent than episodes of loss. The number of items that are lost far outweigh the number that are stolen. Additionally, it is assumed that anything that is not found has been taken by a staff member when in fact residents are known to wander into rooms and "rearrange" other residents' radios, clocks, glasses, dentures, watches, etc. This is especially true in facilities that have residents who are able to walk freely but, due to dementia, lack judgment. In any case, before accusations of any kind are made, a thorough search of the facility is in order.

Another common occurrence is misplaced laundry. Our advice: In the short run, be patient. In the long run, fix the system. Laundry has a way of finding its way back to one's closet although the route can be circuitous, taking several days, even weeks. When that happens, the facility needs to put procedures in place to prevent it from happening again. It can be very difficult to keep track of laundry, but the facility is expected to do it, even the socks and underwear.

Never negate the impact on a family of seeing their mother's clothes on someone else — or vice versa. This is a terrible shock and a very emotional experience when this happens (and all too frequently, it does). Try to prepare both resident and family about this in advance; it may ease the trauma.

If everything fails after an item has been reported missing, time spent in room searches and laundry area forages, families and residents may be entitled to some compensation. The circumstances governing this must be very clearly defined in the facility theft and loss policy using federal and state mandates as guidelines.

Never forget that inherent in all of this is the fact that everything, including items of clothing, has an intrinsic value. We must treat all possessions as prized items because the fewer "treasures" left to us, the greater the trauma associated with any loss.

# Voting

Every individual has the right as both a citizen of the United States and (as a resident) within the Resident Bill of Rights to continue their responsibilities through voting in local and national elections. The information regarding whether a resident is interested and registered is gathered upon admission by either the admissions clerk or through the activity and social service assessment process.

The activity assessment form in the chapter on *Resident Care* has a space on the upper right side for this information.

The Activity Professional needs to know the following information regarding voting:
- Is the resident interested in being registered to vote?
- Is s/he currently registered to vote and if so at what address?
- Would s/he like to vote by absentee ballot?
- Is s/he capable of making this decision or does s/he have a power of attorney?
- Does s/he need any special devices or assistance in order to use voting equipment?
- How many residents in the facility are registered?
- Where do you keep this information and how do you update it?
- Do you know who to contact in the community to assist the residents with current issues and initiatives? (League of Women Voters, Registrar of Voters)
- Would you like the facility to be a Polling Place for the community? If so, contact the Registrar of Voters and request information on this and the guidelines necessary.

As you can see, there are many important issues to address regarding voting. The form on the next page will assist you in keeping this information up to date. Add every resident's name onto the form and identify his/her current voting status.

# VOTING STATUS FORM

Record each resident's name on form. Check off appropriate column and date the last column when completed. List also if they need assistance with voting forms.

| Resident Name | Interested | Registered | Absentee Form |
|---|---|---|---|
| | Yes/No | Yes/No | Yes/No |
| | | | |
| | | | |
| | | | |
| | | | |
| | | | |
| | | | |
| | | | |
| | | | |
| | | | |
| | | | |
| | | | |
| | | | |
| | | | |
| | | | |
| | | | |
| | | | |
| | | | |
| | | | |
| | | | |
| | | | |
| | | | |
| | | | |

# Restraints

Federal law requires that the least invasive approach be tried first before the more invasive approaches to modifying a resident's behavior are tried. This is especially true when one considers restraints. Restraints can be either physical (like geri-chairs or lap belts) or chemical (like Ativan or other psychoactive medications).

While it is usually the physician, in consultation with the nursing staff, who decides if a resident is to be restrained in any manner, *it is not the staff's right to make that decision independent of the resident and his/her guardians.* Any time a restraint is needed, there should be clear documentation as to the path taken to achieve consent from the resident or his/her legal guardian. This documentation should also show a progression of the least restrictive restraints being tried first, before more restrictive ones.

The physician and the nursing staff may be the primary individuals initiating the use of restraint, but all professional staff are expected to be advocates for the resident and notify the treatment care team that a violation of the residents' rights may have occurred. This violation is a very serious violation. Each department head is responsible to ensure that all of his/her staff are aware of the importance of residents' rights and to notify the administrator immediately if there is a potential violation. In some states this may be considered a case of resident abuse and, by law, needs to be called into the appropriate state agency within 24 hours.

# Restraint Reduction

The interdisciplinary team (IDT) needs to look for ways to reduce restraints and find alternatives to guarantee the highest possible quality of life for the residents. Modification of behavior works best when the entire team and environment are working together, in a unified and integrated approach. As a member if the interdisciplinary team, the Activity Professional plays an integral role in providing the best possible quality of life to residents. Because a resident will be in the activity program for some portion of the day, the IDT works together to determine the specific role that the Activity Professional will be playing as part of this program.

A facility should have a set of procedures in place to initiate a restraint program for residents and another set of procedures which allow the frequent review of possible reductions in the use of restraints for every resident who currently is involved in a restraint program. This may include having a specific group of staff (including the Activity Professional and the Social Service Professional) to help identify strategies for restraint reduction. This restraint reduction committee should be well versed in ways to reduce the use of restraints based on each residents abilities and strengths.

After the IDT or restraint reduction committee has tentatively identified a resident as needing a reduction of restraint, six steps are taken. The steps are
1. assessment to determine if the resident would benefit from a restraint reduction program,
2. approval from the resident's physician for a restraint reduction program,
3. identification of the possible levels of reduction,
4. identification of responsibilities,
5. approval from the resident (or surrogate) and
6. inservice for the staff on the specific aspects of the program.

The first step is to assess if the resident is a good candidate for a reduction in his/her restraint program or if the alternatives to the current program are indicated. "Good candidates" usually come from residents who are doing exceptionally well or exceptionally poorly on their current program. If a resident is doing exceptionally well on his/her restraint program, it may mean that s/he could tolerate and even thrive with a less restrictive program. If a resident is not doing well on his/her current program (e.g., the desired results are not being achieved), then a change in the restraint program is definitely called for. A checklist for resident behaviors which make a resident a "good candidate" can be used or other types of assessment forms can be created by staff. The "scoring" or data placed on the assessment tool should include input from all other disciplines.

The second step involves the resident's physician. The physician needs to give approval and orders for any reduction. The orders need to be signed and in the medical chart.

The third step is to identify possible levels of a physical restraint reduction or alternative strategies. There will be different levels of reduction within any restraint reduction program. These include the removal of the restraint (least restrictive), alternatives to provide maximum freedom within safety margins (moderately restrictive) or the identification that a restraint is required (most restrictive). If the team (and resident/surrogate) recognize that some kind of restraint is required, effort can be made to minimize the type and time when the restraint is being used.

The fourth step is to identify who is responsible for implementing the various parts of the resident's restraint/restraint reduction program. It should be clearly defined which staff member is responsible for each duty. Communication is crucial for the security of the resident and success of the program. When the resident participates in an activity, it is important to identify *who* is responsible to release the restraints and *who* will re-secure them at the end of the group.

Informed consent from the resident and/or his/her surrogate is step five. In the ideal situation, the resident and/or his/her surrogate will have helped define the restraint reduction process. Sometimes this is not possible, but at this point, once the restraint reduction program has been formally defined, they must give informed consent.

The sixth and last step of a restraint reduction program is to let all the staff know what they will be expected to do. Each restraint reduction or alternative program will likely follow similar guidelines but vary according to resident needs, team work and individual goals. All staff need to be educated about the goals of the program, the program structure and expectations of staff involved for the specific resident.

In addition to the specifics of each resident's restraint reduction program, the training of Activity and Social Service Professionals needs to include gait belt use, restraint options, use and techniques, positioning, transfer techniques (when included in the policy) during activity times.

The Activity Professional will need to determine which activities are appropriate for this reduction. S/he will supervise and observe responses while the resident is restraint-free in a structured activity. Small groups are better than large groups for evaluating the effect of any restraint reduction on resident performance and affect.

The names of each participant, information regarding his/her restraint reduction needs or goals and seating position should be available for any staff who are assisting in the room in which the activity is held. This could be a diagram posted behind the door or on a clip board for reference. As with the other professionals, the Activity Professional will want to be evaluating, assessing and documenting resident behavior, mood, safety issues and functional levels.

In terms of chemical restraint reduction or alternatives, a Behavior Management Program is often the most successful approach.

# Behavior Management[46]

With the implementation of OBRA and MDS version 2.0, staff are called upon to deal with unwanted behaviors through behavioral interventions first, before using any psychoactive medications. If behavioral interventions fail, then the use of medication to modify behavior may be tried. Gone are the days when we saw an unwanted behavior and called the attending physician for a psychoactive medication to control the behavior. This change is a good thing. It asks us to pay attention to the specific behavior and to be creative and professional in dealing with it. On the MDS we are asked if a behavioral plan has been implemented. This section will provide some ways to deal with managing behavior instead of using psychoactive medications, prior to using psychoactive medications or in conjunction with them.

A behavior is an observable action. Many behaviors are a result of experience, values or beliefs. Others are caused by organic changes within the resident's own body (e.g., psychosis). There are three primary ways we can effect behavioral change: help the resident change his/her own behavior, change the environment that the resident is in or use psychoactive medications (medications that change a person's behavior by changing his/her body chemistry).

Often when we look at behaviors, it is the environment that has created the behavior. For example, a resident who has moved into a facility learns that s/he gets his/her needs met quicker when s/he yells out. After a time s/he begins to yell out just to get attention. By modifying the environment (having staff respond quicker to his/her call bell) and by re-training the resident, we can decrease the yelling.

The first place to begin modifying unwanted resident behaviors is to make sure that the environment within the facility promotes positive, cooperative behaviors. It is also important to train all staff in appropriate behavioral interventions. These interventions are not necessarily part of a formal behavioral management program, but are consistent behaviors used by all staff to encourage appropriate resident behaviors. When the facility is able to offer a positive environment with appropriate staff behaviors, the need for formal behavioral modification programs will drop significantly. This is a win-win situation. The residents have a better, more social place to live and the staff spend less time with the paperwork required of a formal behavioral management plan.

## Environmental Management

Environmental management means changing the environment to affect the behavior. This may be as small a change as playing classical music versus rock and roll in the activity room to painting the double door which leads off the unit to look like a bookshelf. (Painting a mural of a bookshelf across the door which leads off the unit confuses residents with dementia who wander, making it less likely that they will leave the unit.) By using environmental management we may be able to deal with unwanted behaviors without using psychoactive medications. It could mean changing rooms, roommates, the showering schedule, meal times. Be creative and listen to what the resident is telling us through his/her words and actions.

This is an example that happened during one of my consultations. A long time resident of a nursing home became a little more agitated than normal. She had a long history of psychiatric problems. The behaviors associated with her psychiatric diagnosis were generally not disruptive but included episodes of hallucinations. While I was there, the nurse received a phone call from the resident's physician with an order for Haldol 1 mg BID for three days for agitation with delusions. This order was unexpected, as the resident's behavior did not seem significantly different then her normal baseline — a baseline that seemed well within the facility's ability to accommodate without the use of psychoactive medications. As the nurse did some detective work, she found that the resident had called her daughter and told her the nursing home was making her stay in a room with a dead person. Because of the resident's psychiatric history, the

---

[46] This section is by Kay Garrick, LCSW. Used with permission.

daughter assumed the resident was becoming psychotic and called the physician. The nurse came to me with the dilemma of whether to implement the physician's orders or to call the physician back to discuss the situation. The nurse was concerned because she felt the resident was not hallucinating as the resident's roommate was in the process of dying. I suggested we check with the resident to see if she wanted to move to another room. The resident gladly accepted the move. We called the daughter, explained the situation and then called the physician who canceled the medication order. The resident was moved to another room. By being sensitive to the resident's concerns and what was happening in her environment, we were able to solve the problem without using medications.

# Behavioral Intervention

Behavioral intervention is just another term for providing the resident with gentle, normal consequences for inappropriate behavior. Staff frequently create unrealistic "community" standards for social skills within the facility. Instead of ignoring grabbing behavior from a resident, the staff should be taught how to respectfully ask the resident not to grab them and, just as important, figure out why the resident felt the need to grab. Behavioral interventions can be used when the behavior is seen in limited situations — when the behavior is not pervasive. An example would be a resident who yells when s/he is in an activity and not at other times. Talk to the resident about the behavior when the behavior is not happening. If a resident calls out in group, talk to him/her before the group. Tell him/her what behavior you have noticed and then ask what s/he thinks is causing the behavior. (This is for residents who have the mental ability to understand.) Let him/her know that it is affecting other people and how it is affecting others. Ask the resident if s/he has any suggestions to solve the problem. Perhaps his/her hearing is bad and if s/he sits in the front of the group, s/he would not yell out. If s/he has no suitable ways to solve the problem, let the resident know what you will do. If s/he disrupts the group again, you will need to remove him/her from the group.

Remember to maintain the resident's dignity as much as possible. If the situation arises where you must remove a resident from an activity, do not discipline him/her in front of the group. Simply go to the resident and take him/her out of the activity. Outside of the group remind him/her that his/her behavior was disruptive to others. Use a consistent simple phrase that describes the behavior and use it every time the behavior happens. Do not touch, smile sweetly at the resident or show anger. In our guilt at taking this kind of action, our behaviors can reinforce the wrong behavior. Keep your facial expression blank. Later, visit privately with the resident to see how s/he responded to the intervention.

Make a plan to meet the needs of the resident. If you have a resident who consistently yells out in group and not when s/he is in his/her room, why do you continue to bring him/her to group? Perhaps one-on-one visits would be more effective. Often residents with dementia get over-stimulated in large groups. Try smaller, quieter activities for this type of resident. Physical activities may be successful also.

In one facility a newly admitted resident with a diagnosis of dementia called out constantly, "Nurse, nurse, nurse." It was her first admission to a nursing facility and the Director of Nurses was ready to discharge her on her date of admission because of her calling out. The resident loved to receive hugs. I pulled the clock at the nurses station off the wall and went to the resident and put the clock in her lap. I used simple phrases but told her she needed to be quiet for five minutes and that if she is quiet she would get a big hug. I showed her the clock and where the hands of the clock would be when she would get a hug. Her face lit up. I left her in her wheelchair across from the nursing station and sat nearby but out of her range of vision. When she called out, I got her attention and made a quiet signal and verbally cued her to three more minutes until her hug. I kept my face blank and did not touch her. At the end of five minutes she had called out three times and I went to hug her and praised her for the good job she did being quiet. Then I increased the time to ten minutes with the "hug" reward at the end and continued increasing the time in increments of five minutes up to an hour. When the resident was up to an hour, she only called out once.

The Director of Nurses was sold on behavior management along with the rest of the staff. The Maintenance Director found a large kitchen timer that rang at the appropriate amount of time. The certified nurses' aides took the resident to her room, set the timer and when the bell rang they would go to her and give her a big hug and reward her behavior. Initially it took me all morning to work this through with the resident and staff. We were able to eliminate the yelling out behavior so that the resident felt safe and her quality of life was improved. The staff bonded with the resident and gave her attention and praise for appropriate behavior. She was able to be maintained at the facility instead of being placed elsewhere.

# Behavior Management Programs

When a negative behavior is serious and frequent enough to require a systematic change, the team will need to develop a behavior management plan. Behavior management plans should be implemented when the behavior is affecting most aspects of care and the quality of life for other residents is impacted. It is a more complex system that involves all disciplines and the resident and/or family in an organized, planned approach to eliminate the behavior.

The reason that this situation is complex is that it has reached the point where the unwanted behavior is ingrained. Instead of having just isolated occurrences, this behavior has been established as a coping pattern for the resident. To break this pattern, all staff have to work together in a systematic way. Each staff needs to know how to discourage the behavior as well as promote healthy ways of coping.

We can change a behavior *if* there is something a resident *likes*. I prefer to use positive reinforcers rather than negative. Positive reinforcers are more successful with residents. It is often easier for staff to use positive rewards.

Many folks believe that if a resident has a diagnosis of dementia that behavioral management is not effective. That is not my experience. Residents with dementia *can* benefit from behavioral plans. Does the resident really like hugs, candy, to sit outside, time with family/staff? We then use what the resident likes as a reward for the appropriate behavior and behavior can be changed.

Behavioral programs take time initially but, when they are effective, they take less time than responding to the inappropriate behavior. This may be difficult for staff to understand. Just have the staff add up the amount of time they spend answering a person who uses the call light frequently. Changing the behavior will eventually save time. To change a behavior, we must act like a detective and find out the reason for the behavior. The best way to find out the causes is usually at a special care planning conference where all disciplines are represented and can give input related to the behavior. It is very helpful to have the certified nurses' aides who work with the resident present at this meeting. Has something changed in the resident's life that triggered the behavior — a new room, a new roommate, a new nurses' aide, family out of town? What is the resident's diagnosis'? What are the medications the resident is taking? What happens before the behavior occurs? These are called the "antecedents." Is it change of shift? Does the nurses' aide try to provide care? Does the family leave the resident? What exactly is the behavior? We need to be very specific. Is the resident verbally abusive or did they raise their voice and yell at the staff? We cannot change the behavior if we do not know exactly what it is.

What does the resident get by behaving this way — space, distance, control, power, maintaining dignity? This is often called the "consequence." Has anyone told the resident that the behavior is causing a problem for others? Who on the interdisciplinary team has the best relationship with the resident? Would it be better to have a male staff talk to the resident? This often works best with male residents who are physically, verbally or sexually acting out. Could the family help us deal with the behavior? Do they have information about the behavior prior the resident's admission? Can they come in and help at difficult times? Is there anything we can change in the environment to help change the behavior?

Consistency is crucial for a behavioral plan to work. That means all staff must behave the same way — all shifts need to be told of the plan and follow through with it. If we use a verbal phrase, all staff should repeat the same phrase to the resident. Keep your behavioral plan as simple as possible. Only work on one behavior at a time and choose the behavior that causes the most problems for the residents and staff.

Behavioral plans are more difficult for residents with a diagnosis of "borderline personality disorder." These are often the residents who like to stir up tension among staff or family members. They usually do not have anything that is as rewarding to them as the tension they cause, so finding something else they like that will cause them to change can be very difficult.

When behavioral management plans are started, the resident's behavior will often get worse for approximately two weeks. The resident is trying to hold on to what s/he knows, even old coping mechanisms and behaviors which are causing problems. Expect the first two weeks to be difficult, encourage staff to remain consistent, and only change the program during the first two weeks if it is completely clear that the program is going to fail or make matters worse.

# Difficult Behavior

Every facility tends to have at least one resident who exhibits difficult behavior. This part talks about three difficult behaviors that I am often asked to work with: inappropriate sexual behavior, suicidal thoughts and violent behaviors. These behaviors are not often discussed in behavior guides. Use a team approach, define the problem and decide your approach using some of the ideas discussed above.

## Sexual Behavior

One of the most difficult behaviors to deal with is sexually inappropriate behavior. With younger residents being admitted more frequently to facilities, sexually inappropriate behavior is becoming more of an issue for staff to deal with. Remember that this behavior can be exhibited by young and old, as well as male and female.

Sexual behavior is NORMAL. Often what comes up around the behavior is our own judgments, values and religious beliefs. We all have sexual needs and expressing them is part of life for both old and young. It is important for us to define what is "inappropriate" sexual behavior. Staff walking into a resident's room where the curtain is closed to find the resident masturbating is not considered inappropriate behavior on the resident's part. It could be viewed as inappropriate on behalf of the staff. Did you allow the residents the privacy they want it? Did you knock? Did the resident give the staff person permission to enter the room? Married couples have the right to share a room and are entitled to privacy.

It is crucial to know the diagnosis as the approaches will vary depending on whether the resident has mental capacity. Whether the resident has capacity to make health care decisions is determined by the attending physician and can be found in the Advance Directives or in the Physicians Orders.

If a resident becomes sexually aggressive or active with another resident, determine if both residents have capacity. If they do, they can make their own choices and consent as long as privacy is maintained. If the residents have capacity, we are not allowed to discuss this with the residents' families unless the residents gives us permission. To discuss this with the family without the resident's permission is a violation of resident rights. If the resident does not have capacity, the responsible party or agent must be informed and decide if the behavior is acceptable. Cases of sexually aggressive behavior must be reported to the appropriate reporting agency (Ombudsman, Adult Protective Services, Police). Report all episodes of sexually inappropriate behavior to your supervisor.

When a resident without capacity is demonstrating sexually inappropriate behavior you can use the following guidelines. Remember to maintain the resident's dignity. If s/he is exposed, make sure s/he is covered or dressed appropriately. If the resident is in a public place and cannot be distracted, take them to their room and pull the curtain. Make the nursing staff aware so that they respect the resident's privacy. For a resident who exposes himself or urinates in public places, consider ordering the resident a back closure jumpsuit. They are difficult for the residents to remove. A back closure jumpsuit is considered to be a restraint. Before dressing the resident in one, the facility would have to follow the standard procedure for placing a resident in a restraint, including informed consent.

Do not talk down to the resident by saying anything that makes you want to shake your finger at the resident. The resident may not understand what you are saying but they may understand that you are trying to make them feel ashamed of their behavior. You need to look at your values about sexual behavior. Remember that you are the professional and do not personalize the behavior.

Are you doing anything to contribute to the behavior? Watch the "sweetie, honey, baby" phrases. Are you touching the resident or kissing him/her? If a resident displays inappropriate sexual behavior, do not call him/her "sweetie," or kiss him/her. Sometimes residents with this behavior ask for kisses. State professionally, "Mr. Smith I'm the Social Service Director and I will not kiss you but I will shake you hand." Remind the resident of your professional role. "Mr. Jones you must have confused me with someone else. I am the Activity Coordinator and I want to invite you to the piano recital today." Keep your face blank. Do not show shock, displeasure, laughter, smiles, anger. Remember any facial expression could encourage the behavior. If you cannot control your facial expression, turn your face away from the resident.

Do not run to you peers and giggle about the behavior. Someone will always overhear conversations. Again, this means you need to look at your own values around sexuality. Do report the behavior to the charge nurse. Is this new behavior? Is it covered in the care plan? If so, what are our interventions to deal with the behavior?

When a resident with capacity is demonstrating sexually inappropriate behavior, you can use the following guidelines. Refer the resident to the Social Service Director who will talk to the resident about the behavior. Why is it being displayed? Does the resident need more control, power, privacy? What is the resident's solution to the problem? One younger resident consistently exposed himself to older female visitors. When asked why he did this, he said that he had been in prison and that he had more freedom there than in the nursing home. He did this in hopes of being arrested and put back in prison. We were able to give the resident more control over his life and he stopped the behavior. Referral to a therapist, psychologist, social worker or psychiatrist for counseling related to the problem may be helpful. Involve the Ombudsman. Sometimes someone from outside the facility can have more impact on the resident's behavior. And remember, when the resident has been determined to be capable, s/he will need to be involved in the decision-making process.

## Suicidal Behavior

Suicidal behavior is another difficult behavior to deal with. If a resident is displaying suicidal behavior, it must be determined if the facility can provide for the resident's safety. If not, the resident may need to be transferred to an acute psychiatric hospital for appropriate treatment. Suicidal statements are often a cry for help and *must* be taken seriously. Report any suicidal comments to the charge nurse *and* the Social Service Director.

If a resident threatens suicide, states a desire to commit suicide or is known to have been suicidal in the recent past, an assessment to determine whether the resident is currently suicidal will be made by the Social Service Department, possibly in conjunction with any of the following: the Nursing Department, the attending physician, a consulting psychiatrist, consulting psychologist, the Social Work Consultant, the county's mental health specialist or the family. Observe the resident for warning signs of suicide: prolonged depression, marked changes of behavior or personality, a sudden lifting of the mood (e.g., the resident who is depressed suddenly seems happy), making final arrangements as though for a final departure and/or suicide threats or similar statements.

Question resident as to motivation, method and means. If there exists a desire to commit suicide, a plan devised and a viable way to kill oneself, the risk is greater. If a risk exists, the facility interdisciplinary team will formulate an intervention to ensure the safety of the resident. However, if the resident seems to have a clear plan as to how s/he will end her/his life, the staff should questions whether they can keep the resident in the facility. Determine whether there is a need for a temporary transfer. A transfer to a psychiatric unit used to handling this crisis situation is usually a reasonable choice. Check with your county's mental health specialist.

If you decide that the resident can stay in the facility, enlist all staff in monitoring actions of resident, but have one specific staff per shift who is responsible for checking the resident on a regular basis. Institute regular check-ins, usually every 15 minutes. This may require moving the resident closer to the nursing station for observation. To ensure that the frequent checks are done, a sign-off sheet should be available at the nursing station for the staff to document the resident's activity and affect every 15 minutes and then to sign-off, indicating who observed the resident during those last 15 minutes and what the resident was doing.

As much as possible, reduce environmental hazards. Remove sharp objects from resident's room and reach (e.g., matches, razors, scissors). Remove the call light cord and replace it with a tap bell. Remove any belts, cords, etc. from resident's access. Replace silverware with plastic. The nursing staff should be sure that the resident swallows his/her pills and does not hoard or cheek them.

Most residents who feel like taking their own life have mixed feelings about taking action. They frequently feel like life is out of control and want to be able to "grab" onto some strength and stability provided by someone else. Knowing that someone will be there to help gives them a sense of security. Consider using a written contract with the resident (verbal would be fine but written is more powerful). This way the resident knows that someone will be there if s/he feels the need for support. Write a contract that states "I, _____ (resident's name), agree that if I feel like harming myself in any way, I will not take any action to do myself harm. I agree to contact the social service director _____ (name) or the charge nurse _____ (name)." Have a place for the resident to sign and for a staff signature. Give a copy to the resident and put a copy in the chart. Be sure to include this service/intervention in the care plan. Remember to designate staff to cover on the weekends, holidays and during staff illness and be sure the resident knows who the staff are.

Encourage the resident to talk about feelings. Often staff avoid stating the obvious, "Do you feel like killing yourself?" It will not encourage the resident to take this action but may be seen as a relief by the resident that someone will talk about it — that someone understands. Make sure you visit the resident regularly. Often staff avoid seeing the resident because they do not know what to do. All you need to do is let the resident know that you care about them and sit with them for a few minutes. Offer touch when appropriate.

## Violent Behavior

Violent behavior exhibited by one or more residents can be difficult to deal with, can endanger the other residents and staff and can cause a facility to lose its license. Violent behaviors cannot be tolerated and need to be addressed immediately.

This behavior can be a result of inability to control one's impulses or feeling powerless over one's environment. Anger can be directed at others or the environment. The resident may be combative with staff, peers, family or throw things such as food or furniture. This anger can be a result of a feeling of a lack of control or inadequate coping skills. It may also be as a result of impulse control problems which arise after a head injury or stroke. Staff's first responsibility is to assure that residents involved in a violent situation are safe. Do others need to be protected, moved or other staff called to assist?

Staff need to be safe, and you need to insure the safety of other residents. If someone is being violent, stay an arms length away from them. Give the person space to calm down. Take them to a quiet place. If there is no mental decline, let the resident know that the violent behavior will not be tolerated and that staff need to keep others safe. The resident needs to know that staff will protect and set boundaries since they feel out of control. The behavior could lead to eviction if the resident cannot control the violent outbursts. (Although, this may not be the most prudent thing to say during the middle of a resident's violent outburst.)

Staff should avoid areas or topics that cause conflict. Avoid power struggles. Instead of "It's time for your shower." try asking, "When would you like to shower?" This gives the person more control over his/her life.

When interacting with a resident who seems on the edge of losing control, keep a neutral manner. Do not show fear, anger, laughter. Keep your face blank and present a calm professional demeanor. Do not try to shame the resident.

Controlling one's anger requires good coping skills and socially appropriate ways to express one's feelings. The resident may be justified in his/her feeling of anger although his/her way to express it is not appropriate. How would you feel if the same thing happened to you? It is good to identify the feeling and offer acceptance. "I can understand why you felt angry after what happened." Referral to a counselor, psychologist, therapist, psychiatrist or social worker may help the resident explore his/her anger and ways to express it appropriately.

Violence may be a way for the resident to release energy. Offer the resident alternatives and appropriate ways to release his/her anger thereby increasing his/her coping skills. Consider trying workouts with weights, give the resident a pillow to pound on or regular exercise such as walks around the facility.

When the violence is severe and cannot be stopped, staff may have to call 911 to have the police assist the resident. Remember, assault, no matter where it happens, is against the law. If the law is being broken, the facility may need to have professionals who are used to dealing with violent behavior take over the situation.

# Time Management

Time management is the process by which we manage our time to the extent that we feel accomplishment, completion and a personal sense of well-being. Managing our lives — being on time — is something we're always going to do ... tomorrow. As a result, we tend to engage in a lot of "knee-jerk" activity; we react instead of act.

Staying on a schedule seems an especially daunting objective in a profession that deals with people and their problems. In effect, a day is never linear as we are continuously diverted to mend and fix. At the end of the day, even though we have been busy, sometimes it seems that we haven't really done any work! It is only an illusion that we can never really get it all done. In fact, we have a responsibility, an obligation to do just that: to address everything our job description says we must do.

Time management is not a skill that most people are born with, it is an acquired skill that needs attention and practice. Managing time also means that the manager needs systems designed which work for him/her. All people organize their thoughts and schedules in a unique style. For this reason, each person needs to organize in the way that best suits his/her style, type of work and personality.

## Have a Schedule

We have attempted to give you a bird's eye view of the work in the sections entitled "Life of A..." For an Activity Professional, the schedule has some clear responsibilities at set times so this discussion will help you with the less structured times. The Social Service Professional has more schedule freedom so what we say here applies to most of your schedule.

What you need to do is derived directly from your job description. Within those obligations, you need to develop a plan for when you work and decide on your own cues for completion. For example, you might try to do your computer work each morning before 9 am; or do your quarterly notes between 4–5 pm after you have had time in the day to see each of the residents you need to report on, jotting notes as you proceed throughout the day.

Set goals for the week. You can do this on Monday morning for the ensuing week or Friday afternoon in anticipation of the week ahead. Revise these goals each morning before you begin. Of course, no one working with people will ever get from A to B every time but with an idea of your task load, you can do it much of the time.

## Keys to success:

- Prioritize each day's responsibilities.
- Complete the least appealing work first.
- Complete one task at a time. Too much time and energy are spent trying to complete two to three things within the same amount of time. Some people are able to do this but most find that it does not work for them.
- Discourage interruptions by scheduling calls and appointments at a good time for you. Advise staff of this schedule also. When you are leading a group, you should not be answering calls. This leaves the unspoken message to the group participants that your calls are more important than they are.
- Schedule enough time each day to complete all required documentation.
- Schedule enough time each day to visit on a one-on-one basis and record this in the bedside log.
- Keep your desk organized so that you can sort through stacks of papers according to priorities.
- Write a list of all the work responsibilities that you have. By referring to this list, you can better identify a plan and way of organizing all of the different types of duties.

### Make Choices

There will always be more demands than you can possibly respond to. Be realistic as to personal goals and abilities. If the frustration becomes too great because of lack of organization, stress mounts, anxiety occurs and there is a general feeling of loss of control. Break the cycle before this happens. There are four D's in time management: *Drop it, Delay, Delegate, Do it.*

If you are a department head, you will have greater demands and expectations. Not only are you required to provide the services expected of *you,* but you are also responsible for all the other mandated responsibilities of the department, other staff members and volunteers.

When you go about trying to meet all of these demands, the most important thing you can do is to set priorities (act — don't react). Decide what needs to be done first, second and so on. Then write down your decisions so you will remember what you have to do and how soon you plan to do it.

Try to find a balance between never varying your plan and having the plan disrupted by everyone who asks you to do something. A good rule of thumb is if you already have something on your list of things to do, you should do it when you planned to even if someone just asked you how soon it would be done. The only time to change your priorities is when something new comes up. Then you need to decide where it goes in your list of priorities.

When human need arises (and that's why we do what we do), get involved up to your elbows. If you have to decide between addressing a need or writing a quarterly report, the choice is obviously to attend to the need. In fact, addressing a need as it arises is really the action position; ignoring/avoiding creates the need for reaction. However, do not allow diversion to derail you. Act, but return to your schedule of work as soon as possible. Work on your documentation skills so that you say what you need to say in a clear concise manner. Don't waste time writing too much.[47]

Chip away at your schedule and list of goals in order to keep going forward. As you finish one project for the day/week, immediately focus on your next task. There will always be something waiting for your attention; it's the nature of work like ours where we are not only dealing with people but also with paper — lots of it.

### TGIF

Before you leave work for your well-deserved weekend, check the list of goals you started with on Monday (this includes the must do's from your job description, e.g. assessments and quarterlies). Is everything complete? If not, why not? Can it wait until Monday? What will be the consequence if a task remains incomplete?

If you can safely answer that everything is done that needs doing with no ill effect from a job that might be left, then you can leave!! However, you might feel better prepared to face Monday morning if you write a sketch for the coming week; that way, you will not have to dread that day or face decisions first thing in the morning after a relaxing weekend.

# Time Management Calendar

One way to determine how well you are managing your time is to complete a Time Management Calendar for one month and then analyze the results. This has been a helpful tool for many Activity and Social

---

[47] For more information on documentation see Ann Uniak, **Documentation in a Snap for Activity Programs (with MDS Version 2.0)**, 1996, available from Idyll Arbor, Inc.

Service Professionals. Read the codes below. These represent your responsibilities. Be sure to add duties specific to your facility.

**FM** (Facility Management) Any responsibility directly associated with office and departmental functions. In other words, everything related to keeping the department in order. This may also include resident shopping.

**DRC** (Direct Resident Care) Direct leadership and time spent with residents. This would be either in a group setting or on a one-on-one basis. If you are arranging an activity for adult education teachers or a volunteer, this would be listed under coordination and not direct resident care.

**D** (Documentation)

**T** (Transportation) Time bringing residents to and from groups.

**PR** (Public Relations) Time spent explaining your work to the public, press or other agencies.

**TMC** (Time Management Calendar) The time spent in completing this form each day for a month needs to be added on. It will be approximately 15 minutes daily.

**RCC** (Resident Care Conferences) The time spent preparing for and attending care conferences.

**C** (Coordination) This includes calendars, newsletters, interdepartmental functions, fundraising, etc.

**PD** (Personal Development) This is the time spent reviewing program ideas, going to workshops, reading and reviewing guidelines. You should have some of this each week.

**M** (Meetings) These could be staff meetings, MDS meetings, QA meetings. You should note what kind of meeting it was.

**S** (Supervision) Time when you are supervising volunteers and staff in the department.

**CV** (Consultant Visits) Add the time spent with the consultant for the department.

**FC** (Family Concerns) The time spent working with the family and friends of the residents.

**G** (Grievances) The time spent learning about and resolving grievances.

**CL** (Clothing) Making sure residents have appropriate clothing.

**LA** (Lost Articles) Check on lost clothing and other articles.

**DC** (Discharge Planning)

**L** (Lunch)

**O** (Other) Explain how the time was spent.

# How to Complete the Calendar

At the end of each day for one month, record where your time went on any standard wall or notebook calendar. Each category must be in an increment of no less that 15 minutes. If you find that you are doing two things at one time, you must divide the time and show each one separately. Use the codes shown above. These represent the various functions of the work. If you work more than eight hours, this must be reflected on the calendar also. In order for this to be accurate, the calendar needs to be completed each day at the end of the day.

*Example of how an average day will appear on the calendar when completed:*

| | | | | | |
|-----|------------|---|--------|-----|------------|
| DRC | 2 hours    | S | 1 hour | RCC | 1 hour     |
| D   | 1 1/2 hours | L | 1 hour | PD  | 15 minutes |
| T   | 45 minutes | C | 1 hour |     |            |

Total time: 8 1/2 hours.

By reviewing an average day over a period of one month, you will be able to see what takes the longest amount of time to complete, how much direct time is spent with residents in programming, what needs more time and what may be an area of weakness.

# Budgets

Every department has a budget that must be adhered to. This budget is created by the Administrator and/or corporate office and is an integral part of the total facility budget. If you do not have previous experience with budgets and accounting, ask for some advice or reading materials to better educate yourself about protocols and requirements.

When you are looking at budgets, it is important to understand the difference between a supply item and a capital item. The capital items are large items which the department needs to provide a basic service. (In accounting terms, these items are depreciated rather than expensed.) Some of these items may include slide projectors, VCR and monitors, head sets with tape decks and/or radios, large bingo games, reality orientation boards, eraser boards, monthly calendars, typewriters and computers. The money for capital items may not come from the budget you use to get supplies, but you need to check this out with you administrator to be sure how your facility budgets its capital funds.

In some facilities, the activity or social service budget contains *all* costs which are incurred through this department. Some examples could be coffee supplies, paper supplies, consultant costs, entertainment and many more. Other facilities budget some of these things separately. It is important to understand how your individual facility budget works so that you can not only plan ahead but also negotiate when you know the budget will not meet the current resident needs.

As with any business, accountability is extremely important. Accountability in this instance refers to the ability of the department head to identify where every penny has gone, with receipts to back up the expenses. Without the paper backup, there is no record to substantiate purchases and payments.

At least once a year, your facility will plan the budget for the next year. You need to be part of this process. The best way to figure out what you need is to go through your records for the last year (another reason to keep these records) and add up your expenses for each category of expenditure. Make rough schedules for the next year, noting especially differences between the past year and the coming year. (Some important differences are changes in the number of residents, changes in the diagnoses, changes in requirements for consulting or needs for capital items.) Be prepared to defend your proposed budget by showing exactly where the money will go and exactly what kind of programs you will be running. Tie the programs to resident assessments and to OBRA regulations to demonstrate that they need to be run.

Each state varies in their rules about budgets. Some may make no reference to the activity budget. You need to understand facility and state regulations about activity budgets.

Many of the items and supplies you buy should be ordered with a purchase order. Get in the habit of using purchase orders when sending in orders and requesting supplies. If your facility does not already have a purchasing system, you can purchase your own at any office supply store. If there is a delay or question in regards to this order, you can refer back to this transaction by the purchase order number, the date and the items listed.

Each department needs to keep an inventory of all supplies and equipment. The activity department should have an up-to-date inventory identifying all current supply items in the facility. For any of you who have taken a position in an unorganized facility, you know what it is like to try to figure out what you have, where it is, what you need to order and whether you will have enough money to last the year.

Being organized in this way is like leaving a legacy in the facility for those department heads to come. Always keep things in the manner that you would like to find them.

# Policies and Procedures

Policies and procedures are the framework of any organization and any department. Each department head needs to review the current policy and procedure manual in use for the facility and specific departments. Review the policies specific to your department and determine if they are up to date with federal and state, corporate and facility requirements. If not, the department head is responsible for making sure that these policies are written. After policies and procedures are written, they need to be reviewed and approved by the policy review committee in the facility. After approval, committee members sign and date the front page of the manual.

There should be a policy for each aspect of the service provided through the department. When you write policies and procedures, keep in mind the following definitions:

**POLICY:** A policy identifies and defines an administrative decision about *what* needs to be done.

**PROCEDURE:** A procedure describes *how* the policy will be implemented.

Both the policy and procedure need to be written *clearly* enough to define the need while at the same time they need to be *general* enough to encompass a variety of situations. Be sure that the descriptions are realistic as the facility can be cited for not following through with their own policies during a federal or state survey.

Many policies are designed from federal and state regulations. An example would be a residents' right to vote in elections. This is a federal law protecting the rights of the resident as a citizen and as a resident. By writing a policy and procedure, the facility not only is complying with the law, but clearly defining how this regulation will be adhered to and implemented in the facility. An example policy and procedure statement for outings is shown below.

## Outings

**Policy:**
It is the policy of this facility to plan and offer resident outings away from the facility. This meets OBRA Regulations.

**Procedures:**
- Each resident participating in *any* outing needs a doctor's order to leave the facility. This outing order should include both approval for a responsible party and/or activity staff.
- A list of participants needs to be reviewed and approved by the Director of Nursing or Charge Nurse to determine if they are physically, cognitively and emotionally able to leave the facility.
- The Activity Professional will contact the families to update them as to the date and time that their family member will be away from the facility.
- The Activity Professional will arrange for appropriate numbers of staff and volunteers, not to exceed eight residents for each staff.
- All medications will be administered before the departure or after the resident returns. *No medications will be transported unless an RN or LPN goes on the outing to administer them to the residents.*
- Resident who have approval for self-administration will be addressed on a case-by-case basis.
- All residents need to be signed back into the nursing station upon return to the facility. The Activity Professional will also share any information felt to be pertinent in regards to behavior, interaction and/or condition changes which may have occurred during the outing.

There are other special policies that will need attention. An example would be a policy and procedure for a facility pet. Although this is not a required area, the philosophy of many facilities is to encourage homelike environments that includes a facility pet. A sample policy and procedure might look like this:

---

## Facility Pets

**Policy:**
It is the policy of this facility to provide and care for a facility pet.

**Procedures:**
- All veterinary records and vaccination records will be kept on file in the facility.
- A designated staff member will be responsible for the feeding, grooming and general care of the pet.
- The pet will not be in the halls, resident rooms or dining areas during meal times for infection control purposes.
- A schedule will be arranged by the Activity and Social Service departments for in-room pet visits.

---

Notice how the procedures are broadly written. For instance the designated staff member who will be responsible for the grooming and care of the pet. Obviously this individual will have a schedule designed for when and where and how often this will occur. This may be a page attached to the original policy and procedure as additional information.

There is no mystery to writing policies and procedures. Look at your department and see if there is an area that needs a policy. Write the policy to meet either the regulations or current need. Writes the procedures to describe how the policy will be implemented. After completion, have the policy and procedure reviewed and approved by the administrator and committee. **The Professional Activity Manager and Consultant**[48] has a full chapter on how to write policies and procedures. It describes each step in the process in an easy-to-follow way.

---

[48] D'Antonio-Nocera, A., N. DeBolt, and N. Touhey, Eds., 1996, **The Professional Activity Manager and Consultant**, Idyll Arbor, Inc., Ravensdale, WA.

# OBRA Regulations

The OBRA law contains over 180 sections. These sections are called "Tags" and each tag has a number. While there are only two tags dealing directly with activities (Tags F248 and F249) and another two tags dealing directly with Social Services (Tags F250 and F251), there are over 80 other tags which deal indirectly with activities and social services. These other tags cover the general environment and livability of the nursing home and apply to all professionals. The Activity and Social Service Professionals are two of these professionals.

Because the survey process depends largely on the Federal regulations, it is important that the Activity or Social Service Professional understands how to use and interpret the regulations. The regulations are divided into 15 requirements. They are

1.    Resident's Rights
2.    Admission, Transfer and Discharge Rights
3.    Resident Behavior and Facility Practices
4.    Quality of Life
5.    Resident Assessment
6.    Quality of Care
7.    Nursing Services
8.    Dietary Services
9.    Physician Services
10.   Specialized Rehabilitative Services
11.   Dental Services
12.   Pharmacy Services
13.   Infection Control
14.   Physical Environment
15.   Administration

As shown in the boxes under Tags F248 and F250, each section describes the regulation and also contains a set of interpretive guidelines. The guidelines give the surveyor additional information about the meaning of the regulation and provide accepted survey procedures and probes. If you read the regulations, you will have a good idea of how the surveyor will look at this section of the regulations. It will help you prepare for a survey.

It is important to note that the interpretive guidelines are guides only and not requirements. The regulations themselves are used as the basis for survey activities.

When a problem is found during a survey, the problem is written up under the tag number which corresponds to problem. The primary tag numbers that could be used to measure how well the activity and social service staff were meeting the needs of residents are listed below along with a summary of the regulations and surveyor guidelines.

Each resident has the absolute right to be treated with dignity and to exercise his/her rights of citizenship. Just because the resident is no longer in "his/her own home" does not mean that s/he looses the rights associated with being an adult citizen. The resident is guaranteed 10 basic rights: 1. privacy and respect, 2. medical care and treatment, 3. freedom from abuse and restraint, 4. freedom of association and communication in privacy, 5. activities, 6. work, 7. personal possessions, 8. grievances and complaints, 9. financial affairs and 10. transfer and discharge. These rights include services (and recreation programs of their choice) both inside and outside of the facility.

**Tag F151** The resident has the right to exercise his/her rights to make choices concerning the manner and way s/he lives subject to reasonable rules outlined by the facility and by local, state and federal law. The resident also has the right to be free from negative actions or undue pressure from the facility and facility staff when exercising his/her rights in a reasonable manner. This right includes freedom from the reduction of the group activity time of a resident trying to organize a resident group or singling out residents for prejudicial treatment such as isolating residents in activities.

**Tag F152** The federal and state government has set up specific guidelines to follow if the treatment team feel that a resident is no longer cognitively able to make thoughtful, informed choices about his/her care. This part of the OBRA law provides a check and balance for residents who are at risk of well meaning staff "making choices for him/her." The system is meant to be set up so that a guardian can place the resident's needs first when making choices about care (not just what is convenient for the facility). This tag requires the surveyors to make sure that all consents (*including photo release and outing release*) are signed by the legally appointed guardian.

**Tag F153** The resident and/or his/her legal representative have the right to review all of the resident's records within 24 hours or less of the request. This request may be either verbal or in writing; the facility cannot insist that only written requests be accepted. This requirement is for the resident's medical chart as well as trust fund ledgers, contracts with the facility, facility incident reports and any other record which may have been made on behalf of or about the resident. The facility may charge the resident for any copies of the records that s/he may request, however, the amount of that charge may not exceed what is normally charged at places like the public library, the post office or low cost copy shops.

**Tag F154** The staff and consultants at the facility must make sure that the resident is fully informed about his/her health and status in a manner that s/he can easily understand. Total health status includes functional status, activities potential, cognitive status, psychosocial status and sensorial and physical impairments. The resident should be involved in the assessment and care planning process, including the discussion of diagnoses, treatment, options, risks and prognoses. The information must be presented in advance of the treatment and must let the resident know if the treatment will affect the resident's well-being. Unless the resident has been previously determined (legally) to be incompetent or otherwise found to be incapacitated, the resident has the right to participate in planning care and treatment or changes in care and treatment.

**Tag F155** The resident has the absolute right to refuse to participate in any treatment (unless it is court ordered). The resident also has the right to sign an Advanced Directive and have the facility honor that Directive. This tag leads to a philosophical discussion about whether the treatment team — especially the Activity and Social Service Professional — can write up any treatment objective based on participation. If the Activity Professional has the care plan objective that the resident will participate in three activities a week, then the treatment being provided is *participation*. The resident always has the absolute right to refuse all treatment and the right to refuse to participate in facility sponsored activities. When most residents decline the invitation to go to any specific activity, they are not usually refusing treatment in their mind, they just are not interested in going to the activity. If the care plan objective is to participate in activities, the resident says "no-thank you" and yet the staff person still tries to persuade the resident to go — that staff person is violating the resident's right to refuse treatment and is trying to coerce the resident to abandon (even if for a short while) his/her rights. This leads to potential violation of both Tag F155 and Tag F151. The prudent professional will always separate the treatment plan (therapeutic intervention) from the normal leisure pastime of going to activities. Leave participation in the domain of a normalizing activity. When you feel that the resident needs a treatment, the care plan should be based on treating the identified need (e.g., increase frequency of initiation of social communications, increase use of fine motor skills, decrease percentage of time spent alone) and not on going to activities or talking to the Social Service Professional.

**Tag F156** It is hard for a resident to exercise his/her rights if s/he does not know what they are. For this reason, the Federal Government has required that the resident receive a copy of his/her rights written in a language and manner that s/he can read (avoid small print) and understand (native language if necessary). The resident must also be verbally told of his/her rights. This notice of his/her rights (both verbally and in writing) must happen: 1. right before and/or at the time of admission, 2. immediately upon any changes in those rights, 3. upon request and 4. periodically throughout admission. The surveyors are instructed to interview some of the staff to determine if the staff know the rights and rules well enough to help implement them. This tag also covers specific information which the facility must make available to the resident.

**Tag F157** Communication from the facility with the resident, the resident's legal guardian or interested family member and the resident's physician is important. In situations that the resident: 1. has been involved in an accident, 2. has experienced a significant change in health status, 3. has a need to have a change in treatment, 4. is to be discharged, 5. is scheduled to have a change of roommate and/or 6. has a change is his/her rights, the listed parties are to be notified *immediately*. A subsection of this tag requires that the facility must periodically check to make sure that all of the phone numbers and addresses that they have for legal guardians, interested family members and the resident's physician are current.

**Tags F158 – F161** The resident has the right to continue managing his/her finances after s/he is admitted to the long term care facility according to Tag F158. The facility may not require that the resident deposit his/her money with the facility or at a bank of the facility's choosing. Tags F159-F161 specify the manner in which the facility may handle the resident's money if the resident chooses to allow the facility to do so.

**Tag F164** The resident has the right to maintain his/her personal privacy and to have all of his/her records maintained in a confidential manner.

**Tags F165 – F166** The resident has the right to complain (voice grievances) about treatment received or not received or about other things that dissatisfy him/her about the facility. The facility must take these grievances seriously by: 1. listening to the grievances, 2. investigating the complaint, 3. promptly trying to address the cause of the grievance (resolve the grievance if possible) and 4. monitoring to ensure that the cause does not lead to the same situation again. This includes addressing the resident's complaints about the behaviors of other residents and of staff.

**Tag F167** The resident and the public in general have the right to see a copy of the facility's most current survey along with the plan of correction written up by the facility. This copy must be easily available and either the actually survey document or a notice of its availability must be posted in a prominent place for all to see.

**Tag F168** The resident has the right to contact agencies acting as client advocates.

**Tag F169** The resident has the right to be free from the requirement to work for the facility. If the resident elects to work for the facility (e.g., folding clothes, running activity groups, etc.) the facility must have in writing whether the resident is working for a wage or as a volunteer (as well as documentation that the resident is knowledgeable about his/her pay status). If the resident is getting paid for the work being done, s/he must be paid the prevailing wage for the job being done.

**Tags F170 – F171** The resident has the right to receive mail and packages without them first being opened by facility staff. The laws that apply to the individual's right to privacy of mail received applies to residents of the facility just as it would if they were in their own homes. Because many of the residents are not able to go shopping for stationery, writing implements and postage stamps, the facility is expected to provide them for the residents but may attach a reasonable charge to these supplies. These tags also specify that residents must receive their mail in less then 24 hours of it being delivered to the facility and that the residents outgoing mail must be to the post office in less then 24 hours after being given to a staff person.

**Tag F172** The facility may not have visiting hours which apply to any individual whom the resident wishes to visit. Visitors must be admitted 24 hours a day if the resident wishes it to be that way. Certain state and federal officials must be allowed immediate access to any resident at any time.

**Tag F173** The facility must allow the State Appointed Ombudsman access to the resident's records if the resident or his/her legal guardian give permission.

**Tag F174** The resident has the right to have reasonable access to a telephone to receive and place calls in a private manner. This phone must meet ADA (Americans with Disabilities Act) standards for height and volume control.

**Tag F175** Residents who are married to each other have the right to share a room in the facility as long as both partners want to share a room.

**Tags F201 – F206** To help protect the rights of each resident, the Federal government has outlined the acceptable reasons for transfer or discharge and the procedures and required steps to take before, during and after a resident is either discharged or transferred.

**Tag F221 – F222** The resident has the right to be free from any physical restraints imposed; or chemical restraints imposed for purposes of discipline or convenience, not required to treat the resident's medical symptoms. **Physical restraints** are any manual method or physical or mechanical device, material or equipment attached to or adjacent to the resident's body that the individual cannot remove easily which restricts freedom of movement or normal access to one's body. Leg restraints, arm restraints, hand mitts, soft ties or vest, wheelchair safety bars, geri-chairs and bed rails are physical restraints. **Chemical restraints** are psycho pharmacological drugs used for discipline or convenience and not required to treat medical symptoms. **Discipline** is any action taken by the facility for the purpose of punishing or penalizing the resident. **Convenience** is any action taken by the facility to control resident behavior or maintain residents with a lesser amount of effort by the facility and not in the residents' best interest. Before using restraints, a facility must demonstrate the presence of a specific medical symptom that would require the use of restraints and how the restraint would treat the cause of the symptom and assist the resident in reaching his/her highest level of physical and psychosocial well-being. Often appropriate exercise and therapeutic interventions such as orthotic devices, pillows, pads or lap trays will be sufficient. These less restrictive, supportive devices must be considered prior to using physical restraints. If after a trial of less restrictive measures, the facility decides that a physical restraint would enable and promote greater functional independence, then the use of the restraining device must first be explained to the resident, family member or legal representative and if the resident, family member or legal representative agrees to this treatment alternative, then the restraining device may be used for specific periods for which the restraint has been determined to be an enabler. Any resident who requires a restraint must have a **specific intervention in the care plan to ensure maintenance** of his/her physical, mental, psychosocial and functional status. To determine maintenance, the treatment team should administer the appropriate assessments to establish a **baseline**.

**Tag F223** The resident has the right to be free from verbal, sexual, physical or mental abuse, corporal punishment and involuntary seclusion.

**Tags F224 – F225** These two tags say that the facility must have policies and procedures in place to prevent abuse and specify the kind of actions the facility must take to ensure that the resident is not verbally or physically abused, including being free from the risk of being taken care of by individuals known to mistreat residents and the required actions to take if neglect or abuse is suspected.

**Tag F240** The facility must care for its residents in a manner and in an environment that promotes maintenance or enhancement of each resident's quality of life.

**Tag F241** The facility must promote care for residents in a manner and in an environment that maintains or enhances each **resident's dignity and respect** in full recognition of his or her individuality.

**Tag F242** The resident has the right to chose activities, schedules and health care consistent with his or her interests, assessments and plans of care; interact with members of the community both inside and outside of the facility; and make choices about aspects of his or her life in the facility that are significant to the resident.

**Tags F243 – F244** These two tags outline the residents' right to hold meetings in the facility, with adequate space for the meeting provided by the facility. The residents and their families have the right to meet in private and to present a written request to the facility to address grievances and/or recommendations. The facility is then required to address the grievances and/or recommendations presented in a timely manner.

**Tag F245** A resident has the right to participate in social, religious and community activities that do not interfere with the rights of other residents in the facility. The facility, to the extent possible, should accommodate an individual's needs and choices for how s/he spends time, both inside and outside of the facility.

**Tags F246 – F247** These two tags further define the resident's rights to receive the services that s/he wants and to have some control over who his/her roommate is. Residents have the right to refuse to have a specific aide give them a bath if they do not feel comfortable with that aide. They have the right to hire outside services (e.g., their own nursing aide or companion) without interference from the facility unless his/her action places the other residents at risk. Other issues covered under this tag include the requirement that the environment of the facility be set up for the residents, not the staff, and that measures are in place to enable residents with dementia to walk freely, to promote reorientation and remotivation, to encourage conversation and socialization and to increase mobility and independence for disabled residents.

**Tag F248** This tag (provided in its complete form below) outlines the content and scope of activity services required to be provided for the resident by the facility. For non-interviewable residents, the surveyors try to determine if the activities agree with assessed interests and functional level including whether cues/prompts and adapted equipment are provided as needed and according to care plan. The surveyors ask the families to describe the activities before and after becoming a resident of the facility. For interviewable residents and groups of residents, the surveyors are to ask:
- Activities programs are supposed to meet your interests and needs. Do you feels the activities here do that?
- How do you find out about activities that are going on?
- Are there activities available on the weekends?
- Do you participate in activities?
    - (If yes) What kind of activities do you participate in?
    - (If resident participates) Do you enjoy these activities?
    - (If resident does not participate, probe to find out why not.)
- Is there some activity that you would like to do that is not available here?
    - (If yes) Which activity would you like to attend? Have you talked to anybody about this? What was the response?
- Are there enough help and supplies available so that everyone who wants to can participate?
- Do you as a group have input into the selection of activities that are offered?
- How does the facility respond to your suggestions?
- Is there anything about the activities program that you would like to talk about?
- Outside of the formal activities programs, are there opportunities for you to socialize with other residents?
- Are there places you can go when you want to be with other residents?
    - (If the answers are negative) Why do you think that occurs?

# Tag F248 [Activities]

§483.15(f)(1) The facility must provide for an ongoing program of activities designed to meet, in accordance with the comprehensive assessment, the interests and the physical, mental and psychosocial well-being of each resident.

Guidelines: §483.15(f)(1)

Because the activities program should occur within the context of each resident's comprehensive assessment and care plan, it should be multi-faceted and reflect each individual resident's needs. Therefore, the activities program should provide stimulation or solace; promote physical, cognitive and/or emotional health; enhance, to the extent practicable, each resident's physical and mental status; and promote each resident's self-respect by providing, for example, activities that support self-expression and choice.

Activities can occur at any time and are not limited to formal activities provided by the activity staff. Others involved may be any facility staff, volunteers and visitors.

Probes: §483.15(f)(1)

Observe individual, group and bedside activities.

1.  Are residents who are confined or choose to remain in their rooms provided with in-room activities in keeping with life-long interests (e.g., music, reading, visits with individuals who share their interests or reasonable attempts to connect the resident with such individuals) and in-room projects they can work on independently? Do any facility staff members assist the resident with activities he or she can pursue independently?

2.  If the residents sit for long periods of time with no apparently meaningful activities, is the cause:
    a.  Resident choice;
    b.  Failure of any staff or volunteers either to inform residents when activities are occurring or to encourage resident involvement in activities;
    c.  Lack of assistance with ambulation;
    d.  Lack of sufficient supplies and/or staff to facilitate attendance and participation in the activity programs;
    e.  Program design that fails to reflect the interests or ability levels of residents, such as activities that are too complex?

For residents selected for a comprehensive review, or a focused review, as appropriate, determine to what extent the activities reflect the individual resident's assessment. (See especially MDS III.1 and Sections B, C, D and I; MDS version 2.0 sections AC, B, C, D and N.)

Review the activity calendar for the month prior to the survey to determine if the formal activity program:
*   Reflects the schedules, choices and rights of the residents;
*   Offers activities at hours convenient to the residents (e.g., morning, afternoon, some evenings and weekends);
*   Reflects the cultural and religious interests of the resident population; and
*   Would appeal to both men and women and all age groups living in the facility.

Review clinical records and activity attendance records of residents receiving a comprehensive review, or a focused review, as appropriate, to determine if:
*   Activities reflect individual resident history indicated by the comprehensive assessment;

> - Care plans address activities that are appropriate for each resident based on the comprehensive assessment;
> - Activities occur as planned; and
> - Outcomes/responses to activities interventions are identified in the progress notes of each resident.

**Tag F249** This tag outlines the types of credentials required of any person who is employed as the Activity Director.

**Tag F250** This tag outlines the scope of social services to be provided by the facility. The entire text of Tag F250 is shown in the box below.

# Tag F250 [Social Services]

§483.15(g)(1) The facility must provide medically-related social services to attain or maintain the highest practicable physical, mental and psychosocial well-being of each resident.

Intent §483.15(g)

To assure that sufficient and appropriate social services are provided to meet the resident's needs.

Guidelines: §483.15(g)(1)

Regardless of size, all facilities are required to provide for the medically related social services needs of each resident. This requirement specifies that facilities aggressively identify the need for medically-related social services and pursue the provision of these services. It is not required that a qualified social worker necessarily provide all of these services. Rather, it is the responsibility of the facility to identify the medically-related social service needs of the resident and assure that the needs are met by the appropriate disciplines.

"Medically-related social services" means services provided by the facility's staff to assist residents in maintaining or improving their ability to manage their everyday physical, mental and psychosocial needs. These services might include, for example:
- Making arrangements for obtaining needed adaptive equipment, clothing and personal items;
- Maintaining contact with family (with resident's permission) to report on changes in health, current goals, discharge planning and encouragement to participate in care planning;
- Assisting staff to inform residents and those they designate about the resident's health status and health care choices and their ramifications;
- Making referrals and obtaining services from outside entities (e.g., talking books, absentee ballots, community wheelchair transportation);
- Assisting residents with financial and legal matters (e.g., applying for pensions, referrals to lawyers, referrals to funeral homes for preplanning arrangements);
- Discharge planning services (e.g., helping to place a resident on a waiting list for community congregate living, arranging intake for home care services for residents returning home, assisting with transfer arrangements to other facilities);
- Providing or arranging provision of needed counseling services;
- Through the assessment and care planning process, identifying and seeking ways to support resident's individual needs and preferences, customary routines, concerns and choices;
- Building relationships between residents and staff and teaching staff how to understand and support resident's individual needs;
- Promoting actions by staff that maintain or enhance each resident's dignity in full recognition of each resident's individuality;

- Assisting residents to determine how they would like to make decisions about their health care and whether or not they would like anyone else to be involved in those decisions;
- Finding options that most meet the physical and emotional needs of each resident;
- Providing alternatives to drug therapy or restraints by understanding and communicating to staff why residents act as they do, what they are attempting to communicate and what needs the staff must meet;
- Meeting the needs of residents who are grieving; and
- Finding options which most meet their physical and emotional needs.

Factors with a potentially negative effect on physical, mental and psychosocial well-being include an unmet need for:
- Dental/denture care;
- Podiatric care;
- Eye care;
- Hearing services;
- Equipment for mobility or assistive eating devices; and
- Need for homelike environment, control, dignity, privacy.

Where needed services are not covered by the Medicaid State Plan, nursing facilities are still required to attempt to obtain these services. For example, if a resident requires transportation services that are not covered under a Medicaid State Plan, the facility is required to provide these services. This could be achieved, for example, through obtaining volunteer assistance.

Types of conditions to which the facility should respond with social services by staff or referral include:
- Lack of an effective family/social support system;
- Behavioral symptoms;
- If a resident with dementia strikes out at another resident, the facility should evaluate the resident's behavior. (For example, a resident may be re-enacting an activity he or she used to perform at the same time everyday. If that resident senses that another is in the way of his or her re-enactment, the resident may strike out at the resident impeding his or her progress. The facility is responsible for the safety of any potential resident victims while it assesses the circumstances of the resident's behavior);
- Presence of a chronic disabling medical or psychological condition (e.g., multiple sclerosis, chronic obstructive pulmonary disease, Alzheimer's disease, schizophrenia);
- Depression;
- Chronic or acute pain;
- Difficulty with personal interaction and socialization skills;
- Presence of legal or financial problems;
- Abuse of alcohol or other drugs;
- Inability to cope with loss of function;
- Need for emotional support;
- Changes in family relationships, living arrangements and/or resident's condition or functioning; and
- A physical or chemical restraint.

For residents with or who develop mental disorders as defined by the **Diagnostic and Statistical Manual for Mental Disorders (DSM-IV)**, see §483.45, F406.

Probes: §483.15(g)(1)

For residents selected for a comprehensive or focused review as appropriate:
- How do facility staff implement social service interventions to assist the resident in meeting treatment goals?

- How do staff responsible for social work monitor the resident's progress in improving physical, mental and psychosocial functioning? Has goal attainment been evaluated and the care plan changed accordingly?
- How does the care plan link goals to psychosocial functioning/well-being?
- Have the staff responsible for social work established and maintained relationships with the resident's family or legal representative?
- (NFs) What attempts does the facility make to access services for Medicaid recipients when those services are not covered by a Medicaid State Plan?

Look for evidence that social service interventions successfully address residents' needs and link social supports, physical care and physical environment with residents' needs and individuality.

For sampled residents review MDS, Section H.

**Tag F251** This tag specifies the qualifications of the individuals providing social services and the requirement for one full time Social Service Professional for any facility with 120 beds or more.

**Tag F252** All areas of the facility must provide a homelike environment. The resident has the right to keep some of his/her personal possessions in his/her room (including furniture) as long as its presence does not jeopardize the health and safety of the other residents.

**Tags F253 – F258** These six tags provide guidelines for the quality and comfort level of the living space for the residents. For a more in-depth review of these tags the reader should review the OBRA Environmental Review Form in this book.

**Tag F272** The facility is required to conduct a comprehensive assessment on each resident when s/he is admitted and then at intervals during his/her stay. This assessment must done using a standardized assessment (the MDS), the findings must be accurate, the staff who do the assessment must be qualified to do the assessment and a variety of staff must be able to get substantially similar results (reliability). This tag also explains that the testing tools that the staff use (i.e., the nursing assessment, the social service assessment, the activity assessment) must, when put together, measure everything that is required to be written into the MDS. Each facility must use the RAI (which includes both the MDS and the RAPs). The areas measured include:

- medically defined conditions and prior medical history
- medical status measurement
- physical and mental functional status
- sensory and physical impairments
- nutritional status and requirements
- special treatments and procedures
- mental and psychosocial status
- discharge potential
- dental condition
- activities potential (The resident's ability and desire to take part in activities which maintain or improve physical, mental and psychosocial well being. Activity pursuits refer to any activity outside of ADLs which a person pursues in order to obtain a sense of well-being. Also included are activities which provide benefits in the areas of self-esteem, pleasure, comfort, health education, creativity, success and financial or emotional independence. The assessment should consider the resident's normal everyday routines and lifetime preferences.)
- rehabilitation potential
- cognitive status, including the resident's ability to problem solve, decide, remember and be aware of and respond to safety hazards
- drug therapy

**Tags F273 – F276** These four tags specify the timing associated with assessing and reassessing the resident. By Federal law, the first MDS must be completed within 14 days of admission, reassessed quarterly and redone at least once every 12 months. These tags also specify what kind of medical and social events would trigger a complete reassessment prior to the passage of 12 months.

**Tag F278** Assessments must be done accurately and signed by each person who completes a portion of the assessment.

**Tags F279 – F280** Each resident is required to have a comprehensive care plan based on his/her needs that were identified in the assessment process. This care plan must be developed no later then 7 days after the completion of the MDS. This care plan must be developed by the resident (and/or his/her legal guardian or family) working along with the treatment team and must be reviewed periodically to ensure that it is still appropriate.

**Tags F281 – F282** These two tags state that each professional within the facility must provide his/her services in a way that will meet or exceed the standards of practice published by his/her professional group, as well as any other governmental or accrediting standards that apply. For facilities who are surveyed by either the Joint Commission or CARF, the professional will want to comply with the standards of those groups to also comply with this tag.

**Tags F283 – F284** These two tags outline the requirements for discharge summaries.

**Tags F308 – F309** These two tags state that the resident must receive the types and quality of care indicated as needed by the assessment and outlined in the care plan. If the facility has some difficulty meeting this requirement, Tag F309 will be cited. If the facility has significant difficulty meeting this requirement, Tag F308 will be cited.

**Tags F310 – F318** These tags specify the facilities responsibilities related to the resident's activities of daily living, vision and hearing, pressure sores, urinary incontinence and range of motion.

**Tags F319 – F320** These two tags provide the facility with a detailed explanation of the scope and depth of services and treatment expected for the mental and psychosocial functioning of each resident.

**Tags F323 – F324** These tags sets the expectation that the environment will be free of accident hazards and that each resident will receive adequate supervision and assistance to be able to avoid accidental injury.

**Tag F330** This tag sets forth a very rigid set of standards and steps required before any resident admitted to a nursing home is given antipsychotic drugs for the first time. The entire treatment team should be familiar with the steps required to be taken before a resident may receive an antipsychotic medication. The physician, who is seldom in the facility, will need to rely on input from many of the professionals (not just nursing) working with the resident before prescribing such medications.

**Tags F410 – F412** This requirement concerns dental care. The rest of the tags in this section outline the types of dental care that should be available to the resident as well as the kind of help the staff needs to provide to meet the resident's dental needs.

**Tag F464** The facility must provide one or more rooms designed for resident dining and activities. These rooms must be well lighted. Carole B. Lewis in her book **Improving Mobility In Older Persons** (Aspen Publications 1989) states: "The lens of the eye becomes thicker with age and the person needs more light to see correctly. Treatment suggestion: use a lot of light (200 watts) especially in functional areas (e.g., reading spots, kitchens and bathrooms." (page 95)). The facility must have adequate ventilation and if a room is a non-smoking area, the signage indicating such must meet state requirements. The facility's rooms must be adequately furnished. Furnishing are structurally sound and functional (e.g., chairs of varying sizes to meet varying needs of residents, wheelchairs can fit under the dining room table). The activity room must have sufficient space to accommodate all activities. Space should be adaptable to a variety of uses and resident needs. Residents and staff have maximum flexibility in arranging furniture to accommodate residents who use walkers, wheelchairs and other mobility aids. No crowding evident. Space does not limit resident access.

**Tag F514** How often should the professional write in the progress notes? The questions surveyors are instructed to ask themselves is: Is there enough recorded documentation for staff to conduct a care program and to revise the program as necessary to respond to the changing status of the resident as a result of interventions? How is the clinical record used in managing the resident's progress in maintaining or improving functional abilities and psychosocial status?

**Tags F520 – F521** The facility must have a functioning quality assurance committee which meets at least quarterly and develops and implements appropriate plans of action to correct quality deficiencies.

# Surveys

Each one of the settings providing treatment services and health care to elderly, psychiatric and DD clients are governed by federal and state regulations.

HCFA (Health Care Financing Administration) is responsible for issuing the Federal Register (federal regulations). Each state then reviews these federal guidelines and interprets them for state regulation which will be in compliance with the federal government standards. In some cases the state may add regulations. It may not remove regulations.

In order to be a participant in the Medicare/Medicaid program, long term care facilities and other agencies, are reviewed and certified. Also, to receive a license by the state to operate as a business, the facilities need to be reviewed and re-licensed annually.

Every aspect of the facility functions are reviewed for compliance to both Federal and State regulations. Because Activities and Social Services are required and extremely important to the well being of the resident, they are reviewed yearly in this process. The department heads need to be very clear on what the requirements are for these departments. Documentation needs to be presented to the surveyors upon request. You will also have the opportunity to share with them the special programs that you have implemented. The table below outlines some important considerations which will help you do well in the survey process.

---

## Things To Remember About Survey

1.   Know your regulations

2.   Be friendly and welcome conversation about what you do. Surveyors play an important role in assuring quality of care and quality of life.

3.   Have records of participation, bedside logs, resident council (member list and minutes of meetings), calendars and PR available for review. Present a packet of information (approved by your administrator) to the surveyors when they first get to the facility.

4.   Have your office and supplies neatly organized and labeled.

5.   Be responsible for your department but do not involve yourself in issues related to the other departments. They are better trained to do this themselves, just as you are for the service your department.

6.   Discussion and clarity are important in communicating what and why you do something. If your treatments follow from your assessments and you have made sure that the treatments are carried out according to the resident care plans, there should be no problem during survey.

7.   Be yourself.

# Compliance with Regulations

Compliance with health care regulations is required. The goal of the federal government is for every health care facility to be in substantial compliance with all regulations. Substantial compliance means that the facility is providing a reasonable quality of care to its residents. There can be no deficiencies (services or equipment that do not meet standards) that cause actual harm to any resident and no more than the potential for minimal harm.

Prior to the implementation of the OBRA Final Rule in July 1995, there were instances of facilities not caring if one or two tags were out. For repeated minor deficiencies, there were no penalties. The facilities knew that they could implement a plan of correction and stay in business. If they were out of compliance again by the next survey, there was still no penalty.

The OBRA Final Rule changed that. Now there are required penalties for every facility that is out of substantial compliance. The intent of the new process is to have facilities stay in compliance year round and not experience the previous "yo-yo" compliance at survey time.

When deciding on the penalties, the surveyors look at the severity of the deficiency and its scope for deficiencies found in **Quality of Care**, **Quality of Life** or **Resident Behavior and Facility Practices**. Severity measures the level of harm being caused by the deficiency as shown below:

| | |
|---|---|
| **Level 1:** No actual harm with potential for minimal harm | Nothing has happened to a resident and the worst that can happen is a minor negative impact. |
| **Level 2:** No actual harm with potential for more than minimal harm that is not immediate jeopardy. | The resident has been impacted in a minor negative way and/or there is a potential for significant harm that has not actually happened yet. |
| **Level 3:** Actual harm that is not immediate jeopardy | The resident has been significantly harmed by some practice at the facility and has been prevented from reaching his/her highest practicable level of well being. |
| **Level 4:** Immediate jeopardy | Immediate jeopardy is a situation where immediate corrective action is necessary because what the facility is doing either has caused or may cause serious injury, serious harm or death to a resident in the facility. |

Scope refers to the number of residents who are affected by the deficiency. See the table below:

| | |
|---|---|
| Isolated | One or a very limited number of residents, staff or locations are involved. |
| Pattern | More than a limited number of residents, staff or locations are involved or the same resident has been affected by the deficiency on repeated occasions. |
| Widespread | The problems causing the deficiency exist throughout the facility and a large portion of the residents have been affected or might be affected. |

The surveyors look at the cause of the deficiency as well as the number of deficiencies to determine the scope. If the deficiencies are because the facility does not have a policy or system, the deficiency will probably be widespread. If the deficiency results from inadequate implementation, there will probably be a pattern of deficiency. If only one or a very limited number of residents are affected, the scope is isolated.

If the deficiencies are serious enough or widespread enough, the surveyors will find that the facility is providing a Substandard Quality of Care. This is an official term that means a certain level of deficiency is found during survey. Any Immediate Jeopardy is Substandard Quality of Care. Any pattern of Actual Harm or widespread Actual Harm (Level 3) or Potential for More Than Minimal Harm (Level 2) that is widespread is also considered Substandard Quality of Care. In the chart below the white areas are areas of Substantial Compliance, the light gray areas are out of Substantial Compliance, but not considered Substandard Care. The dark gray areas are Substandard Care. The chart also shows the level of penalty required for facilities which are out of substantial compliance.

| | ISOLATED | PATTERN | WIDESPREAD |
|---|---|---|---|
| **Level 4.** Immediate jeopardy to resident health/safety | Plan of Correction Required: Cat. 3 Optional: Cat. 2 Optional: Cat. 1 | Plan of Correction Required: Cat. 3 Optional: Cat. 2 Optional: Cat. 1 | Plan of Correction Required: Cat. 3 Optional: Cat. 2 Optional: Cat. 1 |
| **Level 3.** Actual harm that is not Immediate Jeopardy | Plan of Correction Required*: Cat. 2 Optional: Cat. 1 | Plan of Correction Required*: Cat. 2 Optional: Cat. 1 | Plan of Correction Required*: Cat. 2 Optional: Temporary Management. Optional: Cat. 1 |
| **Level 2.** No actual harm with potential for more than minimal harm that is not immediate jeopardy | Plan of Correction Required*: Cat. 1 Optional: Cat. 2 | Plan of Correction Required*: Cat. 1 Optional: Cat. 2 | Plan of Correction Required*: Cat. 2 Optional: Cat. 1 |
| **Level 1.** No actual harm with potential for minimal harm | No remedies No Plan of Correction Commitment to correct | Plan of Correction | Plan of Correction |

*It is possible to terminate the operation of the facility instead of imposing these penalties. If termination is not chosen, these penalties are required.

The penalties in the chart above increase depending on the category of penalties.

Category 1 penalties include:
- Directed plan of correction;
- State monitor and/or
- Directed inservice training

Category 2 penalties include:
- Denial of payment for new admissions;
- Denial of payment for all residents and/or
- Civil penalties of $50 to $3000 per day

Category 3 penalties include:
- Temporary Management
- Termination
- Optional Civil Money Penalties of $3050 to $10,000 per day

There are two more conditions for compliance in addition to these penalties. They state that:
- Denial of payment for new admissions must be imposed when a facility is not in substantial compliance within three months after being found out of compliance.
- Denial of payment and state monitoring must be imposed when a facility has been found to have provided substandard quality of care on three consecutive standard surveys.

The new penalty structure makes it more important than ever for a facility to be in compliance with regulations. One of the best ways for Activity and Social Service Professionals to do their part is to participate in the quality assurance process at their facility and to regularly check the compliance of their department using the Survey Checklist forms at the end of this section.

# Survey Groups

There are several different survey groups which may be responsible for looking at your facility. The major ones are in the following list:

**HCFA**
Health Care Financing Administration: Responsible for ensuring that minimal federal standards are met. Required of all long term care facilities. Usually sub-contract with state to do their surveys.

**State Department of Health Standards**
State surveys are required at least every twelve months unless the state requests an extension. The surveyors may also survey specific state regulations concerning long term care services.

**JCAHO**
Joint Commission on Accreditation of Healthcare Organizations: This is a private credentialing body that conducts voluntary surveys. Standards are usually more stringent with a different focus than state and federal regulations. The intent of this survey process is to acknowledge a higher level of standards above federal, state and corporate standards. There is a charge to the facility for this survey process. More and more nursing facilities are requesting this accreditation as the services being provided in many facilities are more specialized and resident based.

**CARF**
Commission on Accreditation of Rehabilitation Facilities: This is a private credentialing body that conducts voluntary surveys. CARF Standards apply to rehab services. There is a charge for this survey.

**Peer Review**
The peer review survey process is a voluntary process requested by the facility. The team may be comprised of management staff from the corporation that owns the facility, a peer review team of a sister facility or a survey team comprised of staff members from a professional long term care organization or community group. There are usually no fees associated with this process as it is an assurance review process in preparation for any of the above reviews.

# Federal Regulations

The federal regulations are standard to all states. In 1987 the Omnibus Budget Reconciliation Act (discussed earlier in the chapter) was enacted. (It was last revised in 1995.) All nursing facilities or "long term care facilities" participating in Medicare and Medicaid are subject to the Act. The regulations serve as the basis for survey activities for the purpose of determining whether a facility meets the requirements for participation in Medicare and Medicaid.

# State Regulations

Each state also has regulations for licensing and certification of long term care facilities. These regulations may be stricter than the federal regulations but not more lenient. They will be used in addition to the federal regulations for survey purposes. It is not possible in the scope of this book to review each state's requirements. A copy of the state regulations should be available in the facility. If not, a copy can be reviewed at the county law library.

# Corporate or Facility Policy

Many corporations standardize policies and procedures in all of their facilities across the United States. Others allow facilities to adopt their own policies and procedures. Independently owned facilities adopt standardized procedures or create their own. Again, these policies and procedures can be stricter than federal and state law but may not be more lenient. A copy should be available in the facility and in the Activity and Social Service Departments.

If a policy is no longer applicable or needs to be revised, this should be brought to the attention of the Administrator. Facility policy and procedures must be followed, just as state and federal law must be followed. It is in the best interest of the professional to follow all laws, regulations and policies. They serve as a protection and provide a rationale for any action that may be taken in the care and treatment of the resident.

# Survey Checklists

You should use the survey checklists on the following pages (and the checklists in the *Quality Assurance* section of the *Resident Care* chapter) to see if your program will pass survey.

# OBRA

# Quality of Life Review Form

Facility:_____     Date:_____

| F240 A – Quality of Life |
| :--- |
| "A facility must care for its residents in a manner and in an environment that promotes maintenance or enhancement of each resident's quality of life." |

+ = Met
- = Not Met

| Requirement | Interpretation | |
| :--- | :--- | :--- |
| **F241** Dignity | Focus on a resident as an individual<br>Respect for space and property<br>Treating residents respectfully as adults<br>Promoting independence and dignity in dining | |

| Requirement | Interpretation | |
| :--- | :--- | :--- |
| <u>Self-Determination and Participation.</u><br>The resident has the right to — | | |
| **F242** Choose activities, schedules and health care consistent with his or her interests, assessment and plans of care | Accommodating individual schedules and needs according to resident's requests and previous lifestyle and interests | |
| **F242** Interact with members of the community both inside and outside the facility | Facilitating involvement in community groups and matters which were important to resident before admission | |
| **F242** Make choices about aspects of his or her life in the facility *that are significant to the resident* | Providing smoking areas for residents who smoke<br>Working around the resident's schedule (including television programs) | |

| Requirement | Interpretation | |
| :--- | :--- | :--- |
| **F243-244** Participation in resident and family groups in the facility | Provide a private space for family and resident groups upon requests | |
| **F243** Facility must provide a designated staff person responsible for providing assistance and responding to written requests that result from group meetings | This staff person listens, records and assists administration with following through with grievances and recommendations | |
| **F246** Accommodation of Needs (1)...adaptations of the facility's physical environment and staff behaviors to assist residents in maintaining independent functioning, dignity, well-being and self-determination. | Accommodation of Needs pertains to how well the team is enhancing and maintaining independence vs. dependence on staff and environment including: telephone access, personal property, married couples, activities, social services, psychosocial functioning, homelike environment, Activities of Daily Living and accidents & prevention-assistive devices | |
| **F247** (2)...Receive notice before the resident's room or roommate in the facility changes | Resident must have a say in who his/her roommate is and the timing of any change | |

# OBRA

# Environment Review Form

Facility: _____  Date: _____

| | |
|---|---|
| **F252 — Environment**<br>"The facility must provide a safe, clean, comfortable and homelike environment, allowing the resident to use his or her personal belongings to the extent possible." | Be sure to review the *Environmental Assessment Form* to begin problem solving. |

| Requirements | Interpretation | + = Met<br>- = Not Met |
|---|---|---|
| De-emphasize institutional character | Encourage personal belongings. | |
| Cleanliness | How clean is the facility? Are there odors detected in any of the rooms and halls? | |
| Individuality | Do you get to know who this person is and what their past interests were by observing their room and personal things and style? | |
| Clutter | Are day rooms and private rooms cluttered? Is there space for wheelchair and equipment accessibility? | |
| **F253** Housekeeping and Maintenance services | Assuring cleanliness and an infection-free environment for resident's equipment and supplies: toothbrush, dentures, denture cups, bed pans, urinals, feeding tubes, leg bags, catheter bags, pads and positioning devices. | |
| **F254** Clean bed and bath linens that are in good condition | Are there adequate linens available? Are they in good condition and without stains? | |
| **F255** Private closet space in each room | Closets must be provided with ample space and accessible shelves for resident use. | |
| **F256** Adequate lighting | Lighting suitable to tasks that residents choose to perform or facility staff must perform. Minimal glare and comfortable to the visually impaired.<br>Is lighting accessible to the resident? | |
| **F257** Comfortable and safe temperature levels | Ambient temperature levels to decrease likelihood of temperature changes which could affect well being of residents. Are there any rooms which are noticeably cold or too warm? | |
| **F258** Comfortable sound levels | Is conversation easy or do you have to raise your voice to be heard? Are there many distractions during group events? Are TVs and radios on too loud and too early or late at night? | |

# OBRA

# Activities Potential Review Form

---

**F 272 (x) Activities Potential**
"...The resident's ability and desire to take part in activities which maintain or improve physical, mental and psychosocial well-being."

---

|  |  | + = Met |
| --- | --- | --- |
| **Requirements** | **Interpretation** | **- = Not Met** |
| All activities which are not Activities of Daily Living | These would be activity/leisure involvement which a resident pursues for a sense of well being. | |
| Self-Esteem | Focus on the individual. Meaningful activities which highlight the abilities and uniqueness of each resident. | |
| Health Education | Nutrition related activities, wellness, leisure education, relaxation, understanding medical conditions and treatment plans. | |
| Pleasurable experiences | These can be social activities which encourage passive or active participation. What brings the pleasure is feeling safe, familiar surroundings, rekindling past interests. | |
| Opportunities for creative expression | Art, creative writing, oral histories, poetry, music, drama, gardening, cooking. | |
| Opportunities for achieving success | Can be incorporated in all activities at any level. It must be adapted and broken into stages for success at each level. | |
| Opportunities for achieving financial independence | Money management. Involvement in previous interests such as the stock market, investments and banking. | |
| Opportunities for achieving emotional independence | Problem solving activities and situations. Creative and expressive outlets. Activities which promote self-respect and individuality. Life review. Activities which assist others so that the resident has the chance to continue giving to others. | |

# Medications in the Elderly[49]

In the United States, the use of medications by those who are elderly is far too common. They consume over 30% of all prescription drugs and 40% of all non-prescription drugs. Those who are living in long term care facilities average more than 6 drugs per resident. All medications cause a change in the body. Because of the normal changes in how the body functions as one ages, the additional changes caused by medications may have a significant effect on the person's overall well-being. The chart below outlines some of the typical changes in one's body as one ages which help increase the impact of medications.

## Common Body Changes Associated with Aging

| | |
|---|---|
| **Cardiovascular Function:** Congestive Heart Failure | a. Decreased organ perfusion: as the heart weakens, it is less able to supply blood to the various vital organs. <br> b. Decreased metabolism: decreased blood flow to the liver or to the kidneys may result in decreased drug metabolism and excretion and, in turn, greater drug activity. |
| **Central Nervous System:** Degenerative Changes | a. Over time, the central nervous system (CNS) may exhibit degeneration and also the tissues in the CNS often have an enhanced response to medications. |
| **Kidney and Liver Function** | a. Decreased functional ability: may be a result of decreases in blood perfusion or a long-term disease process such as diabetes mellitus or high blood pressure. <br> b. Decreases in metabolism and excretion. |
| **Body Composition Changes** | a. Decreased lean body mass: decreases in muscle mass and protein stores may influence the response to a medication. <br> b. Contributes to changes in drug activity. |
| **Sensitivity to Drugs** | a. The tissues in the body and various receptor sites where medications exert their pharmaceutical activity may show increased sensitivity resulting in a greater response to a particular drug. This may result in an increased number of side effects. |

## Adverse Drug Reactions

All drugs have the potential to cause a side effect or adverse reaction. The elderly are more likely to experience an adverse effect and are more likely to be hospitalized as a result. Adverse drug reactions fall into three categories: 1. they are as a result of an allergic reaction to the medication, 2. they are as a result of a non-allergic reaction to a medication or 3. they are considered to be an unusual or idiosyncratic reaction to a medication. There are six general risk factors considered to increase the risk of an adverse drug reaction:

1. Age                          3. Duration of Treatment           5. Dosage
2. Number of Drugs              4. Gender (Female)                 6. Underlying Condition

Generally, individuals who are elderly have many of these risk factors present which increase the likelihood of experiencing a side effect to a medication.

Medications are frequently grouped together by "types" because they are prescribed for similar disorders, they change the body in similar ways and they frequently share common side effects. The chart below

---

[49] Written by Gina C. Johnson, Pharm.D.

shows some of the medication types that are most frequently prescribed for those who are older and common side effects.

## Frequently Prescribed Medications and Their Side Effects

| Type of Medication | Some Specific Medications | Potential Side Effects |
|---|---|---|
| **Cardiovascular Medications** | Digoxin<br>Verapamil | a. Dizziness, weakness, syncope due to low blood pressure.<br>b. Abnormal heart rhythm<br>c. Confusion, depression |
| **Diuretics** | Lasix<br>Hydrochlorothiazide | a. Dehydration<br>b. Headache<br>c. Weakness, fatigue<br>d. Nausea, vomiting |
| **Potassium Products** | | a. Stomach distress |
| **Pain Medications** | Tylenol with Codeine<br>Vicodin | a. Stomach: bleeding, nausea, pain<br>b. Dizziness, drowsiness, confusion, depression<br>c. Narcotics: physical and psychological dependence |
| **Antidiabetic Agents** | Insulin<br>Micronase | a. Low blood sugar (Hypoglycemia)<br>b. Chills<br>c. Nausea<br>d. Nervousness<br>e. Confusion<br>f. Hunger<br>g. Rapid, shallow breathing<br>h. Fast heartbeat<br>i. Fatigue |
| **Stomach-Intestinal Medications** | Tagamet<br>Reglan<br>Lomotil | a. Diarrhea<br>b. Confusion<br>c. Dizziness<br>d. Depression |
| **Psychoactive Medications:** Antipsychotic Medications | Haldol<br>Mellaril<br>Thorazine<br>Navane | a. Drowsiness<br>b. Low blood pressure<br>c. Tremors, shaking<br>d. Inability to sit still (akathesia)<br>e. Tardive dyskinesia — irreversible abnormal movements of the mouth and tongue |
| **Psychoactive Medications:** Antidepressants | Elavil<br>Desyrel<br>Imipramine | a. Low blood pressure<br>b. Fast heart rate<br>c. Dry mouth, blurred vision, constipation<br>d. Lethargy |
| **Psychoactive Medications:** Antidepressants | Prozac<br>Paxil<br>Zoloft | a. Insomnia<br>b. Anxiety, nervousness<br>c. Tremors |
| **Psychoactive Medications:** Anti-Anxiety and Sleeping Medications | Valium<br>Ativan<br>Xanax<br>Restoril<br>Dalmane | a. Lethargy, tiredness<br>b. Clumsiness, drunken walk<br>c. Confusion<br>d. Depression |

# Summary

The responsibilities and challenges of Activity and Social Service Professionals keep growing in direct proportion to the increased needs of the residents they serve.

OBRA regulations have changed the face of long term care forever. The regulations have added onto the work responsibilities for all staff members. The beauty of the change is that the focus is on the individual and how we as a team can assist them in meeting goals and projecting outcomes. The medical model focused on the diagnosis and now our functional/holistic model focuses on how a person heals, what gives them the resilience to meet new challenges, how the environment either enhances or negatively impacts their ability to improve and have a high quality of life.

As you have seen in the flow of information in this book, the authors have attempted to bring you full circle with why the services are important, who the residents might be, what the environment offers and how we as staff make a profound difference in individual lives — regardless of cognitive and functional abilities and/or limitations.

The impact of quality programming and teamwork are inspirational and do make a difference in both our lives and the lives of the very special individuals who find themselves in need of our services.

Many things change but, as Socrates observed far back in history, much remains the same:

*I consider the old who have gone before us along a road which we must all travel in our turn and it is good we should ask them of the nature of that road.*

The work that you put your spirit and soul into will not only make an impact on the residents living today in long term care settings, but create increasingly higher standards for the generations of residents in the future.

# Appendix A: Glossary[50]

**Note to Readers:** Whenever possible, the exact definition from federal law, regulations and interpretive guidelines were used. To help identify when the exact wording was used, the abbreviation for the document is placed before the definition.

**Code to Abbreviations Used in this Glossary:**
**ADA:** Americans with Disabilities Act
**OBRA:** Federal laws governing long term care facilities
**RAI:** Resident Assessment Instrument for long term care facilities

**Abduction** The process of moving a body part away from midline. In the case of the digits (the fingers or toes), abduction refers to the process of moving the digit away from the axis of the limb. Most leisure activities require some degree of abduction. These include walking (abduction of lower limbs, arms), cooking (abduction of arms in mixing), etc.

**Abstract Thinking** The ability to look at a situation, picture a variety of actions to take, understand the implications for actions taken and then analyze everything and come to a conclusion or decision.

**Accessibility** The ability of a site or object to be reached and used by individuals. The *Americans With Disabilities Act* (ADA) in the United States is a major piece of legislation which outlines the specific measurements for accessibility designs and accommodations.

**Active** The act of initiating and sustaining involvement in an activity or social interaction. Opposite of passive. Because active is such a general term it is frequently is used as a qualifying adjective, e.g., active treatment, active participation, etc.

**Activities of Daily Living (ADL)** Those skills that are required on a day to day basis. In the broader sense, all health care professionals use treatment interventions to help the resident overcome difficulties in performing ADLs. Activities of Daily Living are usually grouped into seven categories: 1. bathing, 2. dressing, 3. toilet hygiene, 4. grooming, 5. feeding/eating, 6. functional mobility and 7. functional

---

[50] The glossary is by joan burlingame, © 1996 Idyll Arbor, Inc.

communication.[51] The basic ADL skills of dressing, hand function and vocational skills are frequently the treatment domain of occupational therapy — however, in practice, all members of the interdisciplinary team work toward the resident's increased independence in ADLs. (RAI) Personal mastery of ADLs and mobility are as crucial to human existence in the nursing home as they are in the community. The nursing home is unique only in that most residents require help with self-care functions. ADL dependence can lead to intense personal distress — invalidism, isolation, diminished self-worth and a loss of control over one's destiny. As inactivity increases, complications such as pressure ulcers, falls, contractures and muscle-wasting can be expected. It is important for the staff to be able to set positive and realistic goals, weighing the advantages of independence against risks to safety and self-identity. In promoting independence staff must be willing to accept a reasonable degree of risk and active resident participation in setting treatment objectives. Rehabilitative goals of several types can be considered:

- To restore function to maximum self-sufficiency in the area indicated;
- To replace hands-on assistance with a program of task segmentation and verbal cueing;
- To restore abilities to a level that allows the resident to function with fewer supports;
- To shorten the time required for providing assistance;
- To expand the amount of space in which self-sufficiency can be practiced;
- To avoid or delay additional loss of independence; and
- To support the resident who is certain to decline in order to lessen the likelihood of complications (e.g., pressure ulcers and contractures).

**Activity** A term generally meaning doing something, e.g., movement, action, behavior, thought process, progression, development, wakefulness, physiological functions, etc.

**Activity Professional** An individual hired by a facility to provide free-time activities to maintain and/or enhance a resident's life as well as to provide specific activity interventions to decrease the negative impact of illness, injury and institutionalization. The majority of Activity Professional's work in long term care facilities. In the United States the federal legislation which regulates long term care facilities is called OBRA. The qualified Activity Professionals is someone "who is a qualified therapeutic recreation specialist or an activities professional who is licensed or registered, if applicable, by the State in which practicing; and is eligible for certification as a therapeutic recreation specialist or as an activities professional by a recognized accrediting body on or after October 1, 1990; or has 2 years of experience in a social or recreational program within the last 5 years, 1 of which was full-time in a patient activities program in a health care setting; or is a qualified occupational therapist or occupational therapy assistant; or has completed a training course approved by the State." (Tag F248-F249 — OBRA)

**Activity Intolerance** When a resident has insufficient physiological or psychological energy to endure or complete a required task. Some of the measurable/observable characteristics would include the resident's verbal report of fatigue or weakness, an abnormal heart rate or blood pressure in response to activity, discomfort upon exertion or an abnormal change in the resident's heart beat (e.g., arrhythmias).

**Acuity** The level of the resident's involvement in a disease. The higher the acuity, the more serious the disease is.

**Acute Stage** The first of two or more phases of an illness or disease. This stage is usually somewhat severe and short in duration. The acute stage of tissue and bone damage usually involves a decrease in leisure options caused by pain without exertion, inflammation, immobilization (both voluntary and as treatment) and the sedating effects of pain medications. (See *Subacute Stage* and *Chronic Stage*.)

**Adaptability** The ability of an individual to adjust to changes in the environment; to successfully change to enhance one's ability to fit into a specific situation. Adaptability may include the change in muscle

---

[51] American Occupational Therapy Association. 1989. *Uniform Terminology for Reporting Occupational Therapy, 2nd Ed.*

strength or cardiovascular fitness to better meet the physical challenges or the ability to learn new information or the ability to adjust the way one thinks about a situation.

**Adaptive Switches** The controls used to operate equipment needed by the resident. All switches perform the same basic job: they either turn something off or turn something on. Adaptive switches are usually either a single switch (controlling just one action like a light switch on or off) or a dual (multiple) switch (controlling more then one action like a stereo which has one button for the tape player and another button for the radio). Adaptive switches come in two modes: "momentary contact" which is activated only while the switch is being used (like a door bell) or "normally open" which remains on until turned off by the user (like a nursing call light). Switches are used to help a resident control communication devices, objects in the environment, etc.

**Adduction** The process of moving a body part toward midline. In the case of the digits (fingers and toes) adduction refers to the process of moving the digit toward the axis of the limb.

**Adhesions** A reduction in the normal range of motion due to the build up of collagen fibers. Collagen fibers adhere to surrounding structures and cause a reduction in the normal elasticity and movement of those structures. Adhesions are frequently a complication of surgery, trauma or immobilization.

**Advanced Directive** A legal document which outlines the resident's wishes concerning his/her desire for extra-ordinary measures to be taken to prevent his/her death.

**Aerobic** Activities which provide a paced activity which: allows the heart and circulatory system to keep up with oxygen needs of the body, uses a continuous amount of energy for muscle contraction and maintains a heart beat faster than resting rate for a minimum of 10 minutes. When leading exercise activities for residents with heart conditions, the professional should delay arm exercises until after both the warm up exercises and aerobic activities of the lower extremity (e.g., walking, leg raises). This delay will lower the chance of the resident experience angina episodes (chest pain), dysrhythmias (uneven heart beat), muscle soreness and fatigue (Karam, page 8). The safest aerobic schedule for most residents is 10–20 minutes of exercise three or four times a week. Individuals who exercise over 30 minutes at a time and/or five or more days a week do not significantly increase their aerobic ability and significantly increase the risk of orthopedic injury (Karam, pages 16, 17). When using aerobic activities with residents with diabetes, the biggest challenge is to balance the exercise with diet modifications, especially in Type I diabetes mellitus. This balance is the responsibility of the physician and the dietitian. The professional should also limit the aerobic activity to under 40 minutes, even with a resident who has a balanced program (Karam page 63).

**Agitation** The appearance that a resident is anxious because s/he is demonstrating motor restlessness. Agitation is frequently due to neurological damage, interruption in normal sleep patterns or due to a side effect of a medication.

**Altered Body Image** A change in the way that a resident perceives his/her own body image. The resident may actually have a change in his/her body function or structure or it may be a perceived change in his/her body function or structure.

**Alzheimer's Disease** Named after Alois Alzheimer, a German neurologist, this is one kind of organic mental disorder which describes a general loss of cognitive ability. This loss can be observed as a loss in long term memory, judgment, abstract thinking and changes in personality. The length of time that a person lives after developing the first signs of Alzheimer's Disease is usually 5 to 10 years.

**Ambulatory** The ability to walk. This usually refers to the resident's ability to functionally walk to the places s/he needs to get to on a daily basis, whether using a walker, cane, braces or no assistive devices. Lewis (1989) lists seven neurological changes that occur with age which decrease an individual's ability to ambulate safely. They are: 1. decreased proprioception of toes, 2. increased sway, 3. increased reaction time, 4. decreased sense of vibration at the ankles, 5. decreased number of neurons, 6. decreased cerebral blood flow and 7. increased cerebrovascular resistance.

**Ambulatory Status** The current functional level of the resident when walking or moving about.

**Americans with Disabilities Act 1990** The Americans with Disabilities Act (ADA) is a federal civil rights law. This law has five sections, called "Titles." Title I covers equal employment opportunities for individuals with disabilities. Title II covers nondiscrimination on the basis of disability in the receipt and use of state and local government services. Title III covers nondiscrimination on the basis of disability by public accommodations and in commercial facilities. Title IV covers telecommunications relay services for individuals who have a hearing impairment or a speech impairment. Title V covers miscellaneous provisions including construction, (lack of) state immunity, prohibition against retaliation and coercion, regulations by the Architectural and Transportation Barriers Compliance Board, attorney's fees, technical assistance, federal wilderness areas, coverage of Congress and the agencies of the legislative branch, illegal use of drugs, definitions, amendments to the Rehabilitation Act and alternative means of dispute resolution. The ADA opens up many opportunities in recreation and leisure to individuals with disabilities as it helps break down architectural and attitudinal barriers.

**Aneurysm** The dilation or bulging out of the wall of an artery or vein. It may rupture and cause a spontaneous hemorrhage.

**Angina** The feeling of pain in the chest and perception of difficulty in breathing (due to pain) as a result of the heart's reaction to overexertion or excitement. For individuals with *angina pectoris* (occasional lack of flow of blood to the heart) such an event is very frightening, as the resident has the feeling of impending death.

**Annual Care Conference (OBRA)** Long term care facilities are seeing fewer and fewer residents who are living in the facility for over 12 months. For those who do, the federal law in the United States (OBRA) requires that the interdisciplinary team conduct a re-assessment of the resident's needs, then meet as a group with the resident (and family) to outline a general course of treatment for the next year. This annual care conference is in addition to the quarterly and other care conferences that have taken place.

**Anterior** Referring to the front of the body or organ or indicating a location toward the head.

**Anxiety** One of the most common psychological disorders, anxiety is the psychological and physical response to an exaggerated imagined danger or imagined pending discomfort. In response to this imagined or over-emphasized threat, the resident may experience an increased heart rate, a change in breathing rate, sweating, fatigue, weakness, choking, nausea or abdominal distress, numbness, dizziness or unsteadiness, hot flashes or chills and/or trembling. While anxiety is seldom so severe that it makes a normally functional resident non-functional, it can interfere with the resident's ability to integrate into his/her community. Bourne (1990) stresses that successful intervention to reduce anxiety must include three elements: 1. reduction of physiological reactivity, 2. elimination of avoidance behaviors and 3. a change in subjective interpretations (or "self-talk") which perpetuate a state of apprehension and worry (page 2).

**Aphasia** The loss or decrease in the ability to speak, understand, read or write.

**Apraxia** The inability to carry out purposeful, voluntary movements without presence of muscle weakness, paralysis or impaired sensations. This can be found in physical activities and in speech.

**Arteriosclerotic Vascular Disease** The blood flow to the extremities decreases over time because of a narrowing and fibrosis of the medium to large arteries. This disease is most commonly seen in residents who are elderly or have a long history of diabetes mellitus. Some of the clinical signs include: decreased skin temperature in extremities, chalky white coloring of skin and/or with blanching of the skin in the affected limbs decreased hair growth over affected area, increased susceptibility to skin ulceration and pain. The resident may experience a decreased tolerance to temperature extremes leading to discomfort during certain leisure activities. The pain experienced by the resident may fall into two separate categories: pain upon exertion (intermittent claudication) or pain during periods of inactivity.

**Arthritis** A potentially disabling disability which causes inflammation of a joint or joints. While not always degenerative in nature, arthritis affects 50 percent of people over the age of 65 and 75 percent of people over the age of 80. (Rodman, McEwen, Wallace, 1973) The symptoms of arthritis which may interfere with a resident's level of activity include pain, swelling, stiffness and weakness. There are many different types of arthritis.

**Assessment** The process of placing a value on something through measurement and qualification. Assessment is not the same thing as an evaluation. See *Evaluation*.

**Atrophy** A decrease (or wasting away) in the size and function of a body part due to inactivity, disease or disability.

**Attention Deficits** The inability to attend to a task or a thought due to a lack of: 1. duration of attention, 2. appropriate selectivity of attention, 3. appropriate filtering of attention and/or 4. ability to maintain attention.

**Attrition** The wearing away or progressive deterioration of a body part or skill.

**Autonomy** The ability to make decisions for oneself; to be able to decide which activity to engage in along with having the functional skills to be able to complete the activity. Residents who are dependent on others for their care, even if for a short time, experience a great loss in autonomy. This loss frequently causes a situational depression to develop. Health care workers can make a difference in the resident's perceived loss of autonomy and subsequent development of situational depression by allowing the resident as many real choices as possible. Remember, the resident is the consumer of health care services and as such, has the legal right in almost all situations to make the choices.

**Baroreceptor Sensitivity** The baroreceptor nerve detects pressure applied to body parts. An individual with a baroreceptor sensitivity has hypersensitivity (over sensitivity) to touch and pressure. As a person ages s/he may experience a natural loss of baroreceptor sensitivity.

**Bathing** (OBRA) The process of cleaning the resident's body (excluding back and shampooing hair). This includes a full-body bath/shower and/or a sponge bath. In the United States a resident is technically independent in bathing even if they require a "set-up" assistance. Many facilities routinely provide "set-up" assistance to all residents, such as drawing water for a tub bath or laying out bathing materials. If this is the case and the resident requires no other assistance, for survey purposes, this resident is still considered to be independent in bathing. If a resident is to be discharged to home or participate in an aquatics program, the staff may need to evaluate if the resident is actually able to complete the set-up himself/herself.

**Beck Depression Scale** A quick testing tool which helps the professional determine the degree of clinical depression.

**Bedfast** (OBRA) In the United States, this is a technical term referring to a resident who is in a bed or recliner 22 hours or more per day in the past seven days. The resident may have bathroom privileges and still be considered bedfast.

**Bedrate** The amount paid by the insurance company or government for the resident's care. Bedrates are preset daily amounts determined by the typical cost of care within the region. Many of the services provided by the facility are included in the bedrate and may not be billed separately. Most of the services provided by Activity and Social Service Departments are already contained in the bedrate.

**Bedrest** Bedrest is type of activity status order usually determined by the resident's physician. Bedrest should be avoided or shortened whenever possible because of the severe physiological and psychological side effects. When a resident is on bedrest the professional should try to offset some of the negative aspects by using activities. Prior to engaging the resident in activity, the professional needs to know the specific reasons why the resident is on bedrest and to obtain clearance for specific activities and movements.

## Indicated Interventions During Bedrest

| Body System Effected | Activity Interventions Indicated |
|---|---|
| *Psychological Effects* | |
| Decreased Sensory Stimulation | Activities to help maintain central brain processing skills e.g., pattern tracing activities, radio or other auditory stimulation (including emphasizing the need for the resident to wear his/her hearing aid during bedrest), reading and other activities to stimulate color discrimination, object familiarity and social interaction. |
| Altered Body/Self-Image | Activities which reinforce the skills the resident has and can use during bedrest<br>Activities which reinforce who the resident is (e.g., parent, worker, hobbyist, etc.) |
| Altered Sensation of Time | Provision of calendar, clock, television, radio.<br>Social interaction which deals with what the day and time is as well as what is happening in the community/world in general. |
| Increased Dependence | Ensure that all interactions with the resident, whether they are treatment oriented or just social in nature, allow the resident real choices which make a difference in his/her life. |
| *Musculoskeletal Function* | |
| Muscular Atrophy | Activities which promote the frequent, repetitive use of many muscle groups. Atrophy of the muscle will be slowed only if the resident uses the muscle with adequate frequency and duration to promote strength and good circulation. Use appropriate precautions with residents who have arthritis. |
| Joint Stiffness | Activities which promote Range of Motion (passive, assisted or active depending on the resident's orders). |
| *Cardiovascular Function* | |
| Edema | Activities which promote the gentle movement of swollen area.<br>Proper positioning with frequent positioning changes during activity to facilitate good circulation. |
| *Respiratory Function* | |
| Slower, Shallower Respiration | Activities which encourage the resident to take deep breaths; coughing as needed to bring up secretions from the lungs.<br>Activities which promote the resident's turning from side to side in the bed to help with lung drainage. |
| *Gastrointestinal Function* | |
| Constipation | Since bedrest promotes constipation and fecal impaction, activities that promote sitting/bending at the waist, as well as leg movements to exercise the torso and muscles around the abdomen area.<br>Adequate fluids and proper diet (snacks during activity) to promote a healthy level of fluid intake and nitrogen balance. |
| *Decubitus Ulcers* | |
| Skin Break Downs | Activities that promote frequent and proper positioning for each resident depending on their needs and skin tolerance. |

**Behavior** The observable actions that an individual demonstrates during any type of activity.

**Behavior Modification Program** Behavior modification program (BMP) refers to a planned, systematic way of interacting with a resident and structuring the resident's environment to produce a desired change in the resident's behavior. There are many different types of BMPs which work. The two key elements are to select an age appropriate method and then to consistently implement the program.

**Behavior Problem** (RAI) Between 60% and 70% of residents in a typical nursing facility exhibit emotional, social and/or behavioral disorders; about 40% have purely behavioral problems (i.e., wandering, verbal abuse, physically aggressive and/or socially inappropriate behaviors). Residents with behavior problems also frequently have other related problems. Over 80% of those who have behavior problems will have some type of cognitive deficit; about 75% will have mood and/or relationship problems. Problem behaviors are often seen as a source of danger and distress to the residents themselves and sometimes to other residents and staff. Nursing facilities often find such residents difficult to cope with and physicians often seem unaware of the wide range of available treatment and management options. As a result, overuse of physical restraints or psychoactive drugs is too common. About one half of residents who exhibit "problem" behaviors will be physically restrained and about one half will receive psychoactive medications — antipsychotics (neuroleptics), antianxiety agents and to a lesser extent, antidepressants. These interventions, however, have potentially serious negative side-effects and many nurses in nursing facilities report being uncomfortable using only physical restraints and/or psychoactives to manage residents with behavior problems. As a result, there is an increasing trend toward using other interventions and treatment in addressing problem behaviors.

**Behavioral Lability** A resident's inability to regulate his/her moods and behaviors due to cognitive deficits. The resident may fluctuate between being confused/oriented, overly emotional/flat affect, emotional and behavioral outburst/calm, sexually inappropriate behavior/socially and sexually appropriate and fail to recognize behavior as inappropriate/able to recognize inappropriateness of behavior.

**Bowel and Bladder Disorders** The professional may encounter two specific disabilities associated with bowel and bladder disorders. While these disorders in and of themselves do not produce functional ability deficits, the care associated with these disorders cause a resident to experience life differently than his/her peers.

- **Constipation** is the term used to indicate hard bowel movements, pain upon defecation and abdominal cramping.
     Cause: There are three main causes of constipation:
     1. neurogenic bowels (lack of voluntary bowel control)
     2. inactivity
     3. medication side effects

     **Impact on Functional Ability:** Constipation is associated with the development of hemorrhoids (causing pain), increased abdominal discomfort, irritability and decreased appetite. An individual experiencing the discomfort associated with constipation will be less inclined to engage in leisure activity. Irritability induced by the discomfort of constipation may increase the incidence of behavioral outbursts. The ironic consequence is that frequently these individuals are then placed on (higher doses of) medications to control inappropriate behavior. Most of these medications have a side effect of constipation.

| Concern | Intervention |
|---|---|
| decreased activity | Motion through leisure activity is one of the best treatment modalities for constipation. |
| irritability | Prior to providing intervention through medications or other means of behavior modification the professional may want to recommend a trial period of two to three weeks of daily physical activities which are enjoyable to the resident. |
| constipation inducing diets | Provide educational sessions to help the resident identify the satisfying snacks that can be found at many different community recreation centers and which promote bowel health. |

- **Intestinal Ostomies** An ostomy is the surgical placement of an artificial opening from the intestines to the surface of the abdomen. An ostomy may either be a permanent or temporary solution to abnormalities or diseases of the intestine and anus. The bowel movements bypass part of the intestines, allowing the waste products to be collected in a self-adhesive bag (a pouching system). The stoma is the portion of the intestine which is placed outside of the surface of the skin forming the ostomy opening. The stoma has a raw, red to pink appearance though it is not painful. (Intestinal tissue does not sense pain due to the lack of pain receptors.)

**Causes:** A variety of anatomical and neurological disorders require the placement of an ostomy. The most common reasons for an ostomy to be placed in children and youth is either a congenital (from birth) malformation of the anal/rectal structure or Hirschsprung disease (lack of nerves in the intestine to help push along waste). The combined occurrence of Hirschsprung disease or anatomical malformation is approximately one in five thousands live births. Placement in older adults may be due to intestinal cancer.

**Impact on Functional Ability:** The wearing of a pouching system seldom limits physical activity. Swimming is even possible as long as the pouching system is leak free and secured with water proof tape. The collection of gas is common and the resident should be taught how to release gas if s/he is cognitively and physically able to. Adolescents are somewhat put off by having an ostomy and pouching system as the wearing of tight clothing is counter-indicated. Tight pants cause the stoma to become irritated and bleed. Adolescents or adults with poor self-esteem tend to sabotage their pouching system allowing it to leak and smell, increasing the alienation of his/her peers.

| Concerns | Intervention |
|---|---|
| leakage/smell | The bag may leak due to poor technique in applying the bag or due to activity induced dislodgment. Since the smell has obvious social isolation potential, the professional may want to both 1. assess the type of activity and movement which compromises the integrity of the seal and 2. either work with nursing to modify the system (preferable) or work with the resident to modify the activity. |
| skin integrity | The small intestines have 3 primary sections: 1. the duodenum, 2. the jejunum (jejunostomy) and 3. the ileum (ileostomy). An ostomy placed in the large intestines is called a colostomy. The higher up in the intestinal system the ostomy is, the more erosive and fluid the bowel movement is. A leaking ileostomy is at the greatest risk of causing a skin breakdown. Therapy intervention is the same as for leakage/smell concerns. |
| poor self-esteem | Develop self-esteem through successful completion of activity and through self-esteem programs. |

**Brady Kinesia** An abnormal slowness of movement; a sluggishness of a resident's physical or cognitive response.

**Brainstem** The part of the brain that controls breathing, heart beat and involuntary functions. Also known as the Medulla. The brainstem is near the back, lower part of the brain.

**Budget** A budget is the written document which shows how much money (and other resources) will be used during a specific time period (usually a year). A department's operating budget usually provides an overview of where the department will get money (revenue) as well as where the money will be spent (allocation/expenses). Income for activity departments and social service departments in long term care facilities usually comes from three sources: room rate (Medicare and private insurance), donations and earned income (from arts and crafts sales, etc.).

**Capital Expenditure** An expenditure of money for the new purchase or replacement of a room, a building or large, expensive pieces of equipment and/or the development or expansion of services.

**Cardiorespiratory Endurance** The ability of both the heart and lungs to move oxygen efficiently enough to muscle groups to allow normal activity with reasonable endurance over a period of time. May be increased with the systematic use of leisure activities which stress the heart and other muscle tissues usually at least three times a week and without causing undue fatigue. Cardiorespiratory endurance can be significantly hindered when the resident has second and third degree burns or skin breakdowns to the anterior trunk area. After consultation with the physician, the professional may want to encourage the resident's daily involvement in leisure activities which involve diaphragmatic breathing. Fun activities involving the blowing around balloons suspended from overhead or a game of air hockey using a ping pong ball on a table are good places to begin.

**Care Conference** The meeting during which a resident's status is discussed. During this meeting the resident's needs and strengths are outlined or updated, priorities for intervention and service agreed upon and specific outcomes with anticipated dates are determined. The individuals attending the care conference may include the resident and his/her family, nursing, therapists (recreational, occupational, physical, speech — as needed by the resident), Activity Professional, dietitian, physician and Social Service Professional. The length of time spent on each resident may vary depending on the severity/complexity of the resident's needs, the frequency that conferences are held (daily, weekly, monthly, quarterly) and whether the resident and/or family members are present. A care conference may last for as short a time as 5 minutes or as long as 90 minutes for each resident. The shorter care conferences which typically take place on the unit are called "Rounds." When presenting information on a resident during a care conference the staff need to provide the others with information in a clear, concise and condensed manner. Present enough information to get the information across, no more. (The information presented should be found in the progress notes prior to the meeting.) The other members of the team will let you know when they need more information or further clarification. A typical format for presentation might be: 1. presentation of specific problem/need, 2. short summary of reasons why there is a need/problem and 3. what action the professional and/or resident will need to take.

**Care Plan** The written document which outlines how the staff are going to address the resident's measured (assessed) needs. This plan is usually interdisciplinary with stated needs/concerns, specific objectives, treatment plans and services to be delivered to complete the objectives and the anticipated date of completion. The needs/concerns are frequently prioritized and state which staff or disciplines are responsible for monitoring the resident's status.

**Caretaker/Caregiver** In a broad sense, any one involved in the delivery of a resident's health care. It is usually applied to individuals (community workers, paraprofessionals and/or nurses' aides) who provide these services in the community setting.

**CARF** see *Commission on Accreditation of Rehabilitation Facilities.*

**Case History** A summary of the resident's background including information about who, what, where, when and why of a person's past (including any pertinent treatment). When a case history is presented, it usually follows a specific outline:

> (Name of resident) is a (age) year old (male/female) with (list of primary diagnoses — the diagnoses which impact the resident's treatment). Resident was admitted to (service, facility, program) on (list date) and had (list scores of assessments, results of lab work or other important measurements where were taken during the assessment process). (State a brief outline of services/treatments given to resident). Resident has responded (give outcome of services and therapy).

**Case Mix** (OBRA Survey State Operations Manual) When a survey team evaluates a facility, they have a set equation which they follow to determine which resident's care plans and charts to review. This sample includes residents with a variety of care needs to determine compliance with all Quality of Care requirements. There are four categories in a case mix: *Case Group A*: interviewable residents who are relatively physically independent (light care); *Case Group B*: Interviewable residents who are relatively physically dependent (heavy care); *Case Group C*: Non-interviewable residents who require staff supervision or cueing to maintain independent functioning but do not require extensive or total staff assistance to perform activities of daily living (non-interviewable — light care) and *Case Group D*: Non-interviewable residents who require extensive or total assistance to perform activities of daily living (non-interviewable — heavy care). The residents chosen as part of the sample are selected after the orientation tour. The surveyors are to include, if possible: an officer of the resident council, a resident under 55 years of age, a resident initially admitted to the facility during the month preceding the survey and a resident with mental retardation or metal illness.

**Catastrophic Responses** A sudden and unexpected negative reaction to an event — an extreme overreaction. An example would be the complete emotional collapse of an individual upon hearing that s/he was going to be laid off from work.

**Census** The term used to indicate the number of residents currently admitted to the program or facility.

**Cerebral Palsy** (CP) refers to a chronic neurological disorder developed prenatally, at birth or shortly thereafter. A resident with CP has anatomically normal muscles and nerves. The disability originates in the brain's inability to control these muscles and nerves.

The two primary functions impacted by CP are motor and communication. The range of functional impairment varies from resident to resident and, depending upon the location of the damaged brain cells, the resident may have one or more of the following (Blackman 1990): 1. Spasticity (60%), 2. Dyskinesia (20%), 3. Ataxia (1%), 4. Mixed (30%).

> **Spasticity:** When there is damage to the motor cortex (surface of the brain) or damage to the nerves originating on the surface of the brain and passing through either the corticospinal or pyramidal tracks to the spinal cord, the resident will experience a stiffness of his/her muscles. This stiffness is called hypertonia and produces a slowed response.

> **Dyskinesia:** When there is damage to the basal ganglia (which controls motor function) the resident will experience uncontrolled, jerky movements of his/her body. These jerky movements increase when the resident actively tries to execute a controlled movement or when the resident is experiencing emotional stress. Certain body postures will also increase the resident's tone and decrease function. There are three primary types of dyskinesia: 1. athetosis, 2. choreoathetosis and 3. dystonia. "Athetosis" refers to a slow, writhing movement. Athetosis has a marked impact on activities as it affects the hand's and wrist's ability to perform desired movements. The "jerky" abrupt movements seen with this disorder are called "choreoathetosis." Uncontrolled, rhythmic movements are called "dystonia."

**Ataxia:** When there is damage to the cerebellum the resident will exhibit an abnormal gait. Activities that requires a narrow stanced gait (gymnastics), smooth movements (some forms of dance) and good balance (ice skating, skiing) are usually very difficult for residents with ataxia.

**Mixed:** About a third of the residents with CP have damage to more than one area of the brain and therefore exhibit multiple movement disorders.

| Concern: | Intervention |
|---|---|
| muscles/joint contractures | While the neurological damage causing CP is not progressive, its negative impact on the elasticity of the muscles is. The professional should help the resident develop a leisure repertoire which promotes the full ROM of all affected muscles and joints (either through passive and/or active movement). These leisure activities should be varied enough to allow this ROM a minimum of 4x a day. |
| positioning | Ensure that all leisure activities and equipment are modified to reduce spasticity and encourage good posture. |
| constipation | A resident who uses a wheelchair, which reduces activity, has an increased change of having chronic constipation. Encourage out-of-chair gross motor activities on a daily basis. |
| vision, seizures and hearing impairments | Monitor for vision, seizure and hearing impairments. Approximately 50% of the residents with CP also have visual impairments, 45% have a seizure disorder and a smaller percentage have a hearing impairment. |
| developmental delays/MR | Prescriptive activities to increase muscle control and coordination and a purposeful program to encourage normalizing experiences will help increase muscle control later in life and will decrease developmental delays due to physical disability. Approximately 70% of residents with CP (especially those with spastic diplegia) also are mentally retarded. |

**Cerebral Embolism** An occlusion or blockage of a cerebral artery; a type of stroke.

**Cerebral Hemorrhage** The rupturing of a cerebral vessel with bleeding into the brain tissues; a type of stroke.

**Cerebral Thrombosis** The formation of a blood clot within a cerebral artery, leading to an occlusion of the vessel; a type of stroke.

**Cerebrovascular Accident** (CVA) Stroke. Restricted blood supply to some part of the brain.

**Certified Nursing Assistant (CNA)** An individual who has passed the requirements of the state in which s/he works. These requirements usually involve taking both a written and a skill test in the basics of resident care, documentation, infection control and resident rights. The types of decisions that CNA may make independent of a nurse are very limited — they are to be supervised by a nurse, following orders for resident care.

**Certified Therapeutic Recreation Specialist** An individual formally trained in the field of therapeutic recreation (recreational therapy) and credentialed by the National Council for Therapeutic Recreation Certification.

**Chairbound** (OBRA) In the United States this refers to residents who depend on a chair for mobility. This includes residents who can stand with assistance to pivot from bed to wheelchair or to otherwise transfer. The resident cannot take steps without extensive or consistent weight-bearing support from others.

**Chronic** Referring to long term — is not expected to be resolved soon.

**Chronic Obstructive Pulmonary Disease (COPD)** Resident's with COPD may experience asthma, bronchitis and emphysema as a result of this chronic disease. Most residents will be able to tolerate gradually increasing light to moderate activity and exercise as long as there are frequent, regular opportunities for activity (e.g., two 10 minute sessions or four five minute sessions five times a week). The resident will probably experience an improved quality of life if the professional helps the resident increase his/her muscular strength and endurance along with his/her cardiovascular conditioning, even though such activity may not change the course of the disease. Because of the amount and depth of breathing required with many upper body/arm exercise activities, the professional may find that lower body exercises (e.g., walking) are a superior option for residents with COPD. Always clear the resident's activity with his/her physician first.

**Chronic Stage** The third and last stage of healing, maturation and remodeling after an injury or illness is called the chronic stage. For injuries to the musculoskeletal system there are two subclassifications within the chronic stage. The first involves an injury after the 21st day, when inflammation is no longer present but when the resident's functional ability has not returned to normal. The second involves a continuous state of pain or recurring episodes of pain with a suboptimal return to the resident's normal functional ability. The collagen fibers which are thickening as a result of the injury will not mature for up to 14 weeks. Up to that time the fibers and scar tissue are able to be remodeled through therapeutic activity to lessen the severity of the disability. After around 14 weeks the scar tissue resists remodeling and stretching may only be achieved through surgery or the adaptive (over) lengthening of the tissues surrounding the scar. The over lengthening of tissue around the scar should be done only under the direction of a physician or a physical therapist. (See *Acute Stage* and *Subacute Stage*.)

**Claustrophobia** The fear of being closed in or in a small room/space based on non-rational thoughts.

**Clinical Decision Making** Decisions about resident care and the types of services provided based on assessed resident needs, standards of practice, research findings and institutional policies. Diagnoses and treatment protocols based on established scientific evidence, are two kinds of clinical decision making. When the therapist, using his or her knowledge base and experience, but without supporting evidence from research, makes a decision, it is called a clinical opinion.

**Clinical Opinion** The belief or ideas that a professional holds regarding a resident. This opinion may be based on the use of tests and measurements and on the professional's experience and training but cannot be directly supported by evidence relating to those tests and measurements. Clinical opinions should be based on the therapist's evaluation of all available information; clinical decisions based on a therapist's synthesis of information are based on clinical opinions. (Rothstein, et al. 1990, page 925)

**Cochlea** The snail shell shaped tube which forms part of the inner ear.

**Cognition** The brain's ability to process information is what is usually considered "cognition." Obviously it takes quite a few different skills and processes to take in information; identify, classify and organize the information; and to then be able to retrieve that information in a manner that can be used. While there are many different philosophies about what cognition is, the professional will find it useful to group cognition into three functional aspects: 1. information *processes* (which includes the resident's ability to attend to the information being received, understand the information received, remember the information and organize the information to allow for reasoning and problem solving), 2. information *systems* (which includes a resident's ability to utilize his/her memory in a functional manner (both long and short term memory) and being able to utilize executive function skills based on learned information and reasoning) and 3. information *integration* (which includes the resident's ability to use his/her information processes and information systems to interact with the environment around him/her in a meaningful and functional manner).

**Cognitive Deficits** An inability to perform normal cognitive functions (e.g., judgment, problem solving, communication, interpretation of environmental stimuli, insight, ability to follow commands, memory, abstract thought, attention span, etc.).

**Cognitive Retraining** The systematic use of teaching methods to help an individual relearn information after an illness or accident. When a resident loses information that s/he once knew, it is not just a simple task of relearning the information. Frequently the part of the brain that held the information is permanently damaged or changed and cannot relearn the information in the way that it did before. The staff will need to help develop a compensatory strategy for each resident which helps him/her overcome the loss of previously known information. A resident needs to regain many cognitive skills, including the basic skill of recognizing that s/he has a deficit. Other areas of cognitive retraining include generalization training, sequential thought training, processing and filtering training, problem-solving skills, etc.

**Cognitive Stimulation** The purposeful exercising of an individual's thinking skills.

**Cohort** A term used to identify groups of individuals who have many life events and interests in common. Men who grew up in the United States during the depression, who fought together in W.W.II, then engaged in similar activities after the war (e.g., fraternal organizations) would be a cohort group.

**Coma** An abnormal state of consciousness where all or most of the resident's cognitive processes, voluntary behavior and even reflexes are diminished. The most common way to refer to a resident's depth of coma is by referring to the resident's Glasgow Coma Scale score. See *Glasgow Coma Scale*.

**Commission on Accreditation of Rehabilitation Facilities (CARF)** CARF is a private (non-government) accrediting agency which promotes the provision of quality care to residents. The primary rehabilitation services that are credentialed by CARF are comprehensive inpatient rehabilitation, spinal cord injury programs, chronic pain management programs, brain injury programs, outpatient medical rehabilitation and work hardening programs. CARF's address is 101 North Wilmot Road, Suite 500, Tucson, Arizona 85711.

**Communication** (RAI) Good communication enables residents to express emotion, listen to others and share information. It also eases adjustment to a strange environment and lessens social isolation and depression. *Expressive communication* problems include changes/difficulties in: speech and voice production, finding appropriate words, transmitting coherent statements, describing objects and events, using nonverbal symbols (e.g., gestures) and writing. *Receptive communication* problems include changes/difficulties in: hearing, speech discrimination in quiet and noisy situations, vocabulary comprehension, vision, reading and interpreting facial expression. When communication is limited, the resident's assessment should focus on reviewing several factors: underlying causes of the deficit, the success of attempted remedial actions, the resident's ability to compensate with nonverbal strategies (e.g., ability to visually observe nonverbal signs and signals) and the willingness and ability of staff to work with residents to ensure effective communication. As language use recedes with dementia, both staff and the resident must expand their nonverbal communication skills — one of the most basic and automatic of human abilities. Touch, facial expression, eye contact, tone of voice and posture all are powerful means of communicating with the resident with dementia and recognizing and using all practical means is the key to effective communication.

**Communication Board** A board, book or other flat item on which pictures and words/phrases are presented/attached. Individuals who are not able to talk may use a communication board to communicate with caretakers and friends. These boards are very primitive and limited in their nature — allowing the user a very limited means to communicate. All residents with communication boards need extra time scheduled with staff to allow communication broader then the words on the board to take place. If this time is not scheduled on a regular basis, the resident is at an increased risk of depression and sensory deprivation.

**Compensatory Skill** The ability to successfully complete a task using methods which overcome a disability. An example would be an individual with the ability to use sign language (a compensatory skill) to communicate.

**Comprehension** The ability to understand thoughts, ideas and actions.

**Compulsive** The feeling that one *must* act and then taking action before one has thought through the consequences of one's action.

**Concentration** Concentration is the ability to ignore unrelated noises, sounds and thoughts while being able to attend to the task (or thought) at hand. Concentration problems are the result of an inability to focus (visually and cognitively) and to maintain that attention. Functional skills in concentration and attention are required for mental tracking skills such as information processing, pathfinding and other executive functions.

**Concrete Thinking** The ability to understand simple, straight forward ideas or actions. Concrete thinking accepts things just as they are — with little logical thought process of how they got there or why they exist. It is less complex than abstract thinking. The concept of "leisure" or "free-time" is an abstract concept. Asking residents with cognitive impairments what they do for leisure or free time may too complex of a question if they tend to think concretely. Asking those residents if they like to play cards, walk through a mall or plant flowers is a concrete approach to determining a resident's leisure preferences.

**Confabulation** Telling false information without intending to deceive. Unintentional lying.

**Confidentiality** To keep secret; not to share information with those who do not have the right to know. In health care there are strict laws concerning a resident's right to confidentiality. The professional must keep four areas of resident information confidential: 1. the resident's identity, 2. the resident's physical or psychological condition, 3. the resident's emotional status and 4. the resident's financial situation. Confidentiality not only includes who you can talk to about which resident, but also where you may talk. You may not discuss a resident's confidential information where another person who should not hear, can hear. That means that discussing aspects of a resident's care in the elevator, lunch room, restaurant or other locations may not be acceptable. There are only a few situations which allow for the professional to share information without prior approval. The Activity or Social Service Professional may break confidentiality only if s/he is reporting on a medical emergency, reporting on suspected or known abuse, reporting required information on a communicable disease to the health department or when required to for litigation or administrative activities.

**Consent** Voluntary agreement by a resident or representative of an incapacitated resident to accept a treatment or procedure. **Informed consent** is the voluntary agreement by a resident or a representative of an incapacitated resident to accept a treatment or procedure after receiving all information that is material to their decision concerning whether to accept or refuse any proposed treatment or procedure. Three conditions must be met. The resident must:
1.  be capable (or represented by a legally recognized representative),
2.  receive all the necessary information to make an intelligent decision and
3.  not be coerced.

**Conservator** A method to assume control over financial and/or personal affairs for individuals who are determined to be incompetent or disabled to the point of not being able to assume reasonable control themselves. The area of competency is complicated and there is no one standard definition of it as a general legal term. Each state sets their own standard. Ultimately, however, the courts rule on "competency" and assign the conservator.

**Contracture** The reduction of normal mobility and/or flexibility of a body part caused by a shortening or tightening of the skin, fascia, muscle or joint capsule (Kisner and Colby, 1990 page 684). Contractures may be caused by immobility, injury or scarring and, depending on the cause and degree of involvement, may require surgery to correct. The professional's best approach to contractures (especially in long term care settings) is prevention. Assisting the resident in identifying enjoyable leisure activities which allow the daily range of motion of all body parts during various activities reduces the chance of contracture development.

**Coordination** The ability to perform tasks using more than one body part or function in a harmonious manner. To coordinate multiple functions to achieve a desired outcome.

**COPD** see *Chronic Obstructive Pulmonary Disease.*

**Counsel** A general term used to indicate that one individual is helping another individual: 1. identify and define a problem, 2. develop a vision of what it would look like to solve the problem and 3. determine the decisions to be made, skills to be developed and 4. actions to be taken to resolve the problem. A counselor provides information meant to alleviate the emotional strain surrounding placement of a resident in a long term care facility. Counseling may consist of a one time visit to explain the logistics of placement or may involve ongoing contact providing the opportunity for a resident or family to express feelings of loss, sadness, depression, anger and acceptance. There are many different theories and methods used by therapists to help an individual achieve the desired changes and results.

**Counter Indicated** Means that a treatment or action should not be taken because the situation does not call for it, in fact, the treatment or action may actually make the resident's condition worse.

**Cueing** Prompting, usually with words or gestures, for the purpose of stimulating an activity.

**Culture** A group of people who share common origins, customs and living styles. This group usually also shares a common language and has a general sense of common identity. This shared lifestyle and identity help develop a sense of group values, expectations, beliefs and perceptions. Rituals tend to be shared by the group for all major life events from birth to death.

**Curiosity** The desire to find new or novel objects, experiences and thoughts. This desire to experience part or all of one's environment is a critical component to new learning. To be able to demonstrate curiosity, the individual must have: 1. an awareness that his/her environment exists, 2. a knowledge that s/he can influence and interact with the environment, 3. the ability to recognize something as novel, 4. the desire to experience the novel and 5. the ability to derive pleasure from the experience.

**Custodial Care** The care given to individuals who are not capable to meet their own basic needs.

**Data** The assignment of numerical values or symbols to help facilitate the evaluation of an event over a predetermined period of time. The information collected is based on a predetermined set of criteria which describes what is to be measured.

**d/c** Discontinue treatment.

**Decision Making** The process of selecting one option or item over another. This requires the ability to recognize the purpose and use of each option/item, picture the consequences of using each one and weighing the pro's and con's of the possible outcomes of using one against the other(s). (RAI) The resident's ability to make everyday decisions about the tasks or activities of daily living. Examples of daily decisions may be choosing items of clothing; determining mealtimes; using environmental cues to organize and plan (e.g., clocks, calendars, posted listing of upcoming events); using awareness of one's own strength in regulating the day's events (e.g., ask for help when necessary).

**Deconditioning** A decrease in the combined ability of the circulatory system, cognition, neuromuscular movement and metabolic system to function as a direct result of prolonged immobility and/or bedrest (usually two weeks or longer). This decrease is a direct result of inactivity and not a result of an injury or illness. Typical loss of abilities may include:

1. decreased brain wave activity caused by bedrest or chair rest (which produces the same EEG patterns as individuals placed in environments which promote sensory deprivation)
2. noted decrease in cognitive ability including verbal fluency, color discrimination, reversible figures, distorted awareness of time
3. potential decrease in thermoregulation
4. noted increase in anxiety, irritability, depression and possible hallucinatory experiences
5. decrease in balance (after 2 to 3 weeks on bedrest)
6. increase in resting heart rate (by the end of 3 weeks morning heart rate can increase by 21%, evening by 33% or an average of 1 heart beat per 2 days of bedrest)
7. decrease in oxygen uptake (anticipated 15 to 30% decrease in uptake after just 3 weeks bedrest). (from burlingame and Blaschko, 1990, page 3)

**Delirium** A state of cognitive dysfunction where the resident appears confused, has a decreased ability to attend to stimuli in the environment and may experience a disconnection with reality (from a mild inability to correctly interpret events to full hallucinations). Delirium may mimic other types of organically caused brain disorders, however, delirium and dementia are not the same thing. (RAI) Delirium (acute confusional state) is a common indicator or nonspecific symptom of a variety of acute, treatable illnesses. It is a serious problem with high rates of morbidity and mortality, unless it is recognized and treated appropriately. Delirium is never a part of normal aging. Some of the classic signs of delirium may be difficult to recognize and may be mistaken for the natural progression of dementia, particularly in the late stages of dementia when delirium has high mortality. Thus careful observation of the resident and review of potential cause are essential. Delirium is characterized by fluctuating states of consciousness, disorientation, decreased environmental awareness and behavioral changes. The onset of delirium may vary, depending on the severity of the cause(s) and the resident's health status; however, it usually develops rapidly, over a few days or even hours. Even with successful treatment of cause(s) and associated symptoms, it may take several weeks before cognitive abilities return to pre-delirium status.

**Dementia** An illness or condition which is observed by a progressive loss of intellectual functions. The resident will demonstrate an up and down course of cognitive ability on a day to day and even hour to hour basis with an overall decrease in ability month by month. The ability to use information stored in memory will decrease, as will the resident's ability to exercise good judgment, executive function and abstract thinking. Family members are usually the first to identify dementia because they notice a change in the resident's personality and an increased trend to be "forgetful." Dementia, in the past was usually referred to as senile onset (after the age of 65) or presenile onset (under the age of 65). Since the term "senile" is no longer politically correct, the terms "early onset" (before age 65) and "late onset" (after age 65) are now used. Dementia does not include a loss of cognitive ability due to delirium or depression — although both may mimic aspects of dementia. (RAI) Approximately 60% of residents in nursing facilities exhibit signs and symptoms of decline in intellectual functioning. Recovery will be possible for less than 10% of these residents — those with a reversible condition such as an acute confusional state (delirium). For most resident, however, the syndrome of cognitive loss or dementia is chronic and progressive and appropriate care focuses on enhancing quality of life sustaining functional capabilities, minimizing decline and preserving dignity. Confusion and/or behavioral disturbances present the primary complicating care factors. Identifying and treating acute confusion and behavior problems can facilitate assessment of how chronic cognitive deficits affect the life of the resident. For residents with chronic cognitive deficits, a therapeutic environment is supportive rather than curative and is an environment in which licensed and non-licensed care staff are encourage (and trained) to comprehend a resident's experience of cognitive loss. With this insight, staff can develop care plans focused on three main goals: 1. to provide positive experiences for the resident (e.g., enjoyable activities) that do not involve overly demanding tasks and stress; 2. to define appropriate support roles for each staff member involved in a resident's care; and 3. to lay foundation for reasonable staff and family expectations concerning a resident's capacities and needs.

**Dependence** The state of having to rely on another person or a object for emotional support (love, security, definition of self), physical support (ambulation, feeding, dressing, etc.) or cognitive support (reminders, language, problem solving, etc.). There is a psychiatric diagnosis termed *dependent personality disorder*. This diagnosis refers to an individual who passively allows others to make most of the decisions for him/her. Individuals who have dependent personality disorder tend to lack an awareness of the skills they possess to take care of themselves and also a lack of self-esteem/self-confidence in the abilities that they do acknowledge they have. Health care workers can help decrease a resident's likelihood of developing dependent personality disorder not only by allowing a resident to take care of him/herself as much as possible but by supportively encouraging the resident to do so.

**Dependent Position** Referring to the relaxed position of a limb which is hanging downward, held in place by gravity.

**Depression** A feeling of sadness or grief. In residents with strokes, this depression can be psychological or physiological. Studies have found that over 50% of residents with stroke have clinical depression. The closer the stroke to the left frontal pole of the brain, the greater risk for severe depression. Without intervention, this depression will normally last 9 to 12 months.

**Deprivation** The removal or reduction of a desirable or positive object or stimulus. The human body is meant to be bombarded with sensory input from all senses during the waking hours. A short period of sensory deprivation can be very therapeutic for individuals who frequently experience high levels of stimulation. Relaxation techniques are a healthy, self-initiated type of sensory deprivation. For individuals who are restricted to environments that provide an unhealthy sensory environment (e.g., hospitals, nursing homes, other residential institutions), one of the most important treatment interventions for the professional is to offset the harm done by the lack of healthy stimulation in the environment. A resident will be at an increased risk to develop delirium and other cognitive disorders after as little as two days in a sensory unhealthy environment. Fred Rogers ("Mr. Rogers") goes as far as to suggest that every person would be healthier if they were exposed to the natural stimulation found out of doors one to two hours a day, every day of the year.

**Diabetes** Also known as Diabetes Mellitus. A disorder in the body's production and use of insulin and in the body's use of blood sugar (resulting in a high blood glucose level). Diabetes has both short term and long term consequences. Individual with diabetes have a disorder which causes the abnormal metabolism of carbohydrates, fats and proteins. Diabetes Mellitus is divided into three groups: 1. insulin independent also known as "Type II" (the vast majority of individuals), 2. insulin dependent also known as "Type I" and 3. Maturity-onset diabetes of youth, also known as "MODY." All three types of diabetes mellitus are treated through use of an appropriately balanced diet, exercise and, in the case of individuals who are insulin dependent, insulin. There are a few diseases which are a direct result of diabetes mellitus that the professional may want to be familiar with:
1. Macrovascular Disease is the development of enlarged blood vessels. This enlargement effects the metabolism of carbohydrates leading to a significantly increased likelihood of a stroke (CVA) or an increased likelihood of a heart attack.
2. Microvascular Disease is a disorder of the smaller blood vessels in the body. Individuals with diabetes millitus may develop problems with nephropathy (disease of the kidneys), retinopathy (ongoing damage to the small vessels which provide blood to the eyes) and neuropathy (degenerative/pathological changes in the peripheral nervous system which decreases function).

| Concern | Implications |
|---|---|
| decreased ability to assimilate sugars | Exercise is an important component of treatment for individuals with diabetes millitus. To help assist in the balancing of the insulin hormone in the body, the individual should develop a balanced pattern of leisure activities using physical movements. This balance allows for easier control of diet replaced insulin and helps avoid ketoacidosis (serious imbalance of insulin in the body causing dehydration, electrolyte imbalance, acidosis, coma and then death). |
| insulin dependent vs. activity | Insulin is absorbed faster in muscles which are used extensively (therefore putting individual's who depend on insulin therapy at greater risk of depleting the insulin too quickly). The professional may want to evaluate the muscle groups used in any newly learned leisure activity to ensure that any significant increase in the activity of muscles near the typical injection site are not going to increase activity to the area enough to increase risk. A simple solution is to arrange for the insulin site to be changed. |
| decreased sensation | The professional should assess the degree to which decreased sensation in the lower extremities caused by Macrovascular disease will increase the individual's risk during activities. Ill fitted shoes, extreme water or air temperatures or breaks in skin integrity could be hazardous. If there is also a diagnosis of mental retardation or traumatic brain injury, then the individual is at extreme risk. |

**Diagnosis** The art and science of distinguishing one disease or disability from another. Most diagnoses have commonly known, standardized definitions for what symptoms are present (and not present). Once a diagnosis has been assigned, the treatment team will be able to work with a common understanding of the resident's needs, limitations and strengths based on the listed diagnoses. The professional will find it extremely helpful to read the **DSM IV (Diagnostic and Statistical Manual of Mental Disorders, Fourth Edition)** published by the American Psychiatric Association. This book lists the functional skills lacking in individuals with each disorder. After confirming with the DSM IV it may be easier for the professional to formulate assessment plans and treatment objectives. The other publication which lists the standardized definitions is the **ICD 9 CM (International Classification of Diseases 9th Edition Clinical Modification)** published by the US Department of Health and Human Services.

**Diagnostic and Statistical Manual of Mental Disorders, Fourth Edition.** A book published by the American Psychiatric Association which describes the criteria for all psychiatric diagnoses.

**Diet - Prescribed** There are seven primary groupings of diet types prescribed for patients. It is important that the therapist is aware of the type of diet prescribed for each patient, as well as specific dietary and fluid restrictions. See the chart on the following page.

**Dignity** (OBRA) Federal law in the United States requires that all staff treat residents in long term care facilities with dignity. This means that in their interactions with residents, staff carry out activities which assist the resident to maintain and enhance his/her self-worth. For example:
- Grooming residents as they wish to be groomed (e.g., hair combed, beards shaved/trimmed, nails clean and clipped);
- Assisting residents to dress in their own clothes appropriate to the time of day and individual preferences;
- Promoting resident independence and dignity in dining (such as avoidance of day-to-day use of plastic cutlery and paper/plastic dishware, dining room conducive to pleasant dining, aides not yelling);

**Common Types of Prescribed Diets**

| Type | Description |
|------|-------------|
| **Clear Liquid** | A diet limited to liquids that are clear including water, clear broth, clear fruit juices, plain gelatin, tea and coffee. Check to see if caffeine or carbonation is allowed. |
| **Full Liquid** | Thick fluids including different kinds of juices (including pureed vegetable and fruit juices), milk, ice cream, gelatin, custards and other non-alcoholic drinks that generally accompany a meal. |
| **Light or Convalescent** | This diet may include most foods, the difference is in how the food is prepared. Raw and fried foods are usually not allowed. Foods that are high in fat, which produce fat or which are hard to digest are not allowed. |
| **Mechanical Soft** | Similar to the light or convalescent diet, this food differs only in that it needs to be prepared for those individuals who are not likely to be able to chew the food (e.g., those with no teeth). Most forms of meat are avoided unless it can be prepared in such a manner as to not require chewing. |
| **Regular or General** | A diet which allows most kinds of foods, provides a balanced nutritional intake, one which the patient has some selection as to the meals make up and which will add up to 1400 calories in every 24 hour period. |
| **Special Therapeutic** | A diet which is selected to meet the patient's specific needs due to allergies, caloric intake (high or low), diabetes or those needing reduced amounts of specific types of food (e.g., reduced salt, fat, fiber, high or low protein). |

- Respecting resident's private space and property (e.g., not changing radio or television station without resident's permission);
- Respecting resident's social status, speaking respectfully, listening carefully, treating residents with respect (e.g., addressing the resident with a name of the resident's choice); and
- Focusing on residents as individuals when they talk to them. (Guidance to Surveyors, Tag F241)

**Diminished** The loss of a previously gained skill or skills. Individuals with dementia have diminished cognitive skills.

**Directionality** The skill to be able to determine direction — where you just came from, the way back, the way to the activity room; an element of both short and long term memory.

**Director of Nursing Services** The nurse who is the manager over the nursing services in a facility.

**Disability** (ADA) Legally defined, disability means, with respect to an individual, a physical or mental impairment that substantially limits one or more of the major life activities of such an individual; that there is a record of such an impairment; or being regarded as having such an impairment. The term disability does not include 1. transvestitism, transsexualism, pedophilia, exhibitionism, voyeurism, gender identity disorders not resulting from physical impairments or other sexual behavior disorders, 2. compulsive gambling, kleptomania or pyromania; or 3. psychoactive substance use disorders resulting from current illegal use of drugs.

**Discharge** 1. The act of terminating a resident's active status of receiving services. 2. A drainage of fluids from an opening in the body.

**Discharge Summary** A discharge summary is a report that the professional writes when s/he will no longer be treating the resident. This report may be seen by another health care professional the same day that the report is written or it may be reviewed by a health care professional years later. To help make the discharge summary useful and easy to understand, it is recommend that:
- Whenever possible, refer to the specific instead of the general; be concrete instead of abstract.
- Take care with what you say and how you say it. Avoid fancy or obscure words, abbreviations or words which overstate. Avoid qualifiers such as "rather, very, little, pretty."

- When you write be clear, document sequentially. Be brief but do not take short cuts thus leaving out key information.
- Whenever possible, write your statements describing what the resident could do, rather that what s/he couldn't, e.g., "resident was able to ambulate 45 feet between stores before needing to rest" rather than "resident was not able to ambulate 100 feet before needing to rest." The second sentence leaves the reader wondering if the resident completely lacked ambulation skills or if the resident could go 45 feet before needing a rest — two very different cases. While being positive, do not be reluctant to provide realistic or negative findings. ("Resident was unable to ambulate at time of discharge," is an acceptable statement.)
- If the treatment was as a result of a referral, make sure that all issues addressed in the referral are answered in the discharge summary.
- It will not be helpful to future readers of the discharge summary if you include just raw data from your assessments. Include a concise interpretation of all data presented.
- Whenever you make a recommendation, make sure that the justification for that recommendation can be found in your discharge summary.
- Without being long winded, include an alternative recommendation or an alternative course of action, if it is appropriate for the situation.
- Make your recommendations realistic for the resident, his/her cultural, social and economic background and for his/her discharge destination.
- Remember that the discharge summary is just that, a summary. All of the information presented should be brought together in a way that presents the entire picture of all the pertinent information.

**Disease Model** (also known as Medical Model) The theory that states the origin of most psychiatric disorders can be found in disease states. This is generally the opposite of the Behavioral Model which looks at psychological disorders more as a behavioral or thought pattern dysfunction and not a disease state.

**Disease State** Having a disease.

**Disenfranchised** The feeling of being separate from one's culture.

**Disengagement Theory** A theory on aging that was popular in the 1960's which concluded that as a person aged, s/he tended to withdraw from the community and social systems in his/her preparation to die.

**Disorientation** The temporary (due to drugs, alcohol, etc.) or permanent (due to dementia, CVAs, etc.) inability to understand and use informational stimuli in one's environment. This disorientation may be divided into three areas: 1. the inability to tell and use time (time of day, time of year, time of life, etc.) (*temporal*), 2. the inability to distinguish between and use both visual and non visual information (e.g. proprioception, a mental map of where one is in relationship to room, etc.) (*spatial*) and 3. the inability to cognitively process events in the environment and/or identify objects (including oneself) (*contextual*).

**Distal** Opposite of close; away from the center or midline of the body. The fingers are more distal to the chest than the shoulder.

**Dorsiflexion** Moving a body part closer to the center plane of the body by flexing or bending. To dorsiflex the foot, the resident would flex the toes toward the body. To dorsiflex the hand, the resident would cock his/her hand back over the wrist, exposing the palm.

**Dressing** (OBRA) This refers to the resident's ability to put on, fasten and take off all items of street clothing, including donning or removing prostheses (e.g., brace and artificial limbs). In the United States many facilities routinely set out clothes for all residents. If this is the case and this is the only assistance the resident receives, the resident is still considered to be independent in dressing. However, if a resident receives assistance with donning a brace, elastic stocking, a prosthesis and so on, securing fasteners or putting a garment on, this residents is counted as needing assistance in dressing.

**DSM IV** see *Diagnostic and Statistical Manual of Mental Disorders Fourth Edition.*

**Dying (Stages of Dying — Kübler-Ross)** Elisabeth Kübler-Ross developed a theory of the stages that an individual goes through when they know that they are dying. These five stages are: 1. Denial and Isolation, 2. Anger, 3. Bargaining, 4. Depression and 5. Acceptance. These five stages are well laid out in her book called **On Death and Dying** (1969).

**Dysarthria** The loss of function in the muscles used for speech and voice production. The speech produced is difficult to understand. The individual may have all other language and comprehension centers intact, but be unable to physically to produce speech.

**Dysesthesia** Alteration of any sense, but particularly to the sense of touch. This is usually experienced as pain and/or pinpricks.

**Dysphagia** Difficulty swallowing, due to loss of neurological function.

**Dysrhythmia** A change in the normal rhythm. An abnormal change in the resident's speech rate due to illness or disability or a change in a resident's heart beat due to illness or excessive activity are types of dysrhythmias.

**Edema** The excessive accumulation of fluid in the body's soft tissue causing swelling and discomfort. This swelling is controlled by:
1.  positioning (using gravity to drain fluids)
2.  pressure wraps (like ace bandages)
3.  medications

The professional should be aware of the strategies used to reduce edema in the resident and ensure that the leisure activities that the resident engages in are not counter indicated. The use of ace bandages on extremities or pressure clothing (like Jobst) may be required during leisure activities, even passive ones.

**Embolus** Sudden blocking of an artery by a blood clot or a foreign material that has been brought to that site by the blood. (See *Occlusion*.)

**Emotional Baggage** A slang term from the 1980s which refers to the components of personality based on the sum of one's personal and interpersonal experiences which accompany an individual throughout his/her life. People tend to react or act based on their past experiences.

**Empowerment** The feeling that one can influence one's own life and the events surrounding it. Many activity departments are assigned the job of helping the resident to feel empowered. By the nature of empowerment, this cannot be done through talking or self-help programs. Empowerment only comes from the actual experience of being able to control a significant aspect of one's environment.

**Endurance** The ability of: 1. the muscle to resist fatigue even with repeated contractions over a period of time, 2. the cardiovascular system to resist fatigue through efficient delivery of oxygen over a period of time, 3. the neuropsychological system to resist fatigue allowing the performance of cognitive functions over a period of time and/or 4. the general ability to sustain low intensity activity over a period of time.

**Enhance** To make greater. To enhance a resident's skill or environment or positive feelings is an important aspect of all staff who work in long term care. In the United States, OBRA expects all staff to work on the enhancement of a resident's life. This is considered to be a standard service.

**Environment** A term borrowed from the French which means to encircle. A general term which refers to all stimuli and objects in the proximity of the individual.

**Evaluation** A clinical opinion as a result of the professional's review of data and assessment results. Evaluation is not the same as an assessment.

**Eversion** Turning outward of a body part.

**Excess Disability** A decline that is greater than, or in excess of, the decline expected from the illness or disability. The "excess" may appear in a loss of functional abilities, alertness, cognitive status, orientation, communication, physical status and/or socialization. The excess disability is usually attributed to the environment.

**Executive Function** Those cognitive functions that are considered the "higher" functions (problem solving, judgment, interpretation of social cues, etc.). A person's ability to walk and complete other motor activities has been compared to the engine of a car and the ability to decide where to go and what to do (executive function) has been compared to the steering system of a car. The car can still run without the steering system but it does not get where the driver wants to go, safely. The same can be said of a resident who lacks executive function skills (due to a traumatic brain injury, dementia, etc.). The resident may be able to walk about but not in a purposeful manner.

**Extended Survey** (OBRA) In the process of conducting a resident-centered survey (Standard Survey), the surveyors determine that the facility may have provided substandard care in the areas of Resident Behavior and Facility Practices (42 CFR 483.13), Quality of Life (42 CFR 483.15) and/or Quality of Care (42 CFR 483.25). This extended survey must be conducted within fourteen days after the standard survey.

**Extension** Straightening or unbending a flexed limb. Moving two ends of a jointed part away from each other. Opposite of flexion.

**Facilitator** The term used to refer to the individual who is making the group's job easier by suggesting structure and choices as the group process goes along. The facilitator contributes to an activity by promoting an atmosphere that is conducive to productivity: a safe and intimate environment that encourages the sharing of ideas and feelings. In this type of group dynamics the group is as responsible for the outcome of the group process as the leader/facilitator. This leadership role is different then the role of a leader whose job it is to make the decisions and is responsible for the outcome of the group.

**Facility** The buildings(s) in which services are being provided. In health care the term facility usually means the buildings used to provide specific types(s) of services and which are usually accredited or licensed as one entity (e.g., "psych" facility, "long term care" facility, "rehab" facility). It is not uncommon for people to use the term "facility" to mean both the buildings and the services provided.

**Failure to Thrive** Failure to Thrive means that a resident is not able to take in enough fluids and nutrition to sustain life. (RAI) Cognitively impaired residents can reach the point where their accumulated health/neurological problems place them at risk of clinical complications (e.g., pressure ulcers) and death. As this level of disability approaches, staff can review the following:
- Do emotional, social and/or environmental factors play a key role?
- If a resident is not eating, is this due to a reversible mood problem, a basic personality problem, a negative reaction to the physical and interactive environment in which eating activity occurs or a neurological deficit such as deficiency in swallowing or loss of hand coordination?
- Could an identified problem be remedied through improved staff education — trying an antidepressant medication, referral to OT for training or an innovative counseling program?
- If causes cannot be identified, what reversible clinical complications can be expected as death approaches (e.g., fecal impaction, UTI, diarrhea, fever, pain, pressure ulcers)?
- What interventions are or could be in place to decrease complications?

**Falls** (RAI) Falls are a common source of serious injury and death among the elderly. Each year 40% of nursing home residents fall. Up to 5% of falls result in fractures, an additional 15% result in soft tissue injuries. Moreover, most elders are afraid of falling and this fear can limit their activities. In about one third of falls, a single potential cause can be identified; in two thirds, more than on risk factor will be involved. Risk factors that are internal to the resident include the resident's physical health and functional status. External risk factors include medication side effects, use of appliances and restraints and environmental conditions.

**Family Council** An organization within the Long Term Care facility which is run by and for families and friends of the residents. It is independent of the hospital administration, is self-determining and organized to meet the individual's needs and interests of the group.

**Fatigue** The decreased ability of an individual to complete a task because of a lack of oxygen delivery, protective influences of the central nervous system or a depletion of potassium in the elderly. The use of a muscle past the point of fatigue may lead to strain or to overuse syndrome. The idea of "No Pain, No Gain" is a phrase that the professional may want to avoid. Too frequently it leads to over fatigue of a muscle. The intensity of exercise should cause a gentle "pulling" sensation in the tight tissue and not pain (Kisner and Colby, 1990, page 679). With residents who have experienced a recent prolonged reduction in normal leisure activity, the professional may need to help the resident develop a schedule of modified activity until the appropriate level of endurance and strength can be achieved.

**Field Cut** Decrease or loss of a portion of a person's field of vision following a stroke or some other types of brain injury.

**FIM Scale** One of the most common coding systems used in assessment and charting is the Functional Independence Measure or the "FIM." The FIM is a seven point scale which is divided into two basic levels of ability.

---

**Functional Independence Measure (FIM)**

© Copyright 1987 Research Foundation — State University of New York

**Independent** — Another person is not required for the activity (No Helper)

7 **Complete Independence** All of the tasks described as making up the activity are typically performed safely without modification, assistive devices or aids and within reasonable time.

6 **Modified Independence** Activity requires any one or more than one of the following: an assistive device, more than reasonable time or there are safety (risk) considerations.

**Dependent** — Another person is required for either supervision or physical assistance in order for the activity to be performed or it is not performed (Requires Helper).

    **Modified Dependence** The subject expends half (50%) or more of the effort. The levels of assistance required are:

    5 **Supervision or Setup** Subject requires no more help than standby, cueing or coaxing, without physical contact. Or, helper sets up needed items or applies orthoses.

    4 **Minimal Contact Assistance** With physical contact the subject requires no more help than touching and subject expends 75% or more of the effort.

    3 **Moderate Assistance** Subject requires more help than touching or expends half (50%) or more (up to 75%) of the effort.

    **Complete Dependence** — The subject expends less than half (less than 50%) of the effort. Maximal or total assistance is required or the activity is not performed. The level of assistance required are:

    2 **Maximal Assistance** Subject expends less than 50% of the effort, but at least 25%.

    1 **Total Assistance** Subject expends less than 25% of the effort.

---

**Fine Motor** The use of movement which require delicate, well-controlled movement, usually of the hands.

**Flaccid** A muscle or limb that is weak, lacks tone and lacks voluntary control.

**Flexibility** The body's or mind's ability to yield (bend, move, change stance) when required. Muscle and other soft tissues responds when challenged with stretching force, the mind responds when challenged to format thoughts in a different manner. The maintenance of flexibility usually requires an individual's involvement in multiple activities on a regular basis. For residents with a cardiac condition, flexibility is especially important. Being flexible allows the resident to maintain a better posture, decreases the chance of injury and relieves stress (Karam, page 1).

**Flexion** Moving two ends of a joint closer together. Opposite of extension.

**Fluent Aphasia** Speech is fluent with paraphasic errors. Auditory comprehension, reading comprehension and writing comprehension are impaired.

**Focus** The primary interest of one's actions or attention. The ability to focus on one thought or task requires complex skills and is frequently limited or lost with brain damage or dementia. The loss of the ability to focus greatly increases the risk of sensory depravation.

**Functional Ability** The ability to perform a task well enough to have some measured success: to be able to complete enough of a task to achieve the desired outcome.

**Gait** Referring to the body mechanics and movement patterns used by a resident when they ambulate.

**Gestures** The nonverbal actions which are meant to communicate a person's intent or thoughts.

**Glasgow Coma Scale** The Glasgow Coma Scale (GCS) is routinely used to measure the severity of a coma and subsequent injury by grading eye, motor and verbal responses. The numerical values of the scale run from 3 (low) to 15 (normal). The total score of a resident's GCS means: 3–8 = severe coma, 9–12 = moderate coma and 13–15 = mild coma. A newer Glasgow type scale has been developed for children to be able to more accurately measure the early recovery in young children (under the age of three years). This assessment is called the Children's Coma Scale (CCS).

**Graphic Input** (Reading) Damage to the brain often impact a resident's ability to read. Once the resident is able to recognize words and to consistently scan from left to right, s/he is ready to progress to reading safety and other information on community integration outings. Residents tend to progress from being able to find concrete information in reading passages (as found in menus) to being able to figure out implied abstract information (such as satire or subtle meanings found in parks program bulletins). In house therapy along with actual experience on community integration outings with the professional helps the resident understand any visual/spatial deficits that s/he might have and to compensate for them. It is important that reading speed and accuracy increase together.

**Graphic Output** (Writing) Written communication is one of the key skills required of adults. Whether it is writing a check, filling out an insurance form or just writing a letter to a friend, the use of the written word is vital to independence in the community. One of the primary uses of the written word prior to discharge is a memory book. The purpose of the memory book is to provide the resident with a visual reminder of his/her schedule as well as to provide a place to write down thoughts and questions which should not be forgotten. Residents who require the use of a memory book usually have difficulty with spelling, punctuation, sentence formation, paragraph organization. Unless these skills will be required soon (because of vocational or educational needs) it is best to focus on the content of the material and not the manner in which it is written.

**Grievance** The formal process of notifying the long term care facility that an individual feels that s/he has been "wronged" and is seeking a satisfactory resolution to his/her complaint.

**Gross Motor** The use of the large muscle groups for coordinated action and strength to complete a task.

**Guardian** The individual or corporation which has obtained the legal right to make decisions concerning the resident's care because the resident has been determined unable to make his/her own decisions.

**Gustatory** The sense of taste.

**Habilitation** The maintenance of an individual's current health status and functional ability.

**Health Care Financing Administration (HCFA)** The United States Government has divided the funding mechanisms for health care into two divisions. These two division are the Public Health Service and the Health Care Financing Administration. Almost all health care facilities in the United States (with the notable exception of the Veteran's Administration Medical Services) are financed, in part or whole, through the Health Care Financing Administration. Long term care facilities and swing units in hospitals are under the Health Care Financing Administration.

**Hearing Impairment** A hearing loss refers to a decreased ability to hear sounds. The sensation of hearing is made up of two components: 1. the ability to perceive a range of volumes (loud to soft) and 2. the ability to perceive a range of pitches (do-re-mi-fa-so-la-ti-do). When a professional sees an individual with a hearing loss, the loss will be described by the part of the ear which is damaged: 1. conductive (damage to the outer or middle ear resulting in a hearing loss), 2. sensorineural (damage to the inner ear or to the auditory nerve) or 3) mixed ( a combination of both conductive and sensorineural). A sensorineural hearing loss is seldom correctable by medication and/or surgery, requiring instead the use of a hearing aid and/or sign language. A loss of the ability to hear sounds in one's environment is a significant loss. The primary concerns to be addressed by the professional are: 1. social isolation, 2. communication impairment and 3. loss of normal (hearing) development, even with early intervention.

**Helplessness** A term first developed by M. Seligman to describe the loss of functional ability in basic life skills that an individual develops after continual exposure to uncomfortable, noxious situations in which s/he is not able to escape or free himself/herself from. While the noxious situation may be present in only one aspect of the individual's life (e.g., an abusive marriage), the learned helplessness generalizes over all aspects of the resident's life (and skills). This generalization is caused by a chemical reaction inside the body to noxious stimulation. The professional's intervention consists of structuring a situation where the individual has actual control over a part of his/her life that is important to him/her and is able to achieve success with that aspect of his/her life. The chemicals produced inside the resident as a direct result of this honest feeling of success will eventually be able to overcome the chemical/emotional reaction of learned helplessness. This intervention is more successful if the noxious situation can be diminished or removed from the resident's life.

**Hemianopsia** Defective vision or blindness in half of the visual field. This is an anatomical problem. (Also called hemianopia.) *Note:* Do not confuse with neglect.

**Hemiparesis** Weakness of one side of the body.

**Hemiplegia** Paralysis of one side of the body.

**Hemorrhage** The escape of blood from a ruptured vessel.

**Holistic Approach** The awareness that illness is not just a disease state and that an individual's social, emotional, economic and physical states are all connected. When all these elements of an individual's life are taken into account while providing treatment, this treatment is considered to be a holistic approach.

**Huntington's Chorea** A hereditary disease characterized by the progressive deterioration of the resident's cognitive ability and also an erratic deterioration of the resident's involuntary muscle movements. There is no cure for the disease at this point although there is a test to determine if an individual is carrying the gene for the disease.

**Hyperesthesia** Abnormal increased sensitivity of the skin or an organ to sensory stimuli.

**Hyperflexia** Excessive flexion of a joint or joints.

**Hypertension** An elevation in blood pressure. Going above the normal range.

**Hypertonic** An increased level of tension in a muscle or limb.

**Hypoflexia** Less then normal flexion of a joint or joints.

**Hypotension** Blood pressure well below what is considered normal. An individual with hypotension may experience dizziness if s/he stands up quickly.

**Immediate and Serious Threat to Resident Health and Safety** This is the title of a federal regulation which applies to almost all health care settings in the United States. This law supersedes other health care laws, as it is the law that is intended to protect the consumer from the most damaging health care situations. A surveyor may "call" an Immediate and Serious Threat even if no resident has been injured — only the likelihood that one will be injured.

**Impaired Adjustment** A resident's inability to modify his/her style/behavior in a manner that is consistent with a change in his/her health status. The resident may either be purposeful (lack of acceptance) in his/her inability to recognize the change or may be unaware of the change. Due to this impaired adjustment, the resident will probably demonstrate a lack of movement toward independence; experience an extended period of shock, disbelief or anger toward his/her health change; or demonstrate an impaired ability to make plans for the future.

**Impulsivity** The decision to perform an activity without thought of the consequences.

**Incontinence** The inability to control when one urinates (urinary incontinence) or defecates (fecal incontinence). There are many factors which influence incontinence and many degrees of incontinence. Some individuals only have a limited leakage during episodes of coughing or sneezing. Such limited incontinence is usually not a limiting factor for activities. Many of the products on the market work well at providing a barrier to leakage and smell. (RAI) Nationally, 50% of nursing home residents are incontinent. Incontinence causes many problems, including skin rashes, falls, isolation and pressure ulcers and the potentially troubling use of indwelling catheters. In addition, continence is often an important goal to many residents and incontinence may affect residents' psychological well-being and social interactions. Urinary incontinence is curable in many elderly residents but realistically not all will benefit from an evaluation. Catheter use increases the risk of life-threatening infections, bladder stones and cancer. Use of catheters also contributes to resident discomfort and the needless use of toxic medications often required to treat the associated bladder spasms. For many (but not all) resident, urinary incontinence is curable and safer and more comfortable approaches are often practical for residents with indwelling catheters.

**Independent** The state of being able to perform a task or to process a thought without needing the direct help of another person or an adaptive device.

**Ineffective Individual Coping** An impairment in the resident's adaptive behaviors and ability to solve problems related to his/her illness or disability. It is likely that a resident who demonstrates ineffective individual coping related to a newly acquired disability had poor coping skills premorbidly. The professional may want to explore the resident's past coping strategies. This should help the professional identify the specific skills lacking which need to be taught to the resident. A resident with a poor ability to cope with new, distressing situations is not likely to integrate successfully into community based leisure activities.

**Infarct** An area of tissue that has died because of lack of blood supply.

**Informed Consent** see *Consent*

**Inhibition** The internally controlled mechanism which allows an individual to modify behavior or not engage in behavior which s/he considers inappropriate. Residents who lack inhibition will be unable to repress or terminate unwanted behavior appropriately.

**Initial Certification Survey** (OBRA) This survey is for the initial certification of Skilled Nursing Facilities. The surveyors conduct both the Standard and Extended Surveys. Special emphasis is given to the structural requirements that relate to qualification standards and resident rights notification, whether or not problems have been identified during the information gathering process. The surveyors are to gather information to verify compliance with every tag number (e.g., qualifications of the social worker, dietitian and Activity Professional).

**Instrument** A tool used by the professional to obtain a measurement during the assessment process. This instrument may be a questionnaire, a machine or any other device which assists the professional in obtaining the desired measurement.

**Interdisciplinary Team** The health care professionals who work together as a team to help provide the services needed by a resident.

**Intermittent Claudication** Caused by a lack of oxygen to the muscles which are being used and feels like cramping muscles. Because of the nature of some types of heart disease, a progressive conditioning program may do little more than increase the resident's tolerance of activity and to decrease the occurrence of claudication. Residents may be encouraged to exercise through the use of activities multiple times a day to the point of discomfort (and not beyond). Pain subsides slowly with rest. Pain upon rest (which usually has a burning, tingling feeling) is the result of a decreased oxygen flow to the affected limb. This decreased flow may be, in part, caused by positioning (the limb placed above the level of the heart and/or pressure over the arteries leading to the muscles) and/or caused by long periods of rest. (The heart tends to be less productive during sleep and/or during events which lead to deconditioning.) Encouraging the resident to engage in activities which allow the affected limb(s) to be positioned below the heart will help decrease the pain caused by rest.

**Interpretive Guidelines** The detailed explanation of the intent of a regulation or standard.

**Intervention** The act of purposely modifying the environment, an action or thought to influence the outcome.

**Irritability** The emotion combined with action when one is dissatisfied or otherwise bothered by an event or thought. The elements of irritability are: 1. an over reaction to an event, 2. a heightened degree of sensitivity and 3. a decreased ability to use patience.

**Ischemia** A term which means a lack of blood flow and a lack of delivery of oxygen to the cells.

**JCAHO Joint Commission on Accreditation of Healthcare Organizations** This is a private organization (separate from the government) which sets voluntary standards of care for many different types of health care settings. JCAHO's surveys are voluntary and usually take place once every 3 years.

**Judgment** The cognitive ability to make a decision based on a review of various aspects and factors related to the decision as well as being able to reasonably predict the results of an action under consideration.

**Kinesthetic** The use of the muscles, tendons and joints and the corresponding sensations of this movement. Exercise programs which encourage integrative movement using the proprioceptors and equilibrium (balance) are frequently referred to as kinesthetic exercise.

**Knowledge Deficit** An inability to call upon basic information required to survive in one's environment. A resident who has a knowledge deficit may demonstrate an inability to: accurately follow through on instructions given, accurately perform skills needed (although physically able to do so), perform within socially excepted norms for behavior and emotional expression or otherwise function because of missing information.

**Lability** Unable to control inappropriate laughing or crying.

**Lateral** Referring to the side or portion of the body furthest away from the midline of the body.

**Leadership Qualities** Leadership is the ability to have others follow one's lead and instructions. Generally leadership requires the ability to have initiative and the power to direct, drive, instruct and control to achieve the desired outcome. There are two different style of leadership prevalent in health care which are defined by Bradford (1976):

| Traditional Leadership | Group-Centered Leadership |
|---|---|
| • The leader directs, controls, polices the members and leads them to the proper decision. Basically it is his/her group and the leader's authority and responsibility are acknowledged by members. | • The group or meeting, is *owned* by the members, including the leader. All members, with the leader's assistance, contribute to its effectiveness. |
| • The leader focuses his/her attention on the task to be accomplished. S/he brings the group back from any diversions. S/he performs all the functions needed to arrive at the proper decision. | • The group is responsible, with occasional and appropriate help from the leader, for reaching a decision that includes the participation of all and is the product of all. The leader is a servant and helper to the group. |
| • The leader sets limits and uses rules of order to keep the discussion within strict limits set by the agenda. S/he controls the time spent on each item lest the group wander fruitlessly. | • Members of the group should be encouraged and helped to take responsibility for its task productivity, its methods of working, its assignment of tasks, its plans for the use of the time available. |
| • The leader believes that emotions are disruptive to objective, logical thinking and should be discourage or suppressed. S/he assumes it is his/her task to make clear to all members the disruptive effect of emotions. | • Feelings, emotions, conflict are recognized by the members and the leaders as legitimate facts and situations demanding as serious attention as the task agenda. |
| • The leader believes that s/he should handle a member's disruptive behavior by talking to him/her away from the group; it is his/her task to do so. | • The leader believes that any problem in the group must be faced and solved within the group and by the group. As trust develops among members, it is much easier for an individuals to discover ways in which his/her behavior is bothering the group. |
| • Because the need to arrive at a task decision is all important in the eyes of the leader, needs of individual members are considered less important. | • With help and encouragement from the leader, the members come to realize that the needs, feelings and purposes of all members should be met so that an awareness of being a group forms. Then the group can continue to grow. |

**Least Restrictive** When a resident has artificial limitations placed on him/her, it is his/her right to have the restrictions be as little as possible. An example would be a resident who wanders into the rooms of others or off the unit. In the past, residents who wandered were strapped into a wheelchair with its brakes on, even if they did not need a wheelchair to get around. Some facilities have found that placing a wall mural of a set of bookshelves or a mural of a fence caused residents who were cognitively impaired and wandering to not attempt to go out the doors. Other facilities have found that the placement of the upper half of cafe curtains over the door (so that the hem is just below the eye level of the resident who was wandering) caused the resident to stay out of the room.

**Leisure** The concept of leisure is not one shared by all cultures and has two different meanings to those that do share that concept. For those who study leisure in the United States and Canada, leisure is generally considered to be a state of mind. Others view leisure as an absence of work or commitment. Extensive study has been done in Europe and Northern America concerning all of the aspects of leisure as a state of mind, including the study of interests, motivations, attitudes, barriers, boredom, satisfaction, etc.

**Leisure Planning Deficit** An inability to experience self-initiated leisure activities as a result of a lack of knowledge about leisure opportunities, decreased stimulation from or a lack of interest in leisure activities or an inability or unwillingness to use one's leisure time in a manner that is satisfying to the individual.

**Lethargy** An abnormal and undesirable drowsiness or stupor frequently resulting in an increased indifference to one's environment. Lethargy, as a side effect of medication, can place the resident at greater risk of accidents and injury.

**Listening Skills** There are five skills associated with functional listening skills. They are described in the table on the next page (from the book **Messages: The Communication Skills Book** by McKay, Davis, Fanning (1983) which is, in this author's opinion, one of the best written on the subject).

**Locomotion** The action or ability to move from one location to another.

**Major Life Activities** (ADA) Major life activities means functions such as caring for oneself, performing manual tasks, walking, seeing, hearing, speaking, breathing, learning and working.

**Mandate** An action that is required by law.

**Manual Dexterity** The ability to coordinate actions and movements of the hands.

**MDS** See *Minimum Data Set*.

**Medial** Referring to the middle portion or the midline of the body; closest to the midpoint.

**Medicaid** A program of health insurance in the United States for those who are of limited or no income and unable to pay for health care bills. States share in financing the program and determine eligibility and benefits.

**Medical Model Approach** This approach assumes that all illnesses and disabilities originate from a specifically physical cause and that, once that cause can be rooted out and corrected, the resident will experience good health.

**Medical Record** The record of the medical care that a resident has received. Medical records are subject to multiple regulations. Also called a Medical Chart.

**Medical Status** The degree of illness or wellness that a resident is experiencing.

**Medicare** A federal health insurance program for individuals over the age of 65 or for individuals disabled with chronic renal disorders.

**Summary of Listening Skills**[52]

| Listening Skill | Description |
|---|---|
| Basic Total Listening Skills | People want you to listen, so they look for clues to prove that you are. Here's how to be a good listener:<br>1. Maintain good eye contact.<br>2. Lean slightly forward.<br>3. Reinforce the speaker by nodding or paraphrasing.<br>4. Clarify by asking questions.<br>5. Actively move away from distractions.<br>6. Be committed, even if you're angry or upset. to understanding what was said. |
| Active Listening | 1. Paraphrasing: to state in your own words what the other person said.<br>2. Clarifying: to ask questions until you feel that you correctly understand what the person said.<br>3. Feedback: after you have paraphrased and clarified what you heard the other person say you talk about your reactions to what they said — in a non judgmental manner. |
| Listening With Empathy | You do not have to agree with the person talking with you, but realize that they have feelings and worth also. Some questions to ask yourself to help develop empathy:<br>1. What need is the *[anger, etc.]* coming from?<br>2. What danger is this person experiencing?<br>3. What is s/he asking for? |
| Listening With Openness | Your own attitudes and judgment of what the person is saying may get in the way of effective listening. Some of the blocks to listening are:<br>1. Comparing<br>2. Mind Reading<br>3. Rehearsing<br>4. Filtering<br>5. Judging<br>6. Dreaming<br>7. Identifying<br>8. Advising<br>9. Sparring<br>10. Being Right<br>11. Derailing<br>12. Placating |
| Listening With Awareness | Use your own experience and knowledge of history and people and body language to "read" the nonverbal messages being given.<br>Compare what is being said to your own knowledge of history, people and the way things are.<br>Listen to body language and tone. Does the person's tone of voice, emphasis, facial expression and posture fit with the content of his or her communication? |

[52] McKay, Davis, Fanning. 1983. **Messages: The Communication Skills Book**. Oakland. New Harbinger Publications.

**Memory Book** A book, usually made by staff and family for a specific resident, to help him/her remember vital information. A memory book is a type of prosthetic device.

**Memory Deficit** Inability to recall information stored in one's brain, either short (working) or long term. Depending on the cause of the memory deficit, the individual may exhibit a combination of the following symptoms: poor learning ability, reduced self-esteem, short term memory loss, long term memory loss, disorientation, confabulation, poor safety awareness. Short term memory refers to the storage of information that the individual is using or has just used. Thoughts are encoded and organized in short term memory. Because short term memory has limited ability to store large quantities of information, some of the information is selected, encoded and shifted to long term memory. Long term memory contains past learned information, including information related to concepts and words, rules and social/governmental expectations organizational strategies and other memories of past experiences.

**Mental Abuse** As defined by Federal *Immediate and Serious Threat* regulations in the United States: The failure to prevent mental abuse whereby residents suffer psychological harm or trauma. Conditions/Situations which may indicate mental abuse include: 1. residents who appear fearful, suspicious or timid; shake when approached (jittery) or avoid eye contact; are overly obedient or defensive; who are crying or tearful; withdrawn and reclusive; and 2. residents who are treated disrespectfully; i.e., laughed at, called names by staff, etc.

**Milieu** A term meaning environment. In a therapeutic setting, a therapeutic milieu is an environment which is structured to meet the emotional and survival needs of the resident.

**Minimum Data Set** (MDS) The interdisciplinary assessment tool required for every resident admitted to a nursing home in the United States. Also known as the Resident Assessment Instrument.

**Mobility** Mobility refers to the resident's ability to move from one location to another. For a resident to be considered independent in mobility s/he would need to be able to complete the following tasks without cueing or other assistance:
1. ability to move from current position (point A) to desired position (point B). This would include ability to move in bed, with a wheelchair, to transfer and/or to ambulate with prescribed mobility devices (if any),
2. ability to use prescribed mobility techniques and devices in a variety of settings found in the community.

While the resident's initial training in these skills most likely will come from a physical therapist, the Activity Professional or Recreational Therapist will need to supervise, assist and evaluate the resident in his/her skills related to mobility while on community integration outings.

**Modality** The activity and supplies that are used to provide therapeutic services. An example is using a bin of sand with sea shells hidden in the sand for sensory stimulation. The therapeutic intervention is sensory stimulation. The modality is the sand and the sea shells.

**Mood** The emotion that a person is experiencing, usually for a sustained period of time. Mood disorders are those extremes of sustained emotions that interfere with functional ability.

**Mood State** (RAI) About 15% of nursing home residents will have a major depression; about 30% will exhibit noticeable symptomatic signs of a mood state problem. Such signs are often expressed as sad mood, feelings of emptiness, anxiety or uneasiness. They are also manifested in a wide range of bodily complaints and dysfunctions, such as loss of weight, tearfulness, agitation, aches and pains.

**Multi-Infarct Dementia** See *Vascular Dementia*.

**Multi Step Task** A task which takes more than one type of skill or motion to complete. An example of a multiple step task would be asking a resident to finish up his/her project, put away his/her supplies and go to his/her room to clean up for dinner. ("Get ready for Dinner" is the task.)

**Multiple Sclerosis (MS)** Multiple sclerosis is a chronic disabling disease of the central nervous system in which scattered areas of the myelin covering the nerves degenerate. The destruction of this myelin covering causes a "short-circuiting" or blocking of the impulses that control a person's actions. The areas that have the degenerated patches are called plaques. As these areas of plaques combine to make larger holes in the myelin covering, the nerve impulses are not able to function correctly and the message that the nerve was carrying is lost in part or whole. If the nerve was carrying information needed for muscle movement, the movement will be weak or absent. If the nerve was carrying information involving sensation, numbness or tingling may be felt. Treatment includes the use of therapy to reduce muscle spasms, contractures of the muscles and pain. Many residents have noticed that the symptoms get worse when they are under great emotional distress.

**Muscle Tone** Also known as *tonus*, the state of a muscle while resting in a partial contraction.

**Narrative Style of Documenting** Rather than in outline form, this style of documentation is meant to read more like a story, employing figures of speech to paint a word picture. This form of documentation is usually very interesting to write and to read; using the basics of *who, what, when, where, why* can act as a springboard for entries done in this style.

**Nasogastric Tube (NG Tube)** A tube which is placed down the resident's nose into the resident's stomach. This tube is used to help provide nutritional supplement for resident's who cannot eat because of a jaw injury, neurological damage or coma.

**National Association of Activity Professionals** NAAP is a national membership organization which services the needs and interests of professionals and para-professionals who work in activities in long term care, adult day care and residential living settings. It works to promote the advancement of Activity Professionals as well as enhance the quality of services provided to those individuals who live in long term care, adult day care and residential living settings. NAAP's address is P. O. Box 23909, Jackson, MS 39225. Phone 601-853-3722.

**National Certification Council for Activity Professionals (NCCAP)** This is the national credentialing body for Activity Professionals. There are three levels of credentialing: Activity Consultant, Certified (ACC); Activity Director, Certified (ADC); and Activity Assistant, Certified (AAC). NCCAP is independent of the National Association of Activity Professionals (NAAP) and other professional organizations. NCCAP's address is P. O. Box 62589, Virginia Beach, VA 23466-2589. Phone 757-552-0653.

**National Council for Therapeutic Recreation Certification (NCTRC)** The National Council for Therapeutic Recreation Certification (NCTRC) was established in 1981 as the nationally recognized organization in the United States for the certification of therapeutic recreation personnel. NCTRC's mission is to protect the consumer of therapeutic recreation services by promoting the provision of quality services offered by our certificants. This mission is accomplished through: developing, implementing and administering standards for certification and recertification; granting recognition to individuals who meet the standards; monitoring adherence to standards and professional conduct and applying sanctions where warranted; administering a registry of certified therapeutic recreation professionals; promoting the credential; and monitoring changes in practice. There are two paths from which an applicant may apply to receive certification at the professional level. Upon successful review of credentials and passage of the national certification exam, a professional is awarded the "Certified Therapeutic Recreation Specialist™ (CTRS™)" credential. NCTRC's mailing address is 7 Elmwood Drive, New City, NY 10956.

**Neglect (Resident)** As defined by the Federal *Immediate and Serious Threat* regulations in the United States: Neglect is the failure to provide necessary physical or psychological care, attention or treatment, resulting in gross neglect. Situations/Conditions which may indicate neglect include: 1. residents who are dirty, disheveled, inappropriately clothed for the climate, malnourished, lying in urine and/or feces, exhibiting excessive skin break-down/body trauma, incorrect/inappropriate hydration status; and 2. residents who are left alone for excessive amounts of time.

**Neglect (Visual)** Lack of awareness of one side of the body and space, usually seen in individuals with a right CVA who show neglect to the left of midline. (Also called visuospatial neglect or unilateral neglect.)

**Nervous Behaviors** Nervous behaviors are those observable actions that a resident demonstrates when s/he is uncomfortable with a situation. At times these nervous habits become so significant that they reduce a resident's ability to function in his/her environment. Some nervous behaviors include:

| | | |
|---|---|---|
| body swaying | tapping | repetitive movements |
| moistens lips | clearing throat | coughing |
| sits on edge of chair | flashes of smiles | rigid arms |
| pacing | self-grooming | self-hugging |
| can't sit still | rocking | fidgeting |
| leg/arm swinging | clutching hands | twitching |
| nail biting | hands restrained or in pockets | scratching |

**Neuropathy** A measurable disability and/or undesirable change in the peripheral nervous system. Chronic alcoholism and diabetes are two common causes of neuropathy.

**Non Ambulatory** Referring to an individual who is not able to walk a functional distance. An individual is considered to still be functionally ambulatory if s/he is able to move about with the assistance of a cane, walker or braces.

**Nonfluent Aphasia** Speech is effortful and halting. Auditory comprehension is relatively good but not perfect. Reading comprehension is better than written output.

**Normalization** The process of modifying the environment or the resident's skills to allow that resident to better "fit in" to his/her community.

**Noxious Stimuli** Items or actions that irritate. A noxious stimuli response is a nerve reaction to something that is not healthy or produces an undesirable or even damaging result.

**Nursing Supervisor** The nurse who is the supervisor of other nursing staff. Nursing supervisor usually indicates an individual who holds a management position in a health care setting. This individual usually supervises other nurses, nurses' aides and often, the Activity and Social Service Professionals. When the Administrator of a long term care facility is out of the building, the next in charge is usually the Nursing Supervisor. A Nursing Supervisor usually has a bachelors or masters degree in nursing.

**OBRA** The name of the Federal Legislation which outlines the minimum requirements for facilities licensed as Skilled Nursing Facilities in the United States. The full title of the legislation is the **Nursing Home Reform Provisions of the Omnibus Budget Reconciliation Act of 1987**. OBRA was first passed into law in 1987 and modified in 1992 and 1995.

**Occlusion** Closure of a blood vessel, closing off.

**Occupational Therapist** An individual who has completed all of the training and exams required by the American Occupational Therapy Certification Board (AOTCB) or who has met state requirements to be called an "Occupational Therapist."

**Ombudsman** A representative of a government (usually state) program who is appointed to receive and investigate complaints made by individuals (in all licensed and certified facilities) of abuses: physical, sexual, financial and mental. The ombudsman program was mandated and funded by the Older

Americans Act amendments of 1975. Acting as an advocate for the resident, s/he assesses and verifies each complaint and then seeks a way to resolve it. An ombudsman must report findings to the appropriate agencies (law enforcement and Department of Health Services) and help to achieve equitable settlements of issues. The concept of ombudsman programs originated in Scandinavia in the 1800's.

**Organic Brain Syndrome** A general category of disorders of cognitive functioning including dementia, delirium, amnesiac syndrome, delirium organic anxiety syndrome, intoxication and withdrawal, etc. While this term was commonly used prior to 1994, its use should decline. Originally called *Organic Mental Syndrome* in the **DSM-III-R**, it is not found in the **DSM IV**. The types of organically caused brain syndromes once grouped under Organic Mental Syndrome are now re-grouped into different categories.

**Organizational Deficit** The inability to mentally process information in an organized manner. This would include an inability to sequence, classify, prioritize and/or identify relevant features of objects or events.

**Orientation** The ability to be cognitively aware of and express time, place, personal data, relationship(s) of significant others to self, one's own condition and purpose (identity/role).

**Outcome** The results of an action. In health care "outcome" refers to the anticipated and/or actual result expected as a direct result of a treatment intervention. In the 1970's the quality of health care services was frequently measured by evaluating whether a facility has the appropriate policies, procedures and equipment in place (systems approach). It quickly become apparent that a facility could have all appropriate systems in place and not be able to make a meaningful change in a resident's status. During the late 1980's and well into the 1990's, the trend in measuring the quality of services shifted away from the systems approach to the outcomes approach. Facilities are now expected to have functional, workable systems in place which produce meaningful outcomes.

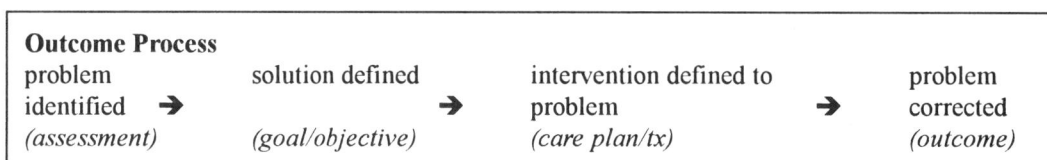

| **Outcome Process** | | | |
|---|---|---|---|
| problem identified → *(assessment)* | solution defined → *(goal/objective)* | intervention defined to problem → *(care plan/tx)* | problem corrected *(outcome)* |

**Over Stimulation** The excitement of nerves to the point that it produces a decreased ability to function in an individual. Since each individual has a different threshold before they are over stimulated and because the amount of sleep or food or illness can affect an individual's threshold, it is hard to indicate the amount of stimulation required before over stimulation is achieved.

**Pain** A generally localized feeling of discomfort brought about by the stimulation of special nerve endings. It is thought that pain is an adapted state to help the individual protect the area that is uncomfortable. The degree of pain that a person "feels" is influenced by three factors (Cailliet, 1988):
1.  biologic factors
2.  psychological factors
3.  social factors

The professional can have a significant impact on the resident's tolerance (or lack there of) for pain and change the degree to which the resident's leisure lifestyle is limited because of pain. Both the prevention of further movement which will actually cause biological damage as well as psychological training to increase tolerance are suitable areas for the professional to work. Also, increasing the resident's social skills to minimize the negative impact of pain is often addressed by the professional. The professional can decrease the resident's need to talk about his/her pain by increasing awareness and interest in other things and by helping the resident redefine his/her role from "victim" to a healthier role. These changes will increase the resident's tolerance for pain.

**Panic Attacks** The primary symptom of anxiety disorders which may occur without an obvious pattern of cause. Typically these attacks are short in duration and cause a severe sense of dread, sweating, heart dysrhythmias and a feeling of not being connected with the world around them.

**Paralysis** Complete loss of voluntary movement.

**Paraphasia** Condition characterized by fluent utterance of speech sounds in which unintended syllables, words or phrases are prominent during speech.

**Paresis** Weakness; partial or incomplete paralysis.

**Paresthesia** An abnormal and frequently intense, feeling of burning and prickling ("biting ants") felt by the resident even though there is little or no pressure on the affected spot.

**Parkinsonian Movements** A term used to refer to a group of physical side effects of psychoactive medications; actually more common then Parkinson's Disease, which it is not related to. See *Tardive Dyskinesia* for more detail.

**Parkinson's Disease** A chronic disease which causes neurological damage. Usually developing later in life, Parkinson's Disease is most commonly known by the muscular tremors and peculiar gait. First described by an English physician named James Parkinson, those with the disease progressively loose sensory-motor coordination and have difficulty initiating activity. Activity requires excessive energy causing individuals to tire quickly.

**Passive** The act of not taking action; of letting others or events in one's life control what happens. It is normal for people to choose to be passive in large group situations.

**Pathfinding** The ability to be able to determine the route one needs to take to reach one's destination.

**Perception Deficit** An inability to recognize objects or to misjudge one object's relationship to another object due to an inability to distinguish:
1. context (figure-ground),
2. significance of an object,
3. intensity of an object and/or
4. the identity of a previously familiar object.

**Perseveration** The person gets "stuck" on the same response. This can be either a verbal or a motor response.

**Phantom Pain** Either a dull or sharp pain felt by a resident that seems to originate from a limb that is no longer present (has been amputated). This pain is very real and frequently limits the resident's ability to concentrate on activities. The professional may want to note the resident's description of the pain (burning, electrical or throbbing) and the duration of the pain. Eventually the resident learns to localize the pain to the stump.

**Phobia** A fear not based on logic or the reality of the situation and that is persistent, intense and causing the individual to run away from the object of fear.

**Physical Abuse** As defined by Federal *Immediate and Serious Threat* regulations in the United States: physical abuse is the failure to protect residents from bodily harm or trauma. Conditions/Situations which indicate resident abuse may include: 1. residents who have bruises, cuts, burns (cigarettes, etc.); 2. residents who state that they have been abused; 3. staff, family or others who state that abuse has occurred; and 4. fractures without adequate explanation or corroborating evidence to support them.

**Physical Restraints** A physical restraint is any mechanical means of restricting a resident's movement, including geri-chairs, seat belts on wheelchairs (when used to restrict standing) and gates across doors. (RAI) Studies of nursing homes show that between 30 and 40% of residents are physically restrained. This is quite serious since negative effects of restraint use include declines in residents' physical functioning (e.g., ability to ambulate) and muscle condition, contractures, increased incidence of infections and development of pressure sores, delirium, agitation and incontinence. Moreover, restraints have been found in some cases to increase the incidence of falls and other accidents (e.g., strangulation). Finally, residents who are restrained face the loss of autonomy, dignity and self-respect. In effect, the use of physical restraints undercuts the major goals of long term care — to maximize independence, functional capacity and quality of life. Thus, the goal of minimizing or eliminating restraint use has become central to both clinical practice and federal law. The primary reason given for applying restraints is to protect residents from falls and accidents. Facilities are also concerned about potential lawsuits and malpractice claims that might result if residents should fall. Other reasons cited for restraint use include providing postural support or positioning for residents, facilitating treatment (e.g., preventing residents from pulling out IV lines or NG tubes) and managing behaviors such as wandering or physical aggressiveness. The experience of many health care providers suggests that facility goals can often be met without the use of physical restraints and their negative side effects. In part, this involves identifying and treating health, functional or psychosocial problems that may be causing the condition for which restraints were ordered (e.g., falls, wandering, agitation). Minimizing use of restraints also involves care management alternative, such as: modifying the environment to make it safer; maintaining an individual's customary routine; using less intrusive methods of administering medications and nourishment; and recognizing and responding to residents' needs for psychosocial support, responsive health care, meaningful activities and regular exercise.

**Pick's Disease** A type of dementia that frequently develops before the age of 65. This type of dementia effects the cerebral cortex and the frontal lobes. The loss of function in this part of the brain causes the resident to loose intellectual functioning and to loose an awareness of social "rules." Both because this disease frequently strikes its victims at an early age and because awareness of social skills and norms vanishes, this is a particularly challenging disability to treat.

**Plaque** A deposit of fatty material in the lining of a blood vessel. Build up of plaque in or near the brain can lead to the blockage of the blood vessel, resulting in a stroke.

**Playfulness (elements of)** Playfulness is a complex skill that goes through many different developmental stages. In general, playfulness requires the ability to be spontaneous, creative, aware of one's environment and imaginative. Being playful is healthy.

**Policy** A formal statement which defines how a facility views a specific topic or event. A sample of a policy might be: *The Activity Professional will conduct an assessment of each resident's activity needs within 7 days of admission.* The policy statement is then followed by a *procedure* which outlines how that policy will be implemented.

**Post Traumatic Stress Response** An individual's response to an unexpected extraordinary life event or events which produces a sustained painful response. The resident may experience an interruption in his/her normal sleep patterns, an inability to concentrate, a increased ability to be startled and a decreased ability to initiate activity.

**Posterior** Referring to the back part of a structure; the dorsal surface of the body.

**Postural Drainage** The use of gravity to help remove unwanted secretions from the airway. Residents frequently show a resistance to postural drainage because of boredom, agitation, pain, etc. The development of enjoyable activities to be engaged in during drainage helps increase compliance.

**Postural Dysfunction** The resident's decreased ability to engage in activities caused by a shortening of soft tissue and muscle weakness. The resident experiences fatigue and a limiting range of motion which can frequently be overcome through the prescriptive use of activities.

**Postural Fault** An abnormal alignment of the body caused by pain, not caused by structural defects or postural dysfunction.

**Potential** The maximum degree of skill or wellness that a resident is judged capable of reaching given the right interventions and environment.

**Powerlessness** A perception that one is unable to influence one's own life; that one is not able to significantly affect an outcome or a perceived lack of control over a current situation. A resident who feels powerless to control the events of his/her life will be less likely to initiate activity.

**Precipitating Factors** A precipitating factor is an event or action which directly causes something else to happen. If an adult in his/her late 80's falls at home and breaks a hip, the fall and resulting hip fracture is considered to be the precipitating factor to his/her being admitted to a nursing home.

**Predictor** A predictor is a specific skill or health status which, based on past experience, means that something else can be expected to happen. An activity assessment which showed that a new resident had chosen to be isolated in his home for the past two years since his wife's death is usually a predictor of difficulty in getting that resident to join in activities at first.

**Premorbid Leisure Lifestyle** The combination of activities that the resident participated in prior to his/her injury or illness.

**Prescription** A prescription is made up of four parts:
1.  the mode of treatment (e.g., type of activity (movement, cognition, etc.) required)
2.  duration of treatment program (e.g., 14 days)
3.  frequency of treatment (e.g., two times a day)
4.  intensity of treatment (e.g., maintenance of 120% resting heart rate for 15 minutes)

**Pressure Release** The lifting or moving of the body to relieve pressure on areas compressed by gravity, constricting garments or appliances.

**Pressure Sore (Also known as "Pressure Ulcers")** A pressure sore is a break down in the normally healthy condition of the skin due to pressure or sheer. A Stage One pressure sore is a red mark that does not fade in 30 minutes after pressure has been relieved. A Stage Two pressure sore is a blister or an open sore which is just skin deep and caused, at least in part, by pressure. A Stage Three pressure sore is an opening in the skin and into the muscle caused, at least in part, by pressure. A Stage Four pressure sore is an opening in the skin and muscle down to the bone caused, at least in part, by pressure. (RAP) Between 3% and 5% of resident in nursing facilities have pressure ulcers (pressure sores, decubitus ulcers, bedsores). Sixty percent or more of residents will typically be at risk of pressure ulcer development. Pressure ulcers can have serious consequences for the elderly and are costly and time consuming to treat. However, they are one of the most common, preventable and treatable conditions among elderly who have restricted mobility. Successful outcomes can be expected with preventative and treatment programs.

**Problem Solving** The process which takes place when an individual is not able to reach a desired goal directly. Some of the skills associated with problem solving include: 1. the ability to identify the desired outcome, 2. the ability to gather and consider relevant information, 3. anticipating potential solutions and 4. the selection of the action(s) which is most likely to get the desired outcome.

**Procedure** The step by step description of how staff are to complete the intent of a policy.

**Processing Deficits** Processing deficits tend to fall into three categories: 1. the inability to *regulate the information being received* (e.g., not being able to handle: the rate of reception, the amount being received, the type of information being received, other noises and input and manage (cope with) information overload in a productive manner); 2. the inability to *organize the information being received* (e.g., not being able to: maintain information in memory, group the information with similar information to allow analysis and problem solving and use internal conversations to help retrieve information — Which way is it to the recreation center?) and 3. the inability to *regulate the manner in which information is expressed* (e.g., not being able to: monitor one's responses to ensure correctness and sequencing that make sense, plan the response to ensure that it is presented in an organized manner and know when one needs more information before a response is appropriate (asking for clarification)).

**Professional** An individual who has attained a high degree of skill and extensive specialized training to be able to perform the tasks of his/her occupational group. A professional has knowledge of the standardized techniques, philosophical base and ethical code of his/her occupation and adheres to them to produce an excellence in service and product. Membership in one's professional organization and regular communication with one's occupational peers is vital for professional growth and development.

**Prognosis** An estimation, based on clinical experience and clinical opinion, on how the resident's health and/or skill level will change over a specific period of time.

**Progress Notes** The section of a resident's medical chart which is used to write information about the resident's ongoing needs and treatment. It is used as the main communication system for the interdisciplinary team. The most successful progress notes tend to be interdisciplinary — each member of the team writes pertinent information as it develops. An often used statement in health care states "If it isn't written down, it didn't happen." While this is obviously not true, it does emphasize the importance of writing key information in the progress notes.

**Progressive Relaxation Technique** E. Jacobson first described the concept that teaching a person to relax his/her muscles in specific groups should then assist the person to relax emotionally.

**Proprioception** A term used to describe the integrated action of all the senses that help a person know their position, location orientation and to sense when and how much his/her body parts have moved.

**Pseudodementia** The temporary loss of cognitive ability, similar to dementia, caused by a distressed emotional state, such as depression or as depressed physical state due to a side effect of medications or other temporary illness.

**Psychiatric Seclusion — Inappropriate** As defined by the Federal *Immediate and Serious Threat* regulation in the United States: A failure to ensure that the removal of residents from their normal environment to an area from which their egress is prevented, is done appropriately and/or failure to ensure that there is adequate and appropriate monitoring of residents while in seclusion. Situation/Conditions which may indicate inappropriate psychiatric seclusion include: 1. use of seclusion room which is unsafe (temperature is too hot/cold, residents cannot be observed at all times, exposed pipes, breakable glass or other harmful materials), 2. incidents of bodily trauma/injury while in seclusion, 3. clinical record reflecting either absence of justification or inappropriate justification for seclusion, 4. incidence reports reflecting injuries during restraint process, 5. seclusion which is used as a punishment, 6. incidence reports which reflect an increase in suicide attempts by residents who are in seclusion.

**Psychoactive Drugs** (OBRA) (Also known as Psychotropic Drugs) A psychoactive drug is a medication that is given to a resident to modify the resident's behavior or thought patterns. If a resident is receiving a psychoactive medication to modify his/her behavior, the facility should be able to show that less invasive behavioral interventions were tried first and failed. (RAI) Psychoactive drugs are among the most frequently prescribed agents for elderly nursing home residents. Studies in nursing facilities suggest that 35%–65% of residents receive psychoactive medications. When used appropriately and judiciously, these medications can enhance the quality of life of residents who need them. However, all psychoactive drugs have the potential for producing undesirable side effects or aggravating problematic signs and symptoms of existing conditions. An important example is postural hypotension, a condition associated with serious and life-threatening side effects. Severity of delirium side effects is dependent on: the class and dosage of drug, interactions with other drugs and the age and health status of the resident.

**Psychosocial Well-Being** (RAI) Well-Being refers to feelings about self and social relationships. Positive attributes include initiative and involvement in life; negative attributes include distressing relationships and concern about loss of status. On average, 30% of residents in a typical nursing facility will experience problems in this area, two thirds of whom will also have serious behavior and/or mood problems. When such problems coexist, initial treatment is often focused on mood and behavior manifestations. In such situations, treatment for psychological distress is dependent on how the resident responds to the primary mood/behavior treatment regiment.

**Quality Assurance** A formal system which 1. identifies (potential) problem(s), 2. establishes indicators and methods to measure change to be able to measure when the problem is corrected, 3. collects data using indicators and methods established to measure, 4. determines solutions including writing an action plan and implementing the plan and 5. determines if the desired change or outcome has been achieved.

**Quality of Life (measurements of/components of)** Quality of Life refers to the degree which the resident perceives that his/her life has meaning and comfort. Quality of Life is considered very important for residents living an a nursing home. OBRA states that (Tag F240) A facility must care for its residents in a manner and in an environment that promotes maintenance or enhancement of each resident's quality of life.

**Quarterly Notes** The information placed in the progress notes of a resident's medical chart which summarizes the resident's treatment and status over the past 90 days.

**RAI** See *Resident Assessment Instrument.*

**Range of Motion (ROM)** Degree of motion (flexion and extension) of a joint. ROM exercises work to increase or maintain the maximum degree of movement. **PROM** — passive range of motion is when a joint is moved by some other person. In nursing homes PROM is usually done by aides and nursing staff. **AROM** — active range of motion is when the resident moves the joint by his/her own efforts. In many states, occupational therapists, physical therapists, physicians, nurses and aides are licensed to perform ROM exercises. However, most regulatory agencies expect all therapists to know enough about range of motion to be able to implement the appropriate type and use the appropriate precautions, while interacting with the resident. An Activity Professional may work with the physical therapist or occupational therapist to develop a set of activities which promote the appropriate range of motion activity for a resident. The professional would then supervise the resident during these activities. There are five primary causes for a loss of ROM (Kisner and Colby 1990, page 109): 1. prolonged immobilization, 2. restricted mobility, 3. connective tissue or neuromuscular disease, 4. tissue pathology due to trauma and 5. congenital or acquired deformities.

**RAP** See *Resident Assessment Protocol.*

**Reality Orientation** A formal or informal program to assist the resident in knowing who they are, where they are and why they are and when. This program includes both verbal and non-verbal cues.

**Reasoning** The ability to consider information presented and then to create inferences and/or conclusions. The skill of reasoning requires that the individual is able to draw upon past experiences and is able to be flexible in the possible interpretations of why an event occurred.

**Receptor** A specialized neural cell which is sensitive to stimulation. Once it receives enough stimulation to make it fire, it will pass on the information to the next neural cell.

**Recognition** The ability to correctly tell if one has seen, experienced or heard an object or event previously. This requires that the individual is able to 1. store information in long/short term memory, 2. to be able to recognize the shape and/or patterns associated with the object or event, 3. recall past events which may be similar, 4. mentally review the possible choices from memory and select the one which matches and 5. feel confident that one's recognition process is accurate.

**Recreational Therapist** A term frequently used instead of the term "therapeutic recreation specialist."

**Referral** The request to add a resident to one's case load. This request may come from a physician, a member of the treatment team, a family member or anyone else who has a legitimate, legal right to make decisions concerning the resident's care.

**Regulation** The term used to indicate that a specific standard is part of a law; a legal requirement to meet or exceed.

**Regulatory Agency** The agency or department which, by law, is responsible to ensure that specific legal standards are being met. Regulatory agencies have individuals called "surveyors" who go to each facility to evaluate the quality of care being delivered. The Health Standards and Quality Bureau (HSQB) (the survey branch of the Department of Health and Human Services in the United States) is an example of a regulatory agency.

**Rehabilitation** The process of improving one's health and functional status through purposeful intervention.

**Relaxation** The purposeful effort to release tension in one or more muscles. A resident's ability to decrease tension in muscles usually becomes more efficient with practice. While some residents may be able to increase this skill through self-directed efforts, most will require some direct training from the professional.

**Reminiscence** The process of recalling events in a resident's past; a normal process as one ages.

**Remotivation** The treatment program which helps bridge the time a resident is concerned only about his/her own problems and the time when s/he is ready once again to help others in the community.

**Resident Assessment Instrument (RAI)** An interdisciplinary assessment tool developed by the Health Care Financing Administration to be administered to every resident admitted to a nursing home in the United States. It includes the Minimum Data Set and the Resident Assessment Protocols.

**Resident Assessment Protocols (RAI)** Outline for organizing MDS (Minimum Data Set) elements, including clinically relevant information concerning the long term care population, to be used in the development of care plans.

**Resident Care Plan** The overall plan of action and treatment which the treatment team developed with the resident's input, based on the assessment of the resident's needs and standards of practice and which is reviewed on a regular basis.

**Resident Council** The governing body made up of residents who discuss concerns about their living environment, propose changes and work with the administrator and staff of the long term care facility to resolve problems.

**Resocialization** As a result of some illnesses and disabilities, the resident may experience a period of time when s/he has lost interest or the ability to interact with others socially. When a resident is emotionally and/or physically ready to enter back into social interactions s/he may need a supportive environment and/or adaptive equipment to build upon the social skills s/he still has. The program and structured environment which promotes this is called a resocialization program.

**Resting Tremors** A jerking or shaking of the muscles when the muscle is not actively being used.

**Restraints** Restraints are objects or systems of limiting a resident's movement. Medications to control a resident's activity level and behavioral patterns are legally considered restraints. At times restraints may be medically indicated but too often they are overused and abused. It is the resident's right not to be restrained unless all other options have been tried and have failed.

**Restraints — Inappropriate** As defined by the Federal *Immediate and Serious Threat* regulation in the United States: Inappropriate restraints are any form of restraint (physical devices, drugs or procedures) that in some way restrict a resident's physical and/or mental independence/autonomy which are inappropriately used and monitored. Situations/conditions which warrant investigation of inappropriate restraints include: 1. clinical records which reflect either an absence of justification or incorrect justification for use of restraints, 2. restraints which are applied as punishment, 3. serious or unexplained injures during the restraint process, 4. restraints which are improperly applied, 5. residents who appear unusually drowsy and/or apathetic and 6. a failure to monitor residents exhibiting symptoms of tardive dyskinesia.

**Right to Appeal (OBRA)** A transfer or discharge from the long term care facility which has not been initiated by the resident may be appealed by the resident or his/her responsible party. The intent of this right to appeal is that no one is discharged from a facility without those parties' consent. The appeal is filed with the Department of Health Services within 10 days of notification of a proposed transfer/discharge and the decision will be made by DHS within 30 days from the date the notice was issued.

**Rigidity** The act of being cognitively, perceptually or socially unbending/inflexible. A muscle is said to have rigidity when it is in a strong contraction.

**Risk** Taking an action even though there may be a possibility of injury or of a loss. In management, a risk is the possibility of a loss or injury in a given situation that is to be controlled to insure the ongoing health of the business.

**Risk Management** In business, risk management is the identification of potential losses and then the controlled management of those losses. The *level of risk* is to be identified to determine which risks are great enough that they need to be addressed. Frequently the degree or level of risk for leisure activities is divided into three levels: 1. high risk, 2. medium risk and 3. low risk. *High risk* are activities which require instruction and lengthy training and practice to perform safely (to control the level of risk). An example of a high risk activity would be ocean kayaking. *Medium risk* activities are activities which require instruction and some supervision and practice prior to engaging the activity. An example of medium risk activity would be cross country skiing. *Low risk* activities are activities which require little to no instruction and practice to reduce risk. An example of a low risk activity would be reading the newspaper.

**Risk Taking** The degree to which an individual is willing to engage in an activity that involves a significant degree of risk.

**Self-Esteem** The feeling that one is of great worth or of high value to others and to self. Self-esteem is earned, not just learned through books and lectures. Actual accomplishment leads to good self-esteem.

**Self-Stimulation** The stimulation of one's own nerves, usually as a result of being in an environment deprived of normal stimulation. Some types of developmental disabilities will decrease the individual's ability to receive or understand stimulation from the environment. These individuals also tend to engage in a high level of self-stimulation. Self-stimulation, in most cases, is not considered to be socially acceptable in public.

**Sensation** A message carried by the nerves as a result of some action or event.

**Sensorimotor** Skills which require the coordination of one's senses with one's movement (motor behavior). Some of the functional skills which require a fair degree of sensorimotor skill are gross and fine motor coordination, muscle control, dexterity, strength and endurance, tactile awareness and range of motion.

**Sensory Deprivation** See *Deprivation*.

**Sensory Integration** The ability to take in stimulation from one's environment using a variety of sensory organs all at the same time. This information is then interpreted and integrated into one's personal knowledge of the world.

**Sensory Overload** The state in which the body is receiving more sensory input then it can handle (or comfortably ignore).

**Sensory Stimulation** A type of treatment intervention used with residents who have a significant cognitive loss and are not able to initiate and produce purposeful interaction with the environment. This intervention involves the frequent (multiple times a day, 5 or more minutes at a time) introduction of objects to stimulate the senses. Sensory stimulation is usually more productive if more than one sense is being stimulated at a time.

**Sequencing Skills** The ability to place objects or events in a logical order: by time, by number or other recognized pattern.

**Short Term Memory** A temporary memory system that will pass information to be remembered on to the long term memory. Short term memory will usually hold about seven or eight items or short ideas for a few seconds to up to a minute or so. The information stored in short term memory can either be forgotten or transmitted to long term memory. For this transfer to happen the information needs to be coded and organized prior to the transfer.

**Significant Change in a Resident's Status** (RAP/OBRA) A significant change means any of the following:
- Deterioration in two or more activities of daily living, communication and/or cognitive abilities that appear permanent. For example, simultaneous functional *and* cognitive decline often experienced by residents with chronic, degenerative illness such as Alzheimer's Disease or pronounced functional changes following a stroke.
- Loss of ability to freely ambulate or to use hands to grasp small objects to feed or groom oneself, such as sponge, toothbrush or comb. Such losses must be permanent and not attributable to identifiable, reversible causes such as drug toxicity from introducing a new medication or an episode of acute illness such as influenza.
- Deterioration in behavior, mood and/or relationships that has not been reversed by current staff interventions.
- Deterioration in a resident's health status, where this change: places the resident's life in danger, e.g., stroke, heart condition or diagnosis of metastatic cancer; is associated with a serious clinical complications, e.g., initial development of a Stage III or Stage IV pressure ulcer, the initial onset of non relieved delirium or recurrent loss of consciousness; or is associated with an initial new diagnosis of a condition that is likely to affect the resident's physical, mental or psychosocial well-being over a prolonged period of time, e.g., Alzheimer's Disease or diabetes.
- A serious clinical complication.
- A new diagnosis of a condition that is likely to affect the resident's physical, mental or psychosocial well-being over a prolonged period of time.
- Onset of significant weight loss (5% in last 30 days or 10% in last 180 days).
- A marked and sudden improvement in the resident's status, for example, a comatose resident regaining consciousness.

**Skill** The ability to demonstrate a refined pattern of movements. Skill requires competence in five areas: 1. coordination, 2. agility, 3. balance, 4. timing and 5. speed. (Kisner and Colby 1990, page 691)

**Skilled Nursing Facility** A subacute health care facility with licensed nurses 24 hours a day but without a physician 24 hours a day.

**Skin Integrity** See *Pressure Sore*.

**Social History (elements of)** One of the essential parts of a resident assessment, the social history presents a biography of the resident beginning with birthplace and proceeding from that point to include number of siblings, important situations from childhood (orphaned, often uprooted, secure and loving), education, religious background, occupation, military experience, marriage(s), children and other important family and friends, retirement and events leading up to hospitalization.

**Social Service Professional** An individual hired by a long term care facility to assist the resident and his/her family adjust to changing health status and functional ability and to assist the resident/family in the application for axillary services and financial support to receive necessary services. In the United States the federal legislation which regulates long term care facilities is called OBRA.

**Spasm** A sudden involuntary contraction of the muscles.

**Spastic** Having a varying stiffness or tightness of a limb caused by spasms.

**Standard Survey** In the United States under the OBRA legislation for long term care facilities a Standard Survey is a resident-centered, outcome-oriented inspection which relies on a case-mix stratified sample of residents to gather information about the facility's compliance with OBRA certification requirements. Based on the specific procedures, the Standard Survey assesses: 1. compliance with residents' rights, 2. the accuracy of residents' comprehensive assessments and the adequacy of care plans based on these assessments, 3. the quality of services furnished, as measured by indicators of medical, nursing, rehabilitative care and drug therapy, dietary and nutrition services, activities and social participation, sanitation and infection control; and 4. the effectiveness of the physical environment to empower residents, accommodate resident needs and maintain resident safety. If a surveyor, in conducting the information gathering tasks of the Standard Survey, identifies a possible noncompliant situation related to any requirement, investigation of the situation is done to determine whether the facility is in full compliance with the requirements. There are three other types of survey in addition to the Standard Survey. They are: 1. extended survey, 2. partial extended survey and 3. initial certification survey.

**Stretching** A prescribed activity designed to lengthen soft tissue which has been pathologically shortened.
- *Passive Stretching* The action of someone else (besides the resident) gently applying force to stretch tight tissue. Passive stretching is usually done by the PT, OT or Certified Nursing Assistant using prescribed ROM (Range of Motion) exercises.
- *Active Stretching* Resident initiated movement designed to increase ROM in affected soft tissue and joints. This is usually carried out in physical therapy using a prescribed exercise program or in therapy/activity programs using a prescribed set of activities designed to achieve the desired outcome.

The professional should encourage activities which involve the slow static stretching of muscles lasting between 10 to 30 seconds. Activities which involve bouncing stretches or ballistic stretches increase the resident's change of injury, especially after a period of immobility (Karam page 1).

**Stretching Selective** Decreased ROM (Range of Motion) for selective muscle groups can greatly increase the level of independence for residents with thoracic and cervical spinal injuries. After a full examination the physician or the physical therapist will determine the amount of tightness for the extensor muscles of the lower back that will be needed to enhance the resident's balance. A slight tightness will allow greater balance while leaning forward in a wheelchair for residents with no active control of the back extensors.

The professional should note the degree of tightness desired and ensure that the resident's leisure activities do not jeopardize that stability.

**Stroke** (also known as a cerebral vascular accident) A stroke is the interruption of the blood supply to the brain. When the brain cells do not receive the oxygen contained in the blood, they start to die. Because different types of brain cells control different actions and thoughts, the type of disability will vary from person to person. The effects of a stroke depends on two factors: 1. the location of the brain affected and 2. the intensity of the interruption (how much blood was cut off from the cells). The National Stoke Association lists four primary warning signs of stroke: 1. numbness, weakness or paralysis of face, arm or leg — especially on one side of the body; 2, loss of balance or coordination when combined with another warning sign; 3. sudden blurred or decreased vision in one or both eyes; and 4. difficulty speaking or understanding language.

**Subacute Stage** The second of three stages of the healing and maturation of an illness or injury. The subacute stage usually begins about the 4th day after an injury and is marked by noted repair of the injured area. The subacute stage usually is over by the 21st day after the onset of an injury, but may last as long as six weeks (Kisner & Colby, 1990, page 216). During this time the remaining blood clots are absorbed and replaced by fibroblastic activity (which produces collagen). Immature connective tissue and granulation tissue form (to speed up the delivery of oxygen to the injured site). These tissues are very susceptible to damage by overstretching, overuse or by being pulled/sheered in the wrong direction. Pain may be experienced by the resident as the immature tissue is stretched just past its normal limit. Some gentle stretching (in consultation with the physical therapist) is recommended to reduce the adherence to surrounding tissues during the healing process. (See *Acute Stage* and *Chronic Stage*.)

**Survey Process** Most facilities are evaluated by an outside agency to measure the quality of services being provided. This evaluation, called a "survey," is usually done by the government and/or a private credentialing agency (e.g., Joint Commission or CARF). A survey team is sent to the facility for a short period of time (usually 2 days to 2 weeks) to evaluate service delivery by sampling approximately 10% of the resident records. The surveyors will frequently evaluate resident records back 6–12 months or more to be able to identify trends in resident care. Just before the survey team leaves the facility, they will have an information "exit" meeting with the administration to give a general overview of their findings. The survey team will then meet after they leave the facility to write up the formal survey document. The time period just before and during a survey tends to produce extreme stress among staff. This is a normal response, however, not a very productive one. The surveyors will be evaluating the services delivered over a long period of time as well as the current treatment environment in the facility; they will be able to tell if the facility has brought in extra staff just for the time of the survey. One element of a survey that tends to produce excessive stress is the fact that most surveys just list areas that need to be improved. (Surveys done by State and Federal agencies are not allowed to put positive comments in the survey document — only citations of substandard care.)

**Syndrome** A group of symptoms, behaviors or disabilities which are interrelated and cause somewhat predictable problems for the person with the syndrome.

**Tactile Defensiveness** The reaction from a resident who is hypersensitive to touch — the withdrawing of a body part when it is touched because the touch is irritating and uncomfortable due to excessive neurological reaction.

**Tags** A tag is the number assigned to each measurable element of a law.

**Tardive Dyskinesia** A movement disorder brought about by a long term use of antipsychotic medications. Prolonged use of antipsychotic medications triggers a heightened sensitivity in the dopamine receptors. Dopamine is a chemical formed by the body as an intermediate product or norepinephrine and acts as a neurotransmitter in the central nervous system. This heightened sensitivity causes the individual to demonstrate abnormal movement patterns. Not only are these abnormal movement patterns a disability in themselves, they also tend to make other people uncomfortable around the individual. Possible early indications of Tardive Dyskinesia include: 1. involuntary repetitious facial movements, 2. lip smacking, 3. tics or spasms, 4. chewing motions with mouth, 5. ocular movements (eyes rolled up and fixed in position, 6. difficulty swallowing (many of these medications suppress the cough reflex) and 7. rocking or swaying. It is important for all staff working with individuals taking antipsychotic medications to continually watch for the onset of these side affects. Discontinuing the use of the medications may stop the process of Tardive Dyskinesia. Symptoms may decrease or disappear after the medication has been discontinued. However, in many cases the individual will continue to exhibit the symptoms at the same level indefinitely. The earlier the syndrome is identified, the better the chances are that the symptoms will subside. In some cases muscle relaxants are prescribed, usually only for short term use during the early stages of the syndrome. It is not unusual for all of the symptoms to subside during sleep. Women, elderly and individuals who have had a long history of taking antipsychotic medications are the three groups most likely to demonstrate the symptoms. However, each individual seems to have his/her own threshold level, so the symptoms may occur in men and women at any age regardless of the dosage taken or the length of time administered.

**Target Heart Rate** The desired heart rate to be achieved during cardiovascular activity. The target heart rate is always determined before the resident is involved in a prescribed program to increase cardiovascular endurance. The professional may want to consult the resident's physician when determining the target heart rate. Some medications may modify the resident's responsive heart rate, making the use of standardized target heart rate scales undesirable.

**Terminal Care** Intervention for residents who are approaching death. Most often these care needs are addressed by a signed advance directive and usually strive to provide comfort for the body (freedom from pain if possible) and provide solace for the mind/soul (religious intervention when requested).

**Test** Measurement of specific skills or knowledge using a predetermined set of questions or tasks; a trial or evaluation.

**Theory** The well defined sets of explanations for why something exists.

**Therapeutic Community** A unit, facility or other structured environment which strives to meet the resident's needs in a holistic manner (physical, social, emotional and psychological). Not all facilities provide a therapeutic community.

**Therapeutic Recreation Specialist** An individual who has finished their college curriculum, graduated, but has not taken and passed the national exam so that they may be called a Certified Therapeutic Recreation Specialist.

**Threshold of Sensation** The point at which a nerve has received enough stimulation to be able to "fire" and send a signal to the next nerve.

**Thrombus** A clot within the heart or a blood vessel that may lead to obstruction.

**Tightness** A term describing a mild contracture of a group of muscles and tendons usually caused by inactivity and easily resolved through gentle, frequent enjoyable activities which promote ROM (Range of Motion) of the involved area.

**Tissue Injury, Degree of** Health care professionals usually divide injury to tissue into three levels or degrees. It is important for the professional to be aware of the three degrees and to be able to make a reasonable determination of the degree of injury received during an activity. Frequently an incident report will need to be written up for any tissue damage of a second or third degree and a continuing quality improvement program will be required to reduce the likelihood of a repeat incident.

**Tolerance** The ability to ignore irritating stimuli.

**Tone** The degree to which the muscles display strength and the ability to recover from normal stretching and contracting.

**Transient Ischemic Attack (TIA)** Temporary symptoms of a stroke. Complete recovery usually results within 24 hours. A clot may have occluded the blood vessel and then released. People having TIAs are advised to seek medical attention immediately because TIAs are signs of future strokes. People who have had a stroke may also have TIAs. Always alert a doctor to these "mini-strokes."

**Traumatic Brain Injury (TBI)** Injury to the brain as a result of a traumatic event. This event may be due to an impact (e.g., being hit on the head by a baseball), due to acceleration/deceleration (e.g., being hit from behind in your car while wearing your seat belt — your head still goes forward then back, as does your brain inside of your skull) or due to a penetrating injury (e.g., gun shot wound). The types of disabilities seen as a result of a TBI would depend on the part of the brain that was injured.

**Treatment** The use of identified methods of intervention to manage the resident's care. This management consists of assessment, specific interventions, reassessment and discharge.

**Treatment Plan** The formally outlined set of treatment interventions and services for a resident to ameliorate an illness or injury. A treatment plan is based on a formal assessment to determine need and using clinical opinion/judgment and pre-established treatment interventions, anticipate an outcome. Also see *Care Plan*.

| problem/need | treatment | outcome | date |
|---|---|---|---|
| ⇓ ability to find room | 1. provide large lettered name on door (service) | ⇑ ability to identify room due to label | 3/2/97 |
| | 2. develop memory book with pictures and directions from activity room to bedroom (service) | ownership of prosthetic device to assist with ⇓ pathfinding ability | 3/5/97 |
| | 3. practice with memory book five days a week, two times a day (therapy) | ⇑ ability/skill in using memory book and residual memory to pathfind to room | 5/6/97 |

**Trigger** A trigger is something which causes action. In the case of long term care facilities in the United States, a "trigger" means that a resident has scored in an unacceptable range on one or more sections of the MDS. This would identify the resident as needing further evaluation using assessment protocols designated either by the State or the Federal government.

**Unilateral Neglect** Lack of awareness of one side of the body. (See *Neglect*.)

**Update** A written report of the resident's response to placement and treatment placed in the medical record based on a reassessment, at least quarterly, of the resident. Updates are to reflect, but are not limited to: health status, psychosocial needs, alteration in ability to participate in activities and new or improved or increased behavior problems with a related program of behavioral interventions.

**Validation** For those individuals who are very disoriented, the validation of the memories and feelings that they have is an important aspect of humane treatment. Validation activities do not focus on orientation; they focus on the resident's perception of what happened in the past (correct or incorrect — it doesn't matter).

**Vascular Dementia** This is a type of dementia that is similar to late onset dementia in the types of cognitive losses demonstrated by the resident, only that the damage to the brain is in measurable step-downs due to strokes and not systematically progressive in a downward flowing manner. (Formally Multi-Infarct Dementia.)

**Vestibular System** The nerves and bony structures of the ears which are responsible for hearing and for being able to discern which way is up (equilibrium).

**Visual Cues** The objects in the environment which when seen, help an individual interpret his/her world. Parking signs, restroom signs and familiar restaurant signs are different type of visual cues which we use everyday. A staff person may use a hand gesture as a visual cue to help a resident remember which way to go back to his/her room.

**Visual Function** (RAP) The aging process leads to a gradual decline in visual acuity; a decreased ability to focus on close objects or to see small print, a reduced capacity to adjust to changes in light and dark and diminished ability to discriminate color. The aged eye requires about 3–4 times more light in order to see well than the young eye. The leading causes of visual impairment in the elderly are macular degeneration, cataracts, glaucoma and diabetic retinopathy. In addition, visual perceptual deficits (impaired perceptions of the relationship of objects in the environment) are common in the nursing home population. Such deficits are a common consequence of cerebrovascular events and are often seen in the late stages of Alzheimer's disease and other dementias. The incidence of all these problems increases with age. In 1974, 49% of all nursing home residents were described as being unable to see well enough to read a newspaper with or without glasses. In 1985, over 100,000 nursing home residents were estimated to have severe visual impairment or no vision at all. Thus vision loss is one of the most prevalent losses of residents in nursing facilities. A significant number of residents in any facility may be expected to have difficulty performing tasks depending on vision as well as problems adjusting to vision loss.

**Visual Impairment** The ability to see is a seven step process. If there is an interruption or malfunction in any of the seven steps, the individual will experience a visual impairment. The degree of impairment, even after treatment, depends on which step is impaired and to what degree. Since information which we receive visually is one of our greatest learning and survival tools, any loss of function changes the way we interact with the world around us.

1. The cornea is a protective covering over the surface of the eye. If this covering is damaged, it distorts the image. A cornea transplant is one means of correction, especially with elderly populations.
2. The anterior chamber is filled with a clear fluid to help the cornea maintain its proper shape.
3. The iris regulates the amount of light allowed into the eye. This regulation of light helps to protect the retina from being "burned" by too much light and helps control the amount of light to allow the best interpretation of objects.
4. The lens adjusts focus to allow better interpretation of images. If the lens becomes cloudy (cataracts), everything appears to be blurred and dimmed.
5. The vitreous body contains a clear jell which helps maintain the correct distance between the lens and the retina. It also helps maintain the correct curvature of the retina, allowing better vision. Glaucoma is a condition where there is an increased fluid build up in the vitreous body. This buildup stretches the outer perimeter of the eye, stretching the optic nerves to the point of failure. This stretching usually impacts the outer optic nerves first (peripheral vision). Untreated, it progressively stretches the optic nerves toward the center. The end result is tunnel vision or total blindness.
6. The retina's function is to change images into electronic signal which can be interpreted by the brain. There are various causes for deterioration or malformation of the retina, but the professional will most frequently see individuals with damage caused by diabetes and/or aging. Diabetes may cause multiple hemorrhages in the retina. These hemorrhages cause dark spots to appear in the individual's vision.
7. The optic nerves transmit the signals from the retina to the vision center of the brain. Youth who have sustained a severe traumatic brain injury (TBI) are at increased risk of damage to these nerves.

Damage to the parts of the brain which interpret vision, may make vision impossible, even if all seven of these steps/body parts are not damaged. The occurrence of severe visual impairment is approximately one in four thousand (Blackman) for the "normal" population. However, that occurrence rate drops to almost 1 in 3 individuals with multiple disorders. Too frequently the professional will over look the importance of training the individual with developmental disabilities, dementia or severe cognitive impairment to wear his/her glasses. The pressure of the glasses on the bridge of the nose or over the ears is difficult to tolerate if you do not understand the reason for the irritation. However, not wearing glasses significantly increases sensory deprivation due to the lack of visual input. The long term prognosis from this deprivation is a greater degree of disability. Staff sometimes become confused about the issue of an individual's right to refuse to wear glasses. An individual, even one with significant cognitive impairment, cannot give an "informed" refusal for treatment (wearing glasses) if the staff have not first informed the individual about the benefits vs. risks. Since few of these individuals learn well via verbal communication, a training program which 1. promotes the wearing of the glasses to allow the individual to experience improved vision and 2. promotes praise, a positive atmosphere and experiences of success resulting from the improved vision should be implemented.

**Visual Neglect** See *Visuospatial Neglect*.

**Visuospatial Neglect** Lack of awareness of one side of the body. (See *Neglect*.)

**Weight Bearing** Refers to the amount of one's own weight that can be supported by one or more body parts. Three levels are usually considered: Non Weight Bearing (NWB), Partial Weight Bearing (PWB), Full Weight Bearing (FWB).

## References

American Psychiatric Association. 1994. **Diagnostic and Statistical Manual of Mental Disorders Fourth Edition**. Washington, DC.

American Psychiatric Association. 1987. **Diagnostic and Statistical Manual of Mental Disorders (Third Edition — Revised)**. Washington, DC.

Armstrong, M., S. Lauzen. 1994. **Community Integration Program**, Second Edition. Idyll Arbor, Inc., Ravensdale, WA.

Blackman, J. A. 1990. **Medical Aspects of Developmental Disabilities in Children Birth to Three**. Aspen Publications, Gaithersburg, MD.

Bradford, Leland P. 1976. **Making Meetings Work: A Guide for Leaders and Group Members**. University Associates, La Jolla, CA.

burlingame, j. and T. M. Blaschko. 1991. **Therapy in Intermediate Care Facilities for the Mentally Retarded**. Idyll Arbor, Inc., Ravensdale, WA.

Health Care Financing Administration. 1990. **Resident Assessment System For Long Term Care Facilities**. US Department of Commerce National Technical Information Service. Springfield, VA.

Health Care Financing Administration. 1992. **State Operations Manual Provider Certification**. US Department of Commerce National Technical Information Service. Springfield, VA.

Hopkins, H. L. and H. D. Smith. 1983. **Willard and Spackman's Occupational Therapy, Sixth Edition**. J. B. Lippincott Company, New York, NY.

Karam, C. 1989. **A Practical Guide to Cardiac Rehabilitation**. Aspen Publications, Gaithersburg, MD.

Kemp, B., K. Brummel-Smith and J. W. Ramsdell. 1990. **Geriatric Rehabilitation**. College Hill Publications, Boston, MA.

Kisner, C. and Colby, L. A. 1990. **Therapeutic Exercise: Foundations and Techniques, Second Edition**. F. A. Davis, Philadelphia, PA.

Kübler-Ross, E. 1969. **On Death and Dying**. Macmillan Publishing Co., Inc., New York, NY.

Lewis, C. B. 1989. **Improving Mobility in Older Persons: A Manual for Geriatric Specialists**. Aspen Publication, Gaithersburg, MD.

McKay, Davis, Fanning. 1983. **Messages: The Communication Skills Book**. New Harbinger Publications, Oakland, CA.

Randall-David, E. 1989. **Strategies for Working With Culturally Diverse Communities and Clients**. Association for the Care of Children's Health, Bethesda, MD.

Reber, A. S. 1985. **Dictionary of Psychology**. Penguin Books, New York, NY.

G. P. Rodman, C. McEwen and S. L. Wallace. 1973. *Primer on the Rheumatic Diseases*. Reprinted from **The Journal of the American Medical Association** 224, no. 5 (April 30, 1973) (Supplement).

US Department of Health and Human Services. 1983. **CDC Guidelines for Isolation Precautions in Hospitals** and **CDC Guidelines for Infection Control in Hospital Personnel**. Centers for Disease Control, Atlanta. GA.

Voelkl, J. E. 1988. Risk Management in Therapeutic Recreation: A Component of Quality Assurance. Venture Publishing, State College, PA.

# Appendix B: Minimum Data Set and the Resident Assessment System

Facilities in the United States which receive Medicare funds are required to use a specific, standardized assessment on every resident admitted to the facility. This standardized assessment, called the Minimum Data Set (MDS), is an interdisciplinary assessment. Each member of the interdisciplinary team is required to conduct their own assessment of the resident, analyze the resident's status and then summarize that information on the MDS form within 14 days of the resident's admission to the facility.

The MDS provides health care workers in long term care settings with two advantages: 1. it standardizes medical vocabulary across the nation and 2. it provides the mechanism for the collection of information: demographic information, morality and morbidity statistics and treatment outcomes. The MDS has been used long enough for us to be able to recognize when a "score" on the MDS indicates health or when it indicates the need to provide some kind of treatment. A book which is used with the MDS, called **Resident Assessment System for Long Term Care**, outlines which scores or combination of scores, point up the need for specific interventions.

A "slang" term has arisen called "RAPs." RAPs (Resident Assessment Protocols) refers to the system of deciding which types of interventions will be needed by scoring the MDS and reviewing the results in the book **Resident Assessment System for Long Term Care.** By reviewing the RAPs each health care professional will be able to determine if there is a specific treatment required for the resident. The treatment interventions "triggered" by using RAPs indicate the basic, minimum standard of treatment for residents in long term care facilities. Not implementing a RAPs treatment intervention (unless otherwise medically indicated) would be providing substandard care.

There are 18 identified RAPs:

- Delirium
- Cognitive Loss/Dementia
- Visual Function
- Communication
- ADL Functional/Rehab Potential
- Urinary Incontinence and Indwelling Catheter
- Psychosocial Well-Being
- Mood State
- Behavior Problem
- Activities
- Falls
- Nutritional Status
- Feeding Tubes
- Dehydration/Fluid Maintenance
- Dental Care
- Pressure Ulcers
- Psychoactive Drug Use
- Physical Restraints

Both the Activity Professional and the Social Service Professional should be familiar with the MDS, the **Resident Assessment System for Long Term Care**, RAPs and how to decide if a treatment intervention is indicated. The chapter on *Resident Care* in this book provides an overview of many of the RAPs that may "trigger" the need for the Activity Professional or Social Service Professional to take action. To help the reader develop a fuller understanding of the MDS and RAPs process a copy of the MDS, the basic instructions for using RAPs and two specific protocols have been included in this appendix. The MDS in this book is used with permission from the Briggs Corporation. The RAPs in this book are from **Resident Assessment System for Long Term Care** published by the US Department of Commerce, National Technical Information Service, Springfield, VA.

Numeric Identifier_____

# MINIMUM DATA SET (MDS) — *VERSION 2.0*
## FOR NURSING HOME RESIDENT ASSESSMENT AND CARE SCREENING
### *BASIC ASSESSMENT TRACKING FORM*

| SECTION AA. IDENTIFICATION INFORMATION |
|---|

| | | |
|---|---|---|
| 1. | RESIDENT NAME ⊛ | a. (First)　　　　b. (Middle Initial)　　　c. (Last)　　　　d. (Jr./Sr.) |
| 2. | GENDER ⊛ | 1. Male　　　2. Female |
| 3. | BIRTHDATE ⊛ | ☐☐ — ☐☐ — ☐☐☐☐<br>Month　　　Day　　　Year |
| 4. | RACE/ ⊛ ETHNICITY | 1. American Indian/Alaskan Native　　4. Hispanic<br>2. Asian/Pacific Islander　　　　　　5. White, not of<br>3. Black, not of Hispanic origin　　　　　Hispanic origin |
| 5. | SOCIAL ⊛ SECURITY AND ⊛ MEDICARE NUMBERS [C in 1st box if non Med. no.] | a. Social Security Number<br>☐☐☐ — ☐☐ — ☐☐☐☐<br>b. Medicare number (or comparable railroad insurance number)<br>☐☐☐☐☐☐☐☐☐☐ |
| 6. | FACILITY PROVIDER NO. ⊛ | a. State No.<br>☐☐☐☐☐☐☐☐☐☐☐☐<br>b. Federal No. ☐☐☐☐☐☐☐☐☐☐☐☐ |
| 7. | MEDICAID NO. ["+" if pending, "N" if not a Medicaid ⊛ recipient] | ☐☐☐☐☐☐☐☐☐☐☐☐ |
| 8. | REASONS FOR ASSESS-MENT | [Note—Other codes do not apply to this form]<br>a. Primary reason for assessment<br>　1. Admission assessment (required by day 14)<br>　2. Annual assessment<br>　3. Significant change in status assessment<br>　4. Significant correction of prior assessment<br>　5. Quarterly review assessment<br>　0. *NONE OF ABOVE*<br>b. *Special codes for use with supplemental assessment types in Case Mix demonstration states or other states where required*<br>　1. 5 day assessment<br>　2. 30 day assessment<br>　3. 60 day assessment<br>　4. Quarterly assessment using full MDS form<br>　5. Readmission/return assessment<br>　6. Other state required assessment |
| 9. | SIGNATURES OF PERSONS COMPLETING THESE ITEMS: | |

| a. Signatures | Title | Date |
|---|---|---|
| b. | | Date |

## GENERAL INSTRUCTIONS
*Complete this information for submission with all full and quarterly assessments (Admission, Annual, Significant Change, State or Medicare required assessments, or Quarterly Reviews, etc.).*

⊛ = Key items for computerized resident tracking

☐ = When box blank, must enter number or letter

|a.| = When letter in box, check if condition applies

**Code "NA" if information unavailable or unknown.**

### TRIGGER LEGEND

1 - Delirium
2 - Cognitive Loss/Dementia
3 - Visual Function
4 - Communication
5A - ADL-Rehabilitation
5B - ADL-Maintenance
6 - Urinary Incontinence and Indwelling Catheter
7 - Psychosocial Well-Being
8 - Mood State
9 - Behavioral Symptoms

10A - Activities (Revise)
10B - Activities (Review)
11 - Falls
12 - Nutritional Status
13 - Feeding Tubes
14 - Dehydration/Fluid Maintenance
15 - Dental Care
16 - Pressure Ulcers
17 - Psychotropic Drug Use
17* - For this to trigger, O4a, b, or c must = 1-7
18 - Physical Restraints

**Form 1748HH** © 1995 Briggs Corporation, Des Moines, IA 50306 (800) 247-2343 PRINTED IN U.S.A.
R196　　Copyright limited to addition of trigger system.

　　　　　　　　　　　MDS 2.0　10/18/94N

Resident _____ Numeric Identifier_____

# MINIMUM DATA SET (MDS) — *VERSION 2.0*
## FOR NURSING HOME RESIDENT ASSESSMENT AND CARE SCREENING
### *BACKGROUND (FACE SHEET) INFORMATION AT ADMISSION*

## SECTION AB. DEMOGRAPHIC INFORMATION

| | | |
|---|---|---|
| 1. | DATE OF ENTRY | *Date the stay began. Note — Does not include readmission if record was closed at time of temporary discharge to hospital, etc. In such cases, use prior admission date.*<br><br>☐☐ — ☐☐ — ☐☐☐☐<br>Month    Day    Year |
| 2. | ADMITTED FROM (AT ENTRY) | 1. Private home/apt. with no home health services<br>2. Private home/apt. with home health services<br>3. Board and care/assisted living/group home<br>4. Nursing home<br>5. Acute care hospital<br>6. Psychiatric hospital, MR/DD facility<br>7. Rehabilitation hospital<br>8. Other |
| 3. | LIVED ALONE (PRIOR TO ENTRY) | 0. No    1. Yes    2. In other facility |
| 4. | ZIP CODE OF PRIOR PRIMARY RESIDENCE | ☐☐☐☐☐ |
| 5. | RESIDENTIAL HISTORY 5 YEARS PRIOR TO ENTRY | *(Check all settings resident lived in during 5 years prior to date of entry given in item AB1 above.)*<br>Prior stay at this nursing home  a.<br>Stay in other nursing home  b.<br>Other residential facility — board and care home, assisted living, group home  c.<br>MH/psychiatric setting  d.<br>MR/DD setting  e.<br>*NONE OF ABOVE*  f. |
| 6. | LIFETIME OCCUPATION(S) (Put "/" between two occupations) | ☐☐☐☐☐☐☐☐☐☐☐☐☐☐☐☐☐ |
| 7. | EDUCATION (*Highest level completed*) | 1. No schooling  5. Technical or trade school<br>2. 8th grade/less  6. Some college<br>3. 9-11 grades  7. Bachelor's degree<br>4. High school  8. Graduate degree |
| 8. | LANGUAGE | *(Code for correct response)*<br>a. Primary Language<br>0. English  1. Spanish  2. French  3. Other<br><br>b. If other, specify ☐☐☐☐☐☐☐☐☐ |
| 9. | MENTAL HEALTH HISTORY | Does resident's RECORD indicate any history of mental retardation, mental illness, or developmental disability problem?<br>0. No    1. Yes |
| 10. | CONDITIONS RELATED TO MR/DD STATUS | *(Check all conditions that are related to MR/DD status that were manifested before age 22, and are likely to continue indefinitely)*<br>Not applicable — no MR/DD (Skip to AB11)  a.<br>MR/DD with organic condition<br>  Down's syndrome  b.<br>  Autism  c.<br>  Epilepsy  d.<br>  Other organic condition related to MR/DD  e.<br>MR/DD with no organic condition  f. |
| 11. | DATE BACKGROUND INFORMATION COMPLETED | ☐☐ — ☐☐ — ☐☐☐☐<br>Month    Day    Year |

☐ = When box blank, must enter number or letter

☐a. = When letter in box, check if condition applies

**Code "NA" if information unavailable or unknown.**

## SECTION AC. CUSTOMARY ROUTINE

| 1. CUSTOMARY ROUTINE | *(Check all that apply. If all information UNKNOWN, check last box only)* | |
|---|---|---|
| *(In year prior to DATE OF ENTRY to this nursing home, or year last in community if now being admitted from another nursing home)* | **CYCLE OF DAILY EVENTS** | |
| | Stays up late at night (e.g., after 9 pm) | a. |
| | Naps regularly during day (at least 1 hour) | b. |
| | Goes out 1+ days a week | c. |
| | Stays busy with hobbies, reading, or fixed daily routine | d. |
| | Spends most of time alone or watching TV | e. |
| | Moves independently indoors (with appliances, if used) | f. |
| | Use of tobacco products at least daily | g. |
| | *NONE OF ABOVE* | h. |
| | **EATING PATTERNS** | |
| | Distinct food preferences | i. |
| | Eats between meals all or most days | j. |
| | Use of alcoholic beverage(s) at least weekly | k. |
| | *NONE OF ABOVE* | l. |
| | **ADL PATTERNS** | |
| | In bedclothes much of day | m. |
| | Wakens to toilet all or most nights | n. |
| | Has irregular bowel movement pattern | o. |
| | Showers for bathing | p. |
| | Bathing in PM | q. |
| | *NONE OF ABOVE* | r. |
| | **INVOLVEMENT PATTERNS** | |
| | Daily contact with relatives/close friends | s. |
| | Usually attends church, temple, synagogue (etc.) | t. |
| | Finds strength in faith | u. |
| | Daily animal companion/presence | v. |
| | Involved in group activities | w. |
| | *NONE OF ABOVE* | x. |
| | **UNKNOWN** — Resident/family unable to provide information | y. |

**END**

## SECTION AD. FACE SHEET SIGNATURES

SIGNATURES OF PERSONS COMPLETING FACE SHEET:

| | | | |
|---|---|---|---|
| a. Signature of RN Assessment Coordinator | | | Date |
| b. Signatures | Title | Sections | Date |
| c. | | | Date |
| d. | | | Date |
| e. | | | Date |
| f. | | | Date |
| g. | | | Date |

**NOTE:** Normally, the MDS Face Sheet is completed once, when an individual first enters the facility. However, the face sheet is also required if the person is reentering this facility after a discharge where return had not previously been expected. It is **not** completed following temporary discharges to hospitals or after therapeutic leaves/home visits.

Form 1748HH   © 1995 Briggs Corporation, Des Moines, IA 50306 (800) 247-2343 PRINTED IN U.S.A.<br>Copyright limited to addition of trigger system.

Resident _____  Numeric Identifier _____

# MINIMUM DATA SET (MDS) — *VERSION 2.0*
## FOR NURSING HOME RESIDENT ASSESSMENT AND CARE SCREENING
### *FULL ASSESSMENT FORM*
(Status in last 7 days, unless other time frame indicated)

## SECTION A. IDENTIFICATION AND BACKGROUND INFORMATION

**1. RESIDENT NAME**

a. (First)   b. (Middle Initial)   c. (Last)   d. (Jr./Sr.)

**2. ROOM NUMBER**

**3. ASSESS-MENT REFERENCE DATE**

a. *Last day of MDS observation period*

Month — Day — Year

b. Original (0) or corrected copy of form (enter number of correction)

**4a. DATE OF REENTRY**

Date of reentry from most recent temporary discharge to a hospital in last 90 days (or since last assessment or admission if less than 90 days)

Month — Day — Year

**5. MARITAL STATUS**

1. Never married   3. Widowed   5. Divorced
2. Married   4. Separated

**6. MEDICAL RECORD NO.**

**7. CURRENT PAYMENT SOURCES FOR N.H. STAY**

*(Billing Office to indicate; check all that apply in last 30 days)*

| | | | |
|---|---|---|---|
| Medicaid per diem | a. | VA per diem | f. |
| Medicare per diem | b. | Self or family pays for full per diem | g. |
| Medicare ancillary part A | c. | Medicaid resident liability or Medicare co-payment | h. |
| Medicare ancillary part B | d. | Private insurance per diem (including co-payment) | i. |
| CHAMPUS per diem | e. | Other per diem | j. |

**8. REASONS FOR ASSESS-MENT**

*[Note—If this is a discharge or reentry assessment, only a limited subset of MDS items need be completed]*

a. Primary reason for assessment
1. Admission assessment (required by day 14)
2. Annual assessment
3. Significant change in status assessment
4. Significant correction of prior assessment
5. Quarterly review assessment
6. Discharged—return not anticipated
7. Discharged—return anticipated
8. Discharged prior to completing initial assessment
9. Reentry
0. NONE OF ABOVE

b. *Special codes for use with supplemental assessment types in Case Mix demonstration states or other states where required*
1. 5 day assessment
2. 30 day assessment
3. 60 day assessment
4. Quarterly assessment using full MDS form
5. Readmission/return assessment
6. Other state required assessment

**9. RESPONSI-BILITY/ LEGAL GUARDIAN**

*(Check all that apply)*

| | | | |
|---|---|---|---|
| Legal guardian | a. | Durable power of attorney/ financial | d. |
| Other legal oversight | b. | Family member responsible | e. |
| Durable power of attorney/health care | c. | Patient responsible for self | f. |
| | | NONE OF ABOVE | g. |

**10. ADVANCED DIRECTIVES**

*(For those items with supporting documentation in the medical record, check all that apply)*

| | | | |
|---|---|---|---|
| Living will | a. | Feeding restrictions | f. |
| Do not resuscitate | b. | Medication restrictions | g. |
| Do not hospitalize | c. | Other treatment restrictions | h. |
| Organ donation | d. | NONE OF ABOVE | i. |
| Autopsy request | e. | | |

## SECTION B. COGNITIVE PATTERNS

**1. COMATOSE**

*(Persistent vegetative state/no discernible consciousness)*

0. No   1. Yes *(If yes, skip to Section G)*

**2. MEMORY**

*(Recall of what was learned or known)*

a. Short-term memory OK—seems/appears to recall after 5 minutes
0. Memory OK   1. Memory problem **2**

b. Long-term memory OK—seems/appears to recall long past
0. Memory OK   1. Memory problem **2**

☐ = When box blank, must enter number or letter.

a.☐ = When letter in box, check if condition applies

Code "NA" if information unavailable or unknown.

**3. MEMORY/ RECALL ABILITY**

*(Check all that resident was **normally able to recall during last 7 days**)*

| | | | |
|---|---|---|---|
| Current season | a. | That he/she is in a nursing home | d. |
| Location of own room | b. | NONE OF ABOVE are recalled | e. |
| Staff names/faces | c. | | |

**4. COGNITIVE SKILLS FOR DAILY DECISION-MAKING**

*(Made decisions regarding tasks of daily life)*
0. INDEPENDENT—decisions consistent/reasonable
1. MODIFIED INDEPENDENCE—some difficulty in new situations only **2**
2. MODERATELY IMPAIRED—decisions poor; cues/ supervision required **2**
3. SEVERELY IMPAIRED—never/rarely made decisions **2, 5B**

**5. INDICATORS OF DELIRIUM— PERIODIC DISOR-DERED THINKING/ AWARENESS**

*(Code for behavior in the last 7 days.)* [Note: Accurate assessment requires conversations with staff and family who have direct knowledge of resident's behavior over this time.]
0. Behavior not present
1. Behavior present, not of recent onset
2. Behavior present, over last 7 days appears different from resident's usual functioning (e.g., new onset or worsening)

a. EASILY DISTRACTED—(e.g., difficulty paying attention; gets sidetracked) 2 = **1, 17\***

b. PERIODS OF ALTERED PERCEPTION OR AWARE-NESS OF SURROUNDINGS—(e.g., moves lips or talks to someone not present; believes he/she is somewhere else; confuses night and day) 2 = **1, 17\***

c. EPISODES OF DISORGANIZED SPEECH—(e.g., speech is incoherent, nonsensical, irrelevant, or rambling from subject to subject; loses train of thought) 2 = **1, 17\***

d. PERIODS OF RESTLESSNESS—(e.g., fidgeting or picking at skin, clothing, napkins, etc.; frequent position changes; repetitive physical movements or calling out) 2 = **1, 17\***

e. PERIODS OF LETHARGY—(e.g., sluggishness; staring into space; difficult to arouse; little body movement) 2 = **1, 17\***

f. MENTAL FUNCTION VARIES OVER THE COURSE OF THE DAY—(e.g., sometimes better, sometimes worse; behaviors sometimes present, sometimes not) 2 = **1, 17\***

**6. CHANGE IN COGNITIVE STATUS**

Resident's cognitive status, skills, or abilities have changed as compared to status of **90 days ago** (or since assessment if less than 90 days)
0. No change   1. Improved   2. Deteriorated **1, 17\***

## SECTION C. COMMUNICATION/HEARING PATTERNS

**1. HEARING**

*(With hearing appliance, if used)*
0. HEARS ADEQUATELY—normal talk, TV, phone **4**
1. MINIMAL DIFFICULTY when not in quiet setting **4**
2. HEARS IN SPECIAL SITUATIONS ONLY—speaker has to adjust tonal quality and speak distinctly **4**
3. HIGHLY IMPAIRED/absence of useful hearing **4**

**2. COMMUNI-CATION DEVICES/ TECH-NIQUES**

*(Check all that apply during last 7 days)*

| | |
|---|---|
| Hearing aid, present and used | a. |
| Hearing aid, present and not used regularly | b. |
| Other receptive comm. techniques used (e.g., lip reading) | c. |
| NONE OF ABOVE | d. |

**3. MODES OF EXPRESSION**

*(Check all used by resident to make needs known)*

| | | | |
|---|---|---|---|
| Speech | a. | Signs/gestures/sounds | d. |
| Writing messages to express or clarify needs | b. | Communication board | e. |
| American sign language or Braille | c. | Other | f. |
| | | NONE OF ABOVE | g. |

**4. MAKING SELF UNDER-STOOD**

*(Expressing information content—however able)*
0. UNDERSTOOD
1. USUALLY UNDERSTOOD—difficulty finding words or finishing thoughts **4**
2. SOMETIMES UNDERSTOOD—ability is limited to making concrete requests **4**
3. RARELY/NEVER UNDERSTOOD **4**

**5. SPEECH CLARITY**

*(Code for speech in the last 7 days)*
0. CLEAR SPEECH—distinct, intelligible words
1. UNCLEAR SPEECH—slurred, mumbled words
2. NO SPEECH—absence of spoken words

**6. ABILITY TO UNDER-STAND OTHERS**

*(Understanding verbal information content—however able)*
0. UNDERSTANDS
1. USUALLY UNDERSTANDS—may miss some part/ intent of message **2, 4**
2. SOMETIMES UNDERSTANDS—responds adequately to simple, direct communication **2, 4**
3. RARELY/NEVER UNDERSTANDS **2, 4**

**7. CHANGE IN COMMUNI-CATION/ HEARING**

Resident's ability to express, understand, or hear information has changed as compared to status of **90 days ago** (or since last assessment if less than 90 days)
0. No change   1. Improved   2. Deteriorated **17\***

MDS 2.0   10/18/94N

Resident _____      Numeric Identifier _____

## SECTION D. VISION PATTERNS

| 1. | VISION | *(Ability to see in adequate light and with glasses if used)* |
|---|---|---|
| | | 0. *ADEQUATE*—sees fine detail, including regular print in newspapers/books |
| | | 1. *IMPAIRED*—sees large print, but not regular print in newspapers/books **3** |
| | | 2. *MODERATELY IMPAIRED*—limited vision; not able to see newspaper headlines, but can identify objects **3** |
| | | 3. *HIGHLY IMPAIRED*—object identification in question, but eyes appear to follow objects **3** |
| | | 4. *SEVERELY IMPAIRED*—no vision or sees only light, colors, or shapes; eyes do not appear to follow objects |

| 2. | VISUAL LIMITATIONS/ DIFFICULTIES | Side vision problems—decreased peripheral vision (e.g., leaves food on one side of tray, difficulty traveling, bumps into people and objects, misjudges placement of chair when seating self) | a. |
|---|---|---|---|
| | | Experiences any of following: sees halos or rings around lights; sees flashes of light; sees "curtains" over eyes | b. |
| | | *NONE OF ABOVE* | c. |

| 3. | VISUAL APPLIANCES | Glasses; contact lenses; magnifying glass |
|---|---|---|
| | | 0. No      1. Yes |

## SECTION E. MOOD AND BEHAVIOR PATTERNS

| 1. | INDICATORS OF DEPRESSION, ANXIETY, SAD MOOD | *(Code for indicators observed in last 30 days, irrespective of the assumed cause)* |
|---|---|---|
| | | 0. Indicator not exhibited in last 30 days |
| | | 1. Indicator of this type exhibited up to five days a week |
| | | 2. Indicator of this type exhibited daily or almost daily (6, 7 days a week) |

**VERBAL EXPRESSIONS OF DISTRESS**
a. Resident made negative statements—e.g., "Nothing matters; Would rather be dead; What's the use; Regrets having lived so long; Let me die" 1 or 2 = **8**
b. Repetitive questions—e.g. "Where do I go; What do I do?" 1 or 2 = **8**
c. Repetitive verbalizations— e.g., calling out for help ("God help me") 1 or 2 = **8**
d. Persistent anger with self or others—e.g., easily annoyed, anger at placement in nursing home; anger at care received 1 or 2 = **8**
e. Self deprecation—e.g., "I am nothing; I am of no use to anyone" 1 or 2 = **8**
f. Expressions of what appear to be unrealistic fears—e.g., fear of being abandoned, left alone, being with others 1 or 2 = **8**
g. Recurrent statements that something terrible is about to happen—e.g., believes he or she is about to die, have a heart attack 1 or 2 = **8**

h. Repetitive health complaints—e.g., persistently seeks medical attention, obsessive concern with body functions 1 or 2 = **8**
i. Repetitive anxious complaints/concerns (non-health related) e.g., persistently seeks attention/reassurance regarding schedules, meals, laundry/clothing, relationship issues 1 or 2 = **8**
**SLEEP-CYCLE ISSUES**
j. Unpleasant mood in morning 1 or 2 = **8**
k. Insomnia/change in usual sleep pattern 1 or 2 = **8**
**SAD, APATHETIC, ANXIOUS APPEARANCE**
l. Sad, pained, worried facial expressions— e.g., furrowed brows 1 or 2 = **8**
m. Crying, tearfulness 1 or 2 = **8**
n. Repetitive physical movements—e.g., pacing, hand wringing, restlessness, fidgeting, picking 1 or 2 = **8, 17\***
**LOSS OF INTEREST**
o. Withdrawal from activities of interest—e.g., no interest in longstanding activities or being with family/ friends 1 or 2 = **7, 8**
p. Reduced social interaction 1 or 2 = **8**

| 2. | MOOD PERSISTENCE | One or more indicators of depressed, sad or anxious mood were not easily altered by attempts to "cheer up", console, or reassure the resident over last 7 days |
|---|---|---|
| | | 0. No mood indicators   1. Indicators present, easily altered **8**   2. Indicators present, not easily altered **8** |

| 3. | CHANGE IN MOOD | Resident's mood status has changed as compared to status of 90 days ago (or since last assessment if less than 90 days) |
|---|---|---|
| | | 0. No change   1. Improved   2. Deteriorated **1, 17\*** |

| 4. | BEHAVIORAL SYMPTOMS | *(A) Behavioral symptom frequency in last 7 days* |
|---|---|---|
| | | 0. Behavior not exhibited in last 7 days |
| | | 1. Behavior of this type occurred 1 to 3 days in last 7 days |
| | | 2. Behavior of this type occurred 4 to 6 days, but less than daily |
| | | 3. Behavior of this type occurred daily |
| | | *(B) Behavioral symptom alterability in last 7 days* |
| | | 0. Behavior not present OR behavior was easily altered |
| | | 1. Behavior was not easily altered    (A) (B) |

a. WANDERING (moved with no rational purpose, seemingly oblivious to needs or safety) A = 1, 2, or 3 = **9, 11**
b. VERBALLY ABUSIVE BEHAVIORAL SYMPTOMS (others were threatened, screamed at, cursed at) A = 1, 2, or 3 = **9**
c. PHYSICALLY ABUSIVE BEHAVIORAL SYMPTOMS (others were hit, shoved, scratched, sexually abused) A = 1, 2, or 3 = **9**
d. SOCIALLY INAPPROPRIATE/DISRUPTIVE BEHAVIORAL SYMPTOMS (made disruptive sounds, noisiness, screaming, self-abusive acts, sexual behavior or disrobing in public, smeared/threw food/feces, hoarding, rummaged through others' belongings) A = 1, 2, or 3 = **9**
e. RESISTS CARE (resisted taking medications/injections, ADL assistance, or eating) A = 1, 2, or 3 = **9**

| 5. | CHANGE IN BEHAVIORAL SYMPTOMS | Resident's behavior status has changed as compared to **status of 90 days ago** (or since last assessment if less than 90 days) |
|---|---|---|
| | | 0. No change   1. Improved **9**   2. Deteriorated **1, 17\*** |

## SECTION F. PSYCHOSOCIAL WELL-BEING

| 1. | SENSE OF INITIATIVE/ INVOLVEMENT | At ease interacting with others | a. |
|---|---|---|---|
| | | At ease doing planned or structured activities | b. |
| | | At ease doing self-initiated activities | c. |
| | | Establishes own goals **7** | d. |
| | | Pursues involvement in life of facility (e.g., makes/keeps friends; involved in group activities; responds positively to new activities; assists at religious services) | e. |
| | | Accepts invitations into most group activities | f. |
| | | *NONE OF ABOVE* | g. |

| 2. | UNSETTLED RELATIONSHIPS | Covert/open conflict with or repeated criticism of staff **7** | a. |
|---|---|---|---|
| | | Unhappy with roommate **7** | b. |
| | | Unhappy with residents other than roommate **7** | c. |
| | | Openly expresses conflict/anger with family/friends **7** | d. |
| | | Absence of personal contact with family/friends | e. |
| | | Recent loss of close family member/friend | f. |
| | | Does not adjust easily to change in routines | g. |
| | | *NONE OF ABOVE* | h. |

| 3. | PAST ROLES | Strong identification with past roles and life status **7** | a. |
|---|---|---|---|
| | | Expresses sadness/anger/empty feeling over lost roles/status **7** | b. |
| | | Resident perceives that daily routine (customary routine, activities) is very different from prior pattern in the community **7** | c. |
| | | *NONE OF ABOVE* | d. |

## SECTION G. PHYSICAL FUNCTIONING AND STRUCTURAL PROBLEMS

**1. (A) ADL SELF-PERFORMANCE—*(Code for resident's PERFORMANCE OVER ALL SHIFTS during last 7 days—Not including setup)***

0. *INDEPENDENT*—No help or oversight—OR—Help/oversight provided only 1 or 2 times during last 7 days
1. *SUPERVISION*—Oversight, encouragement or cueing provided 3 or more times during last 7 days—OR—Supervision (3 or more times) plus physical assistance provided only 1 or 2 times during last 7 days
2. *LIMITED ASSISTANCE*—Resident highly involved in activity; received physical help in guided maneuvering of limbs or other nonweight bearing assistance 3 or more times—OR—More help provided only 1 or 2 times during last 7 days
3. *EXTENSIVE ASSISTANCE*—While resident performed part of activity, over last 7-day period, help of following type(s) provided 3 or more times:
—Weight-bearing support
—Full staff performance during part (but not all) of last 7 days
4. *TOTAL DEPENDENCE*—Full staff performance of activity during entire 7 days
8. *ACTIVITY DID NOT OCCUR* during entire 7 days

**(B) ADL SUPPORT PROVIDED—*(Code for MOST SUPPORT PROVIDED OVER ALL SHIFTS during last 7 days; code regardless of resident's self-performance classification)***

0. No setup or physical help from staff
1. Setup help only
2. One person physical assist
3. Two+ persons physical assist
8. ADL activity itself did not occur during entire 7 days

| | | | (A) SELF-PERF | (B) SUPPORT |
|---|---|---|---|---|
| a. | BED MOBILITY | How resident moves to and from lying position, turns side to side, and positions body while in bed A = 1 = **5A**; A = 2, 3, or 4 = **5A, 16**; A = 8 = **16** | | |
| b. | TRANSFER | How resident moves between surfaces—to/from: bed, chair, wheelchair, standing position (EXCLUDE to/from bath/toilet) A = 1, 2, 3, or 4 = **5A** | | |
| c. | WALK IN ROOM | How resident walks between locations in his/her room A = 1, 2, 3, or 4 = **5A** | | |
| d. | WALK IN CORRIDOR | How resident walks in corridor on unit A = 1, 2, 3, or 4 = **5A** | | |
| e. | LOCOMOTION ON UNIT | How resident moves between locations in his/her room and adjacent corridor on same floor. If in wheelchair, self-sufficiency once in chair A = 1, 2, 3, or 4 = **5A** | | |
| f. | LOCOMOTION OFF UNIT | How resident moves to and returns from off unit locations (e.g., areas set aside for dining, activities, or treatments). If facility has only one floor, how resident moves to and from distant areas on the floor. If in wheelchair, self-sufficiency once in chair A = 1, 2, 3, or 4 = **5A** | | |
| g. | DRESSING | How resident puts on, fastens, and takes off all items of **street clothing**, including donning/removing prosthesis A = 1, 2, 3, or 4 = **5A** | | |
| h. | EATING | How resident eats and drinks (regardless of skill). Includes intake of nourishment by other means (e.g., tube feeding, total parenteral nutrition) A = 1, 2, 3, or 4 = **5A** | | |
| i. | TOILET USE | How resident uses the toilet room (or commode, bedpan, urinal); transfers on/off toilet, cleanses, changes pad, manages ostomy or catheter, adjusts clothes A = 1, 2, 3, or 4 = **5A** | | |
| j. | PERSONAL HYGIENE | How resident maintains personal hygiene, including combing hair, brushing teeth, shaving, applying makeup, washing/ drying face, hands, and perineum (EXCLUDE baths and showers) A = 1, 2, 3, or 4 = **5A** | | |

**Form 1748HH**    © 1995 Briggs Corporation, Des Moines, IA 50306 (800) 247-2343   PRINTED IN U.S.A.
Copyright limited to addition of trigger system.

    MDS 2.0   10/18/94N

Resident _____    Numeric Identifier _____

| | | | |
|---|---|---|---|
| 2. | BATHING | How resident takes full-body bath/shower, sponge bath, and transfers in/out of tub/shower (EXCLUDE washing of back and hair). **Code for most dependent** in self-performance and support.<br>A = 1, 2, 3 or 4 = **5A**<br>(A) BATHING SELF-PERFORMANCE codes appear below.<br>0. Independent—No help provided<br>1. Supervision—Oversight help only<br>2. Physical help limited to transfer only<br>3. Physical help in part of bathing activity<br>4. Total dependence<br>8. Activity itself did not occur during entire 7 days<br>*(Bathing support codes are as defined in **Item 1, code B above**)* | **(A)  (B)** |

| 3. | TEST FOR BALANCE <br>(See training manual) | *(Code for ability during test in the last 7 days)*<br>0. Maintained position as required in test<br>1. Unsteady, but able to rebalance self without physical support<br>2. Partial physical support during test; or stands (sits) but does not follow directions for test<br>3. Not able to attempt test without physical help<br><br>a. Balance while standing<br>b. Balance while sitting–position, trunk control 1, 2, or 3 = **17*** | |
|---|---|---|---|

| 4. | FUNCTIONAL LIMITATION IN RANGE OF MOTION <br>(see training manual) | *(Code for limitations during last 7 days that interfered with daily functions or placed resident at risk of injury)*<br>**(A)** *RANGE OF MOTION*   **(B)** *VOLUNTARY MOVEMENT*<br>0. No limitation   0. No loss<br>1. Limitation on one side   1. Partial loss<br>2. Limitation on both sides   2. Full loss   **(A)  (B)**<br><br>a. Neck<br>b. Arm—Including shoulder or elbow<br>c. Hand—Including wrist or fingers<br>d. Leg—Including hip or knee<br>e. Foot—Including ankle or toes<br>f. Other limitation or loss | |
|---|---|---|---|

| 5. | MODES OF LOCOMOTION | *(Check all that apply during last 7 days)*<br>Cane/walker/crutch a.   Wheelchair primary mode of locomotion d.<br>Wheeled self b.<br>Other person wheeled c.   NONE OF ABOVE e. |
|---|---|---|

| 6. | MODES OF TRANSFER | *(Check all that apply during last 7 days)*<br>Bedfast all or most of time **16** a.   Lifted mechanically d.<br>Bed rails used for bed mobility or transfer b.   Transfer aid (e.g., slide board, trapeze, cane, walker, brace) e.<br>Lifted manually c.   NONE OF ABOVE f. |
|---|---|---|

| 7. | TASK SEGMEN-TATION | Some or all of ADL activities were broken into subtasks during **last 7 days** so that resident could perform them<br>0. No   1. Yes |
|---|---|---|

| 8. | ADL FUNCTIONAL REHABILITA-TION POTENTIAL | Resident believes he/she is capable of increased independence in at least some ADLs **5A**  a.<br>Direct care staff believe resident is capable of increased independence in at least some ADLs **5A**  b.<br>Resident able to perform tasks/activity but is very slow  c.<br>Difference in ADL Self-Performance or ADL Support, comparing mornings to evenings  d.<br>NONE OF ABOVE  e. |
|---|---|---|

| 9. | CHANGE IN ADL FUNCTION | Resident's ADL self-performance status has changed as compared to status of **90 days ago** (or since last assessment if less than 90 days)<br>0. No change   1. Improved   2. Deteriorated |
|---|---|---|

## SECTION H. CONTINENCE IN LAST 14 DAYS

| 1. | CONTINENCE SELF-CONTROL CATEGORIES<br>*(Code for resident's PERFORMANCE OVER ALL SHIFTS)*<br><br>0. **CONTINENT**—Complete control *(includes use of indwelling urinary catheter or ostomy device that does not leak urine or stool)*<br>1. **USUALLY CONTINENT**—BLADDER, incontinent episodes once a week or less; BOWEL, less than weekly<br>2. **OCCASIONALLY INCONTINENT**—BLADDER, 2 or more times a week but not daily; BOWEL, once a week<br>3. **FREQUENTLY INCONTINENT**—BLADDER, tended to be incontinent daily, but some control present (e.g., on day shift); BOWEL, 2-3 times a week<br>4. **INCONTINENT**—Had inadequate control. BLADDER, multiple daily episodes; BOWEL, all (or almost all) of the time |
|---|---|

| a. | BOWEL CONTI-NENCE | Control of bowel movement, with appliance or bowel continence programs, if employed 1, 2, 3 or 4 = **16** | |
|---|---|---|---|
| b. | BLADDER CONTI-NENCE | Control of urinary bladder function (if dribbles, volume insufficient to soak through underpants), with appliances (e.g., foley) or continence programs, if employed 2, 3 or 4 = **6** | |

| 2. | BOWEL ELIMIN-ATION PATTERN | Bowel elimination pattern regular—at least one movement every three days a. | Diarrhea c. |
|---|---|---|---|
| | | Constipation **17*** b. | Fecal impaction **17*** d.<br>NONE OF ABOVE e. |

| 3. | APPLIANCES AND PROGRAMS | Any scheduled toileting plan a. | Did not use toilet room/ commode/urinal f. |
|---|---|---|---|
| | | Bladder retraining program b. | Pads/briefs used **6** g. |
| | | External (condom) catheter **6** c. | Enemas/irrigation h. |
| | | Indwelling catheter **6** d. | Ostomy present i. |
| | | Intermittent catheter **6** e. | NONE OF ABOVE j. |

| 4. | CHANGE IN URINARY CONTI-NENCE | Resident's urinary continence has changed as compared to status of **90 days ago** (or since last assessment if less than 90 days)<br>0. No change   1. Improved   2. Deteriorated |
|---|---|---|

## SECTION I. DISEASE DIAGNOSES

Check only **those diseases that have a relationship** to current ADL status, cognitive status, mood and behavior status, medical treatments, nursing monitoring, or risk of death. (Do not list inactive diagnoses.)

| 1. | DISEASES | *(If none apply, CHECK the NONE OF ABOVE box)* | | |
|---|---|---|---|---|
| | | **ENDOCRINE/METABOLIC/ NUTRITIONAL** | Hemiplegia/Hemiparesis | v. |
| | | Diabetes mellitus a. | Multiple sclerosis | w. |
| | | Hyperthyroidism b. | Paraplegia | x. |
| | | Hypothyroidism c. | Parkinson's disease | y. |
| | | **HEART/CIRCULATION** | Quadriplegia | z. |
| | | Arteriosclerotic heart disease (ASHD) d. | Seizure disorder | aa. |
| | | Cardiac dysrhythmias e. | Transient ischemic attack (TIA) | bb. |
| | | Congestive heart failure f. | Traumatic brain injury | cc. |
| | | Deep vein thrombosis g. | **PSYCHIATRIC/MOOD** | |
| | | Hypertension h. | Anxiety disorder | dd. |
| | | Hypotension **17*** i. | Depression **17*** | ee. |
| | | Peripheral vascular disease **16** j. | Manic depression (bipolar disease) | ff. |
| | | Other cardiovascular disease k. | Schizophrenia | gg. |
| | | **MUSCULOSKELETAL** | **PULMONARY** | |
| | | Arthritis l. | Asthma | hh. |
| | | Hip fracture m. | Emphysema/COPD | ii. |
| | | Missing limb (e.g., amputation) n. | **SENSORY** | |
| | | Osteoporosis o. | Cataracts **3** | jj. |
| | | Pathological bone fracture p. | Diabetic retinopathy | kk. |
| | | **NEUROLOGICAL** | Glaucoma **3** | ll. |
| | | Alzheimer's disease q. | Macular degeneration | mm. |
| | | Aphasia r. | **OTHER** | |
| | | Cerebral palsy s. | Allergies | nn. |
| | | Cerebrovascular accident (stroke) t. | Anemia | oo. |
| | | Dementia other than Alzheimer's disease u. | Cancer | pp. |
| | | | Renal failure | qq. |
| | | | NONE OF ABOVE | rr. |

| 2. | INFECTIONS | *(If none apply, CHECK the NONE OF ABOVE box)* | | |
|---|---|---|---|---|
| | | Antibiotic resistant infec-tion (e.g., Methicillin resistant staph) a. | Septicemia | g. |
| | | Clostridium difficile (c. diff.) b. | Sexually transmitted diseases | h. |
| | | Conjunctivitis c. | Tuberculosis | i. |
| | | HIV infection d. | Urinary tract infection in last 30 days **14** | j. |
| | | Pneumonia e. | Viral hepatitis | k. |
| | | Respiratory infection f. | Wound infection | l. |
| | | | NONE OF ABOVE | m. |

| 3. | OTHER CURRENT OR MORE DETAILED DIAGNOSES AND ICD-9 CODES | Dehydration 276.5 = **14** |
|---|---|---|
| | | a. _____ |
| | | b. _____ |
| | | c. _____ |
| | | d. _____ |
| | | e. _____ |

## SECTION J. HEALTH CONDITIONS

| 1. | PROBLEM CONDITIONS | *(Check all problems present in last 7 days unless other time frame is indicated)* | | |
|---|---|---|---|---|
| | | **INDICATORS OF FLUID STATUS** | Dizziness/Vertigo **11, 17*** | f. |
| | | Weight gain or loss of 3 or more pounds within a 7 day period **14** a. | Edema | g. |
| | | | Fever **14** | h. |
| | | Inability to lie flat due to shortness of breath b. | Hallucinations **17*** | i. |
| | | Dehydrated; output exceeds input **14** c. | Internal bleeding **14** | j. |
| | | | Recurrent lung aspirations in last 90 days **17*** | k. |
| | | Insufficient fluid; did NOT consume all/almost all liquids provided during last 3 days **14** d. | Shortness of breath | l. |
| | | | Syncope (fainting) **17*** | m. |
| | | **OTHER** | Unsteady gait **17*** | n. |
| | | Delusions e. | Vomiting | o. |
| | | | NONE OF ABOVE | p. |

**Form 1748HH** © 1995 Briggs Corporation, Des Moines, IA 50306 (800) 247-2343 PRINTED IN U.S.A.<br>Copyright limited to addition of trigger system.

5 of 10

MDS 2.0  10/18/94N

Resident _____   Numeric Identifier_____

| | | |
|---|---|---|
| 2. | PAIN SYMPTOMS | *(Code the **highest level of pain** present in **the last 7 days**)* <br> **a. FREQUENCY** with which resident complains or shows evidence of pain <br> 0. No pain *(skip to J4)* <br> 1. Pain less than daily <br> 2. Pain daily <br> **b. INTENSITY** of pain <br> 1. Mild pain <br> 2. Moderate pain <br> 3. Times when pain is horrible or excruciating |

| 3. | PAIN SITE | *(If pain present, **check all sites** that apply in **last 7 days**)* | | |
|---|---|---|---|---|
| | | Back pain | a. | Incisional pain | f. |
| | | Bone pain | b. | Joint pain (other than hip) | g. |
| | | Chest pain while doing usual activities | c. | Soft tissue pain (e.g., lesion, muscle) | h. |
| | | Headache | d. | Stomach pain | i. |
| | | Hip pain | e. | Other | j. |

| 4. | ACCIDENTS | *(Check all that apply)* | | | |
|---|---|---|---|---|---|
| | | Fell in **past 30 days** **11, 17***  | a. | Hip fracture in **last 180 days 17*** | c. |
| | | Fell in **past 31-180 days 11, 17*** | b. | Other fracture in **last 180 days** | d. |
| | | | | *NONE OF ABOVE* | e. |

| 5. | STABILITY OF CONDITIONS | Conditions/diseases make resident's cognitive, ADL, mood or behavior patterns unstable—(fluctuating, precarious, or deteriorating) | a. |
|---|---|---|---|
| | | Resident experiencing an acute episode or a flare-up of a recurrent or chronic problem | b. |
| | | End-stage disease, 6 or fewer months to live | c. |
| | | *NONE OF ABOVE* | d. |

## SECTION K. ORAL/NUTRITIONAL STATUS

| 1. | ORAL PROBLEMS | Chewing problem | a. |
|---|---|---|---|
| | | Swallowing problem 17* | b. |
| | | Mouth pain 15 | c. |
| | | *NONE OF ABOVE* | d. |

| 2. | HEIGHT AND WEIGHT | Record *(a.) height in inches* and *(b.) weight in pounds*. Base weight on most recent measure in *last 30 days; measure weight consistently in accord with standard facility practice— e.g., in a.m. after voiding, before meal, with shoes off, and in nightclothes.* <br><br> **a. HT (in.)**       **b. WT (lb.)** |

| 3. | WEIGHT CHANGE | **a. Weight loss**—5% or more in **last 30 days**; or 10% or more in **last 180 days** <br> 0. No    1. Yes 12 | |
|---|---|---|---|
| | | **b. Weight gain**—5% or more in **last 30 days**; or 10% or more in **last 180 days** <br> 0. No    1. Yes | |

| 4. | NUTRI-TIONAL PROBLEMS | Complains about the taste of many foods 12 | a. | Leaves 25% or more of food uneaten at most meals 12 | c. |
|---|---|---|---|---|---|
| | | Regular or repetitive complaints of hunger | b. | *NONE OF ABOVE* | d. |

| 5. | NUTRI-TIONAL APPROACH-ES | *(Check all that apply in last 7 days)* | | | |
|---|---|---|---|---|---|
| | | Parenteral/IV 12, 14 | a. | Dietary supplement between meals | f. |
| | | Feeding tube 13, 14 | b. | Plate guard, stabilized built-up utensil, etc. | g. |
| | | Mechanically altered diet 12 | c. | On a planned weight change program | h. |
| | | Syringe (oral feeding) 12 | d. | *NONE OF ABOVE* | i. |
| | | Therapeutic diet 12 | e. | | |

| 6. | PARENTERAL OR ENTERAL INTAKE | *(Skip to Section L if neither 5a nor 5b is checked)* <br> **a.** Code the proportion of **total calories** the resident received through parenteral or tube feedings in the **last 7 days** <br> 0. None    3. 51% to 75% <br> 1. 1% to 25%    4. 76% to 100% <br> 2. 26% to 50% | |
|---|---|---|---|
| | | **b.** Code the average **fluid intake** per day by IV or tube in **last 7 days** <br> 0. None    3. 1001 to 1500 cc/day <br> 1. 1 to 500 cc/day    4. 1501 to 2000 cc/day <br> 2. 501 to 1000 cc/day    5. 2001 or more cc/day | |

## SECTION L. ORAL/DENTAL STATUS

| 1. | ORAL STATUS AND DISEASE PREVEN-TION | Debris (soft, easily movable substances) present in mouth prior to going to bed at night 15 | a. |
|---|---|---|---|
| | | Has dentures or removable bridge | b. |
| | | Some/all natural teeth lost—does not have or does not use dentures (or partial plates) 15 | c. |
| | | Broken, loose, or carious teeth 15 | d. |
| | | Inflamed gums (gingiva); swollen or bleeding gums; oral abscesses; ulcers or rashes 15 | e. |
| | | Daily cleaning of teeth/dentures or daily mouth care—by resident or staff Not ✓ – 15 | f. |
| | | *NONE OF ABOVE* | g. |

## SECTION M. SKIN CONDITION

| 1. | ULCERS (Due to any cause) | *(Record the number of ulcers at each ulcer stage— regardless of cause. If none present at a stage, record "0" (zero). Code all that apply during **last 7 days**. Code 9 = 9 or more.) [**Requires full body exam.**]* | Number at Stage |
|---|---|---|---|
| | | **a. Stage 1.** A persistent area of skin redness (without a break in the skin) that does not disappear when pressure is relieved. | |
| | | **b. Stage 2.** A partial thickness loss of skin layers that presents clinically as an abrasion, blister, or shallow crater. | |
| | | **c. Stage 3.** A full thickness of skin is lost, exposing the subcutaneous tissues—presents as a deep crater with or without undermining adjacent tissue. | |
| | | **d. Stage 4.** A full thickness of skin and subcutaneous tissue is lost, exposing muscle or bone. | |

| 2. | TYPE OF ULCER | *(For each type of ulcer, **code for the highest stage in the last 7 days** using scale in item M1—i.e., 0=none; stages 1, 2, 3, 4)* | |
|---|---|---|---|
| | | **a.** Pressure ulcer—any lesion caused by pressure resulting in damage of underlying tissue <br> 1 = **16**; 2, 3, or 4 = **12, 16** | |
| | | **b.** Stasis ulcer—open lesion caused by poor circulation in the lower extremities | |

| 3. | HISTORY OF RESOLVED ULCERS | Resident had an ulcer that was resolved or cured in **LAST 90 DAYS** <br> 0. No    1. Yes **16** | |
|---|---|---|---|

| 4. | OTHER SKIN PROBLEMS OR LESIONS PRESENT | *(Check all that apply during last 7 days)* | |
|---|---|---|---|
| | | Abrasions, bruises | a. |
| | | Burns (second or third degree) | b. |
| | | Open lesions other than ulcers, rashes, cuts (e.g., cancer lesions) | c. |
| | | Rashes—e.g., intertrigo, eczema, drug rash, heat rash, herpes zoster | d. |
| | | Skin desensitized to pain or pressure 16 | e. |
| | | Skin tears or cuts (other than surgery) | f. |
| | | Surgical wounds | g. |
| | | *NONE OF ABOVE* | h. |

| 5. | SKIN TREAT-MENTS | *(Check all that apply during last 7 days)* | |
|---|---|---|---|
| | | Pressure relieving device(s) for chair | a. |
| | | Pressure relieving device(s) for bed | b. |
| | | Turning/repositioning program | c. |
| | | Nutrition or hydration intervention to manage skin problems | d. |
| | | Ulcer care | e. |
| | | Surgical wound care | f. |
| | | Application of dressings (with or without topical medications) other than to feet | g. |
| | | Application of ointments/medications (other than to feet) | h. |
| | | Other preventative or protective skin care (other than to feet) | i. |
| | | *NONE OF ABOVE* | j. |

| 6. | FOOT PROBLEMS AND CARE | *(Check all that apply during last 7 days)* | |
|---|---|---|---|
| | | Resident has one or more foot problems—e.g., corns, calluses, bunions, hammer toes, overlapping toes, pain, structural problems | a. |
| | | Infection of the foot—e.g., cellulitis, purulent drainage | b. |
| | | Open lesions on the foot | c. |
| | | Nails/calluses trimmed during **last 90 days** | d. |
| | | Received preventative or protective foot care (e.g., used special shoes, inserts, pads, toe separators) | e. |
| | | Application of dressings (with or without topical medications) | f. |
| | | *NONE OF ABOVE* | g. |

## SECTION N. ACTIVITY PURSUIT PATTERNS

| 1. | TIME AWAKE | *(Check appropriate time periods over last 7 days)* Resident awake all or most of time (i.e., naps no more than one hour per time period) in the: | | | |
|---|---|---|---|---|---|
| | 10B only if BOTH N1a = ✓ and N2 = 0 | Morning 10B | a. | Evening | c. |
| | | Afternoon | b. | *NONE OF ABOVE* | d. |

**(IF RESIDENT IS COMATOSE, SKIP TO SECTION O)**

| 2. | AVERAGE TIME INVOLVED IN ACTIVITIES | *(When awake and not receiving treatments or ADL care)* <br> 0. Most—more than 2/3 of time **10B**    2. Little—less than 1/3 of time **10A** <br> 1. Some—from 1/3 to 2/3 of time    3. None **10A** | |
|---|---|---|---|

| 3. | PREFERRED ACTIVITY SETTINGS | *(Check all settings in which activities are preferred)* | | | |
|---|---|---|---|---|---|
| | | Own room | a. | | |
| | | Day/activity room | b. | Outside facility | d. |
| | | Inside NH/off unit | c. | *NONE OF ABOVE* | e. |

| 4. | GENERAL ACTIVITY PREFER-ENCES (Adapted to resident's current abilities) | *(Check all PREFERENCES whether or not activity is currently available to resident)* | | | |
|---|---|---|---|---|---|
| | | Cards/other games | a. | Trips/shopping | g. |
| | | Crafts/arts | b. | Walking/wheeling outdoors | h. |
| | | Exercise/sports | c. | Watching TV | i. |
| | | Music | d. | Gardening or plants | j. |
| | | Reading/writing | e. | Talking or conversing | k. |
| | | Spiritual/religious activities | f. | Helping others | l. |
| | | | | *NONE OF ABOVE* | m. |

**Form 1748HH**    © 1995 Briggs Corporation, Des Moines, IA 50306 (800) 247-2343 PRINTED IN U.S.A. <br> Copyright limited to addition of trigger system.

MDS 2.0   10/18/94N

Resident _____          Numeric Identifier _____

| 5. | PREFERS CHANGE IN DAILY ROUTINE | Code for resident preferences in daily routines<br>0. No change    1. Slight change    2. Major change<br>a. Type of activities in which resident is currently involved 1 or 2 = **10A**<br>b. Extent of resident involvement in activity 1 or 2 = **10A** | |

## SECTION O. MEDICATIONS

| 1. | NUMBER OF MEDICATIONS | *(Record the number of different medications used in the last 7 days;* enter "0" if none used) | |
|----|----|----|----|
| 2. | NEW MEDICA-TIONS | *(Resident currently receiving medications that were initiated during the last 90 days)*<br>0. No        1. Yes | |
| 3. | INJECTIONS | *(Record the number of DAYS injections of any type received during the last 7 days;* enter "0" if none used) | |
| 4. | DAYS RECEIVED THE FOLLOWING MEDICATION | *(Record the number of DAYS during last 7 days;* enter "0" if not used. *Note*—enter "1" for long acting meds used less than weekly)<br>(NOTE: For **17** to actually be triggered, O4a, b, or c MUST = 1-7 AND at least one additional item marked **17*** must be indicated. See sections B, C, E, G, H, I, J, and K.) | |

|  | | | |
|---|---|---|---|
| a. Antipsychotic 1-7 = **17** | | d. Hypnotic | |
| b. Antianxiety 1-7 = **11, 17** | | e. Diuretic 1-7 = **14** | |
| c. Antidepressant 1-7 = **11, 17** | | | |

## SECTION P. SPECIAL TREATMENTS AND PROCEDURES

| 1. | SPECIAL TREAT-MENTS, PROCE-DURES, AND PROGRAMS | a. SPECIAL CARE—*Check treatments or programs received during the last 14 days* |

| TREATMENTS | | | | |
|----|----|----|----|----|
| Chemotherapy | a. | Ventilator or respirator | l. | |
| Dialysis | b. | **PROGRAMS** | | |
| IV medication | c. | Alcohol/drug treat-ment program | m. | |
| Intake/output | d. | Alzheimer's/dementia special care unit | n. | |
| Monitoring acute medical condition | e. | Hospice care | o. | |
| Ostomy care | f. | Pediatric unit | p. | |
| Oxygen therapy | g. | Respite care | q. | |
| Radiation | h. | Training in skills required to return to the community (e.g., taking medications, house work, shopping, transportation, ADLs) | r. | |
| Suctioning | i. | | | |
| Tracheostomy care | j. | | | |
| Transfusions | k. | NONE OF ABOVE | s. | |

b. THERAPIES—*Record the number of days and total minutes each of the following therapies was administered (for at least 15 minutes a day) in the last 7 calendar days (Enter 0 if none or less than 15 min. daily)* [Note—count only post admission therapies]

(A) = # of days administered for **15 minutes or more**

(B) = total # of minutes provided in last 7 days

| | DAYS (A) | MINUTES (B) |
|----|----|----|
| a. Speech-language pathology and audiology services | | |
| b. Occupational therapy | | |
| c. Physical therapy | | |
| d. Respiratory therapy | | |
| e. Psychological therapy (by any licensed mental health professional) | | |

| 2. | INTERVEN-TION PROGRAMS FOR MOOD, BEHAVIOR, COGNITIVE LOSS | (Check all interventions or strategies used in **last 7 days**—no matter where received) | |
|----|----|----|----|
| | | Special behavior symptom evaluation program | a. |
| | | Evaluation by a licensed mental health specialist in **last 90 days** | b. |
| | | Group therapy | c. |
| | | Resident-specific deliberate changes in the environment to address mood/behavior patterns—e.g., providing bureau in which to rummage | d. |
| | | Reorientation—e.g., cueing | e. |
| | | NONE OF ABOVE | f. |

| 3. | NURSING REHABILI-TATION/ RESTOR-ATIVE CARE | Record the NUMBER OF DAYS each of the following rehabilitation or restorative techniques or practices was **provided to the resident for more than or equal to 15 minutes** per day in the **last 7 days** (Enter 0 if none or less than 15 min. daily.) |

| a. Range of motion (passive) | | f. Walking | |
|----|----|----|----|
| b. Range of motion (active) | | g. Dressing or grooming | |
| c. Splint or brace assistance | | h. Eating or swallowing | |
| TRAINING AND SKILL PRACTICE IN: | | i. Amputation/prosthesis care | |
| d. Bed mobility | | j. Communication | |
| e. Transfer | | k. Other | |

| 4. | DEVICES AND RESTRAINTS | *(Use the following codes for last 7 days:)*<br>0. Not used<br>1. Used less than daily<br>2. Used daily | |
|----|----|----|----|
| | | Bed rails<br>a. —Full bed rails on all open sides of bed | |
| | | b. —Other types of side rails used (e.g., half rail, one side) | |
| | | c. Trunk restraint 1 = **11, 18**; 2 = **11, 16, 18** | |
| | | d. Limb restraint 1 or 2 = **18** | |
| | | e. Chair prevents rising 1 or 2 = **18** | |
| 5. | HOSPITAL STAY(S) | Record number of times resident was admitted to hospital with an overnight stay in **last 90 days** (or since last assessment if less than 90 days). *(Enter 0 if no hospital admissions)* | |
| 6. | EMERGENCY ROOM (ER) VISIT(S) | Record number of times resident visited ER without an overnight stay in **last 90 days** (or since last assessment if less than 90 days). *(Enter 0 if no ER visits)* | |
| 7. | PHYSICIAN VISITS | In the **LAST 14 DAYS** (or since admission if less than 14 days in facility) how many days has the physician (or authorized assistant or practitioner) examined the resident? *(Enter 0 if none)* | |
| 8. | PHYSICIAN ORDERS | In the **LAST 14 DAYS** (or since admission if less than 14 days in facility) how many days has the physician (or authorized assistant or practitioner) changed the resident's orders? *Do not include order renewals without change.* (Enter 0 if none) | |
| 9. | ABNORMAL LAB VALUES | Has the resident had any abnormal lab values during the **last 90 days** (or since admission)?<br>0. No        1. Yes | |

## SECTION Q. DISCHARGE POTENTIAL AND OVERALL STATUS

| 1. | DISCHARGE POTENTIAL | a. Resident expresses/indicates preference to return to the community<br>0. No        1. Yes | |
|----|----|----|----|
| | | b. Resident has a support person who is positive toward discharge<br>0. No        1. Yes | |
| | | c. Stay projected to be of a short duration—discharge projected **within 90 days** (do not include expected discharge due to death)<br>0. No                    2. Within 31-90 days<br>1. Within 30 days    3. Discharge status uncertain | |
| 2. | OVERALL CHANGE IN CARE NEEDS | Resident's overall self sufficiency has changed significantly as compared to status of **90 days ago** (or since last assessment if less than 90 days)<br>0. No change<br>1. Improved—receives fewer supports, needs less restrictive level of care<br>2. Deteriorated—receives more support | |

## SECTION R. ASSESSMENT INFORMATION

| 1. | PARTICI-PATION IN ASSESSMENT | a. Resident:        0. No    1. Yes |
|----|----|----|
| | | b. Family:        0. No    1. Yes    2. No family |
| | | c. Significant other:    0. No    1. Yes    2. None |

2. SIGNATURES OF PERSONS COMPLETING THE ASSESSMENT:

a. Signature of RN Assessment Coordinator (sign on above line)

b. Date RN Assessment Coordinator signed as complete

| | | | — | | | — | | | | |
|---|---|---|---|---|---|---|---|---|---|---|

Month          Day          Year

| c. Other Signatures | | Title | Sections | Date |
|----|----|----|----|----|
| d. | | | | Date |
| e. | | | | Date |
| f. | | | | Date |
| g. | | | | Date |
| h. | | | | Date |

### TRIGGER LEGEND

| | | | |
|----|----|----|----|
| 1 - Delirium | 5B - ADL-Maintenance | 10A - Activities (Revise) | 14 - Dehydration/Fluid Maintenance |
| 2 - Cognitive Loss/Dementia | 6B - Urinary Incontinence and Indwelling Catheter | 10B - Activities (Review) | 15 - Dental Care |
| 3 - Visual Function | 7 - Psychosocial Well-Being | 11 - Falls | 16 - Pressure Ulcers |
| 4 - Communication | 8 - Mood State | 12 - Nutritional Status | 17 - Psychotropic Drug Use |
| 5A - ADL-Rehabilitation | 9 - Behavioral Symptoms | 13 - Feeding Tubes | 17* - For this to trigger, O4a, b, or c must = 1-7 |
| | | | 18 - Physical Restraints |

MDS 2.0  10/18/94N

Resident _____     Numeric Identifier _____

## SECTION T. SUPPLEMENT — CASE MIX DEMO

| 1. | SPECIAL TREAT-MENTS AND PROCE-DURES | a. RECREATION THERAPY—*Enter number of days and total minutes of recreation therapy administered (**for at least 15 minutes a day**) in the **last 7 days** (Enter 0 if none)* |
|---|---|---|

| | | | DAYS | MINS. |
|---|---|---|---|---|
| (A) = # of days administered for 15 minutes or more | | | (A) | (B) |
| (B) = total # of minutes provided in last 7 days | | | | |

*Skip unless this is a Medicare 5 day or initial admission assessment*

b. ORDERED THERAPIES—*Has physician ordered any of following therapies to begin in FIRST 14 days of stay—physical therapy, occupational therapy, or speech pathology service?*

   0. No             1. Yes

*If not ordered, skip to item 2*

c. Through day 15, provide an estimate of the number of days when at least 1 therapy service can be expected to have been delivered.

d. Through day 15, provide an estimate of the number of therapy minutes (across the therapies) that can be expected to be delivered.

| 2. | WALKING WHEN MOST SELF-SUFFICIENT | *Complete item 2 if ADL self-performance score for TRANSFER (G.1.b.A) is 0, 1, 2, or 3 AND at least one of the following are present:* |
|---|---|---|

- Resident received physical therapy involving gait training (P.1.b.c)
- Physical therapy was ordered for the resident involving gait training (T.1.b)
- Resident received nursing rehabilitation for walking (P.3.f)
- Physical therapy involving walking has been discontinued within the past 180 days

*Skip to item 3 if resident did not walk in last 7 days*

*(FOR FOLLOWING FIVE ITEMS, BASE CODING ON THE EPISODE WHEN THE RESIDENT WALKED THE FARTHEST WITHOUT SITTING DOWN. INCLUDE WALKING DURING REHABILITATION SESSIONS.)*

a. **Farthest distance walked** without sitting during this episode.

   0. 150+ feet       3. 10-25 feet
   1. 51-149 feet    4. Less than 10 feet
   2. 26-50 feet

b. **Time walked** without sitting down during this episode.

   0. 1-2 minutes     3. 11-15 minutes
   1. 3-4 minutes      4. 16-30 minutes
   2. 5-10 minutes    5. 31+ minutes

c. **Self-Performance in walking** during this episode.

   0. *INDEPENDENT*—No help or oversight
   1. *SUPERVISION*—Oversight, encouragement or cueing provided
   2. *LIMITED ASSISTANCE*—Resident highly involved in walking; received physical help in guided maneuvering of limbs or other nonweight bearing assistance
   3. *EXTENSIVE ASSISTANCE*—Resident received weight bearing assistance while walking

d. **Walking support provided** associated with this episode (code regardless of resident's self-performance classification).

   0. No setup or physical help from staff
   1. Setup help only
   2. One person physical assist
   3. Two+ persons physical assist

e. **Parallel bars** used by resident in association with this episode.

   0. No           1. Yes

| 3. | CASE MIX GROUP | Medicare [ ][ ][ ][ ][ ]    State [ ][ ][ ][ ][ ] |
|---|---|---|

**Form 1748HH**    © 1995 Briggs Corporation, Des Moines, IA 50306 (800) 247-2343 PRINTED IN U.S.A.
Copyright limited to addition of trigger system.

MDS 2.0   10/18/94N

Resident _____    Numeric Identifier _____

## SECTION U. MEDICATIONS

List all medications that the resident **received** during the last 7 days. Include scheduled medications that are used regularly, but less than weekly.

1. **Medication Name and Dose Ordered.** Record the name of the medication and dose ordered.
2. **Route of Administration (RA).** Code the Route of Administration using the following list:

   1 = by mouth (PO)           5 = subcutaneous (SQ)        8 = inhalation
   2 = sublingual (SL)         6 = rectal (R)               9 = enteral tube
   3 = intramuscular (IM)      7 = topical                  10 = other
   4 = intravenous (IV)

3. **Frequency (Freq.).** Code the number of times per day, week, or month the medication is administered using the following list:

   PR = (PRN) as necessary         2D = (BID) two times daily          QO = every other day
   1H = (QH) every hour                 (includes every 12 hours)      4W = four times each week
   2H = (Q2H) every two hours      3D = (TID) three times daily       5W = five times each week
   3H = (Q3H) every three hours    4D = (QID) four times daily        6W = six times each week
   4H = (Q4H) every four hours     5D = five times daily              1M = (Q month) once every month
   6H = (Q6H) every six hours      1W = (Q week) once each week       2M = twice every month
   8H = (Q8H) every eight hours    2W = two times every week          C = continuous
   1D = (QD or HS) once daily      3W = three times every week        O = other

4. **Amount Administered (AA).** Record the number of tablets, capsules, suppositories, or liquid (any route) **per dose** administered to the resident. Code 999 for topicals, eye drops, inhalants and oral medications that need to be dissolved in water.
5. **PRN-number of days (PRN-n).** If the frequency code for the medication is "PR", record the number of times during the last 7 days each PRN medication was given. Code STAT medications as PRNs given once.
6. **NDC Codes.** Enter the National Drug Code for each medication given. Be sure to enter the correct NDC code for the drug name, strength, and form. The NDC code must match the drug dispensed by the pharmacy.

| 1. Medication Name and Dose Ordered | 2. RA | 3. Freq | 4. AA | 5. PRN-n | 6. NDC Codes |
|---|---|---|---|---|---|
| | | | | | |
| | | | | | |
| | | | | | |
| | | | | | |
| | | | | | |
| | | | | | |
| | | | | | |
| | | | | | |
| | | | | | |
| | | | | | |
| | | | | | |
| | | | | | |
| | | | | | |
| | | | | | |
| | | | | | |
| | | | | | |

**SECTION V. RESIDENT ASSESSMENT PROTOCOL SUMMARY**   Numeric Identifier_____

| Resident's Name: | Medical Record No.: |
|---|---|

1. Check if RAP is triggered.
2. For each triggered RAP, use the RAP guidelines to identify areas needing further assessment. Document relevant assessment information regarding the resident's status.
   - Describe:
     - Nature of the condition (may include presence or lack of objective data and subjective complaints).
     - Complications and risk factors that affect your decision to proceed to care planning.
     - Factors that must be considered in developing individualized care plan interventions.
     - Need for referrals/further evaluation by appropriate health professionals.
   - Documentation should support your decision-making regarding whether to proceed with a care plan for a triggered RAP and the type(s) of care plan interventions that are appropriate for a particular resident.
   - Documentation may appear anywhere in the clinical record (e.g., progress notes, consults, flowsheets, etc.).
3. Indicate under the Location of RAP Assessment Documentation column where information related to the RAP assessment can be found.
4. For each triggered RAP, indicate whether a new care plan, care plan revision, or continuation of current care plan is necessary to address the problem(s) identified in your assessment. The Care Planning Decision column must be completed within 7 days of completing the RAI (MDS and RAPs).

| A. RAP Problem Area | (a) Check if Triggered | Location and Date of RAP Assessment Documentation | (b) Care Planning Decision—check if addressed in care plan |
|---|---|---|---|
| 1. DELIRIUM | | | |
| 2. COGNITIVE LOSS | | | |
| 3. VISUAL FUNCTION | | | |
| 4. COMMUNICATION | | | |
| 5. ADL FUNCTIONAL/ REHABILITATION POTENTIAL | | | |
| 6. URINARY INCONTINENCE AND INDWELLING CATHETER | | | |
| 7. PSYCHOSOCIAL WELL-BEING | | | |
| 8. MOOD STATE | | | |
| 9. BEHAVIORAL SYMPTOMS | | | |
| 10. ACTIVITIES | | | |
| 11. FALLS | | | |
| 12. NUTRITIONAL STATUS | | | |
| 13. FEEDING TUBES | | | |
| 14. DEHYDRATION/FLUID MAINTENANCE | | | |
| 15. ORAL/DENTAL CARE | | | |
| 16. PRESSURE ULCERS | | | |
| 17. PSYCHOTROPIC DRUG USE | | | |
| 18. PHYSICAL RESTRAINTS | | | |

B. _____
1. Signature of RN Coordinator for RAP Assessment Process   2. ☐☐ – ☐☐ – ☐☐☐☐ Month Day Year

_____
3. Signature of Person Completing Care Planning Decision   4. ☐☐ – ☐☐ – ☐☐☐☐ Month Day Year

Form 1748HH   © 1995 Briggs Corporation, Des Moines, IA 50306 (800) 247-2343 PRINTED IN U.S.A.
Copyright limited to addition of trigger system.
10 of 10   MDS 2.0  10/18/94N

## Resident Assessment Protocols

Each of the 18 resident assessment protocols (RAPs) organizes comprehensively clinical information to assist long term care facility staff in thinking about care planning and treatment decisions. A RAP has two parts: 1. a RAP KEY that summarizes all MDS elements applicable to thinking about assessment and care planning in that particular clinical area; and 2. instructions, including clinical background information and suggested approaches to additional assessment. Upon completing a RAP, staff will have:

- Identified the unique problems the resident has that may affect adversely his/her highest practicable physical, mental and psychosocial functioning.
- Identified factors that place the resident's highest practicable physical, mental and psychosocial functioning at risk.
- Considered whether the identified problems and risk factors could be prevented or reversed and evaluated the extent to which the resident is able to attain a higher level of well-being and functional independence.
- Evaluated ongoing care practices for that resident by, for example, considering alternative therapies and the need for medical consultation or consultation(s) by other health professionals such as occupational or physical therapists.

To use RAPs, long term care facility staff shall follow these steps:

- As specified in the utilization guidelines, complete MDS elements, using common definitions.
- Review MDS information. Use the Resident Assessment Protocol Trigger Legend Worksheet that shows which MDS elements serve as triggers for each RAP.
- If MDS item(s) and code(s) trigger a RAP(s), circle those RAP(s) that have been triggered.
- Complete triggered RAPs following instructions for each RAP. Delegate completion of a particular RAP to the facility staff who can address that care area most knowledgeably, whether it be nursing personnel, therapists, social workers, activity specialist or physicians. Whenever possible, get the person(s) who completed the MDS trigger(s) for that RAP to apply the full RAP.
- After competing a RAP, use the Resident Assessment Protocol Summary to document decisions about care planning and to specify where in the resident's record summary information gained from the assessment has been noted, for example, progress note or care plan.
- This summary information must include, as appropriate to the individual resident, documentation of problems, complications and risk factors, the need for referral to appropriate health professionals and the reasons for deciding to proceed or not to proceed to care planning for the specific problems identified.
- The registered nurse coordinating the assessment must sign and date the Resident Assessment Protocol Summary verifying that the triggered RAPs have been applied.

## Resident Assessment Protocol: Psychosocial Well-Being

### I.  Problem

Well-being refers to feelings about self and social relationships. Positive attributes include initiative and involvement in life; negative attributes include distressing relationships and concern about loss of status. On average, 30% of residents in a typical nursing facility will experience problems in this area, two-thirds of whom will also have serious behavior and/or mood problems. When such problems coexist, initial treatment is often focused on mood and behavior manifestations. In such situations, treatment for psychosocial distress is dependent on how the resident responds to the primary mood/behavior treatment regimen.

### II.  Triggers

Well-being problem or need to maintain psychosocial strengths suggested if one or more of the following present:

- Withdrawal from activities of interest (problem)* [E1o = 1,2]
- Conflict with staff (problem) [F2a = checked]
- Unhappy with roommate (problem) [F2b = checked]
- Unhappy with other resident (problem) [F2c = checked]
- Conflict with family or friends (problem) [F2d = checked]
- Grief over lost status or roles (problem) [F3b = checked]
- Daily routine is very different from prior pattern in the community (problem) [F3c = checked]
- Establishes own goals (strength) [F1d = checked]
- Strong identification with past (strength) [F3a = checked]

*Note: This item also triggers on the Mood State RAP.*

### III.  Guidelines

Sequentially review the items found on the RAP key.

**Confounding Problems.**

Treatment for mood or behavior problems are often immediately beneficial to well-being.

---
- Does the resident have an increasing or persistently sad mood?
- Does the resident have increasing frequency or daily disturbing behavior?
- Did the mood or behavior problems appear before the reduced sense of well-being?
- Has the resident's condition deteriorated since last assessment?
- Have ongoing treatment programs been effective?
---

**Situational Factors That May Impede Ability to Interact With Others.**

Environmental and situational problems are often amenable to staff intervention without the burden of staff having to "change the resident."

---
- Have key social relationships been altered or terminated (e.g., loss of family member, friend or staff)?
- Have changes in the resident's environment altered access to others or to routine activities — for example, room assignment, use of physical restraints, assignment to new dining area?
---

**Resident Characteristics That May Impede Ability to Interact With Others.**

These items focus on areas where the resident may lack the ability to enter freely into satisfying social relationships. They represent substantial impediments to easy interaction with others and highlight areas where staff intervention may be crucial.

- Do cognitive or communication deficits or a lack of interest in activities impeded interactions with others?
- Does resident indicate unease in social relationships?

**Lifestyles Issues:**

Residents can withdraw or become distress because they feel life lacks meaning.

- Was life more satisfactory prior to entering the nursing facility?
- Is resident preoccupied with the past, unwilling to respond to the needs of the present?
- Has the facility focused on a daily schedule that resembles the resident's prior lifestyle?

**Additional Information to Clarify the Nature of the Problem.**

Supplemental assessment items can be used to specify the nature of the well-being problem for residents for whom a well-being care plan is anticipated. These items represent topics around which to phrase questions and to establish a trusting exchange with the resident. Each item includes the positive and negative end of a continuum, representing the possible range that staff can use in thinking about these issues. Staff can use or not use the items in this list. For those items selected, the following issues should be considered:

- How do staff or resident perceive the severity of the problem?
- Has the resident ever demonstrated (while in the facility) strengths in the area under review?
- Are corrective strategies now being used? Have they been used in the past? To what effect?
- Is this an area that might be improved?

## PSYCHOSOCIAL WELL-BEING RAP KEY *(for MDS Version 2.0)*

### Triggers

Well-being problem or need to maintain psychosocial strengths suggested if one or more of the following present:

- Withdrawal from activities of interest (problem)* [E1o = 1,2]
- Conflict with staff (problem) [F2a = checked]
- Unhappy with roommate (problem) [F2b = checked]
- Unhappy with other resident (problem) [F2c = checked]
- Conflict with family or friends (problem) [F2d = checked]
- Grief over lost status or roles (problem) [F3b = checked]
- Daily routine is very different from prior pattern in the community (problem) [F3c = checked]
- Establishes own goals (strength) [F1d = checked]
- Strong identification with past (strength) [F3a = checked]

*Note: This item also triggers on the Mood State RAP.*

### Guidelines

Confounding Problems:

- Increasing/persistent sad mood [E2, E3]
- Increasing or daily disturbing behavior [E4, E5]
- Resident's condition deteriorated since last assessment [Q2]

Situational Factors That May Impede Ability To Interact With Others:

- Loss of family member, friend or staff close to resident [F2f; from record]
- Initial use of physical restraints [P4]
- New admission [AB1, A4a], change in room assignment [A2] or change in dining location or table mates [from record]

Resident Characteristics That May Impeded Ability To Interact With Others:

- Delirium or cognitive decline [B5, B6]
- Communication deficit or decline [C4, C5, C6, C7]
- Not at ease interacting with others [F1a]
- Locomotion deficit or use of wheelchair [G1c, G1d, G1f, G5b, G5c, G5d]
- Diseases that impede communication — mental retardation [AB10], Alzheimer's [I1q], aphasia [I1r], other dementia [I1u], depression [I1ee]
- Uninvolved in activities [N2, N4]

Lifestyle Issues:

- Incongruence of current and prior style of life [AC, F3c]
- Strong identification with past roles or status [F3a]
- Length of time problem existed [from record]

Supplemental Problem Clarification Issues [from resident or family if necessary]:

- *Ability to relate to others.* Skill or unease in dealing with others; reaches out or distances self; friendly or unapproachable; flexible or ridiculed by others.
- *Relationships resident could draw on.* Supported or isolated; many friends or friendless.
- *Dealing with grief.* Moving through grief or bitter and inconsolable; religious faith or feels punished.

## Resident Assessment Protocol: Activities

### I. Problem

The Activities RAP targets residents for whom a revised activity care plan may be required to identify those residents whose inactivity may be a major complication in their lives. Resident capabilities may not be fully recognized: the resident may have recently moved into the facility or staff may have focused too heavily on the instrumental needs of the resident and may have lost sight of complications in the institutional environment.

Resident involvement in passive as well as active activities can be as important in the nursing home as it was in the community. The capabilities of the average resident have obviously been altered as abilities and expectations change, disease intervenes, situational opportunities become less frequent and extended social relationships less common. But something that should never be overlooked is the great variability within the resident population: many will have ADL deficits, but few will be totally dependent; impaired cognition will be widespread, but so will the ability to apply old skills and learn new ones; and sense may be impaired, but some type of two-way communication is almost always possible.

For the nursing home, activity planning is a universal need. For this RAP, the focus is on cases where the system may have failed the resident, or where the resident has distressing conditions that warrant review of the activity care plan. The types of cases that will be triggered are: (1) residents who have indicated a desire for additional activity choices; (2) cognitively intact, distressed residents who may benefit from an enriched activity program; (3) cognitively deficient, distressed residents whose activity levels should be evaluated; and (4) highly involved residents whose health may be in jeopardy because of their failure to slow down,

In evaluating triggered cases, the following general questions may be helpful:

- *Is inactivity disproportionate to the resident's physical/cognitive abilities or limitations?*
- *Have decreased demands of nursing home life removed the need to make decisions, to set schedules, to meet challenges? Have these changes contributed to resident apathy?*
- *What is the nature of the naturally occurring physical and mental challenges the resident experiences in everyday life?*
- *In what activities is the resident involved? Is he/she normally an active participant in the life of the unit? Is the resident reserved, but actively aware of what is going on around him/her? Or is he/she unaware of surroundings and activities that take place?*
- *Are there proven ways to extend the resident's inquisitive/active engagement in activities?*
- *Might simple staff actions expedite resident involvement in activities? For example: Can equipment be modified to permit greater resident access of the unit? Can the resident's location or position be changed to permit greater access to people, views or programs? Can time and/or distance limitations for activities be made less demanding without destroying the challenge? Can staff modes of interacting with the resident be more accommodating, possibly less threatening, to resident deficits?*

### II. Triggers

**ACTIVITIES TRIGGER A (Revise)**

Consider revising activity plan if one or more of following present:

Involved in activities little or none of time
    [N2 = 2, 3]

Prefers change in daily routine
    **[N5a = 1, 2][N5b = 1, 2]**

**ACTIVITIES TRIGGERS B (Review)**

<u>Review of activity plan suggested if both of following present:</u>

Awake all or most of time in morning
    **[N1a = checked]**
involved in activities most of time
    **[N2 = 0]**

### III.     Guidelines

The follow up review looks for factors that may impede resident involvement in activities. Although many factors can play a role, age as a valid impediment to participation can normally be ruled out. If age continues to be linked as a major cause of lack of participation, a staff education program may prove effective in remedying what may be overprotective staff behavior.

**Issues to be Considered as Activity Plan is Developed.**

<u>Is Resident Suitably Challenged, Overstimulated?</u> To some extent, competence depends on environmental demands. When the challenge is not sufficiently demanding, a resident can become bored, perhaps withdrawn, may resort to fault-finding and perhaps even behave mischievously to relieve the boredom. Eventually, such a resident may become less competent because of the lack of challenge. In contrast, when the resident lacks the competence to meet challenges presented by the surroundings, he or she may react with anger and aggressiveness.

- *Do available activities correspond to resident lifetime values, attitudes and expectations?*
- *Does resident consider leisure activities a waste of time — he/she never really learned to play or to do things just for enjoyment?*
- *Have the resident's wishes and prior activity patterns been considered by activity and nursing professionals?*
- *Have staff considered how activities requiring lower energy levels may be of interest to the resident — e.g., reading a book, talking with family and friends, watching the world go by, knitting?*
- *Does the resident have cognitive/functional deficits that either reduce options or preclude involvement in all/most activities that would otherwise have been of interest to him/her?*

**Confounding Problems to be Considered**

<u>Health-related factors that may affect participation in activities.</u> Diminished cardiac output, an acute illness, reduced energy reserves and impaired respiratory function are some of the many reasons that activity level may decline. Most of these conditions need not necessarily incapacitate the resident. All too often, disease-induced reduction of activity may lead to progressive decline through disuse and further decrease in activity levels. However, this pattern can be broken: many activities can be continued if they are adapted to require less exertion or if the resident is helped in adapting to a lost limb, decreased communication skills, new appliances and so forth.

- *Is the resident suffering from an acute health problem?*
- *Is resident hindered because of embarrassment/unease due to presence of health-related equipment (tubes, oxygen tank, colostomy bag, wheelchair)?*
- *Has the resident recovered from an illness? Is the capacity for participation activities greater?*
- *Has an illness left the resident with some disability (e.g., slurred speech, necessity for use of cane/walker/wheelchair, limited use of hands)?*
- *Does resident's treatment regimen allow little time or energy for participation in preferred activities?*

## Other Issues to be Considered

Recent decline, in resident status — cognition, communication, function, mood or behavior. When pathologic changes occur in any aspect of the resident's competence, the pleasurable challenge of activities may narrow. Of special interest are problematic changes that may be related to the use of psychoactive medications. When residents or staff overreact to such losses, compensatory strategies may be helpful — e.g., impaired residents may benefit from periods of both activity and rest; task segmentation can be considered; or available resident energies can be reserved for pleasurable activities (e.g., using usual stamina reserves to walk to the card room, rather than the bathroom) or activities that have individual significance (e.g., sitting unattended at a daily prayer service rather than at group activity program).

- *Has staff or the resident been overprotective? Or have they misread the seriousness of resident cognitive/functional decline? In what ways?*
- *Has the resident retained skills, or the capacity to learn new skills, sufficient to permit greater activity involvement?*
- *Does staff know what the resident was like prior to the most recent decline? Has the physician/other staff offered a prognosis for the resident's future recovery, or chance of continued decline?*
- *Is there any substantial reason to believe that the resident cannot tolerate or would be harmed by increased activity levels? What reasons support a counter opinion?*
- *Does resident retain any desire to learn or master a specific new activity? Is this realistic?*
- *Has there been a lack of participation in the majority of activities which he/she stated as preference, even though these types of activities are provided?*

Environmental factors. Environmental factors include recent changes in resident location, facility rules, season of the year and physical space limitations that hinder effective resident involvement.

- *Does the interplay of personal, social and physical aspects of the facility's environment hamper involvement in activities? How might this be addressed?*
- *Are current activity levels affected by the season of the year or the nature of the weather during the MDS assessment period?*
- *Can the resident choose to participate in or to create an activity? How is this influenced by facility rules?*
- *Does resident prefer to be with others, but the physical layout of the unit gets in the way? Do other features in the physical plant frustrate the resident's desire to be involved in the life of the facility? What corrective actions are possible? Have any been taken?*

Changes in availability of family/friends/staff support. Many residents will experience not only a change in residence but also a loss of relationships. When this occurs, staff may wish to consider ways for resident to develop a supportive relationship with another resident, staff member or volunteer that may increase the desire to socialize with others and/or to participate in activities with this new friend.

- *Has a staff person who has been instrumental in involving a resident in activities left the facility/been reassigned?*
- *Is a new member in a group activity viewed by a resident as taking over?*
- *Has another resident who was a leader on the unit died or left the unit?*
- *Is resident shy, unable to make new friends?*
- *Does resident's expression of dissatisfaction with fellow residents indicate he/she does not want to be a part of an activities group?*

Possible Confounding Problems to be Considered for Those Now Actively Involved in Activities. Of special interest are cardiac and other diseases that might suggest a need to slow down.

## ACTIVITIES RAP KEY *(For MDS Version 2.0)*

### TRIGGERS - REVISION

ACTIVITIES TRIGGER A (Revise)

*Consider revising activity plan if one or more of the following present.*

- involved in activities little or none of time
  [N2 = 2,3]

- Prefers change in daily routine
  [N5a = 1,2] [N5b = 1,2]

ACTIVITIES TRIGGERS B (Review)

*Review of activity plan suggested if both of following present.*

Awake all or most of time in morning
  [N1a = checked]

Involved in activities most of time
  [N2 = 0]

### GUIDELINES

*Issues to be considered as activity plan is developed.*

- Time in facility [AB1]
- Cognitive status [B2, B4]
- Walking/locomotion pattern [Glc, d, e, f]
- Unstable/acute health conditions [J5a,b]
- Number of treatments received [P1]
- Use of Psychoactive medications [O4a,b,c,d]

*Confounding problems to be considered.*

- Performs tasks slowly and at different levels (reduced energy reserves) [G8c,d]
- Cardiac dysrhythmias [I1e]
- Hypertension [I1h]
- CVA [I1t]
- Respiratory diseases [I1hh, I1ii]
- Pain [J2]

*Other issues to be considered.*

- Customary routines [AC]
- Mood [E1, E2] and Behavioral Symptoms [E4]
- Recent loss of close family member/friend or staff [F2f, from record]
- Whether daily routine is very different from prior pattern in the community [F3c]

# Appendix C: References and Further Reading

Allen-Burket, Gayle, 1988. **Time Well-Spent: A Manual for Visiting Older Adults.** BiFolkal Productions, Inc., Madison, WI.

American Occupational Therapy Association. 1989. **Uniform Terminology for Reporting Occupational Therapy, 2nd Ed.,** Bethesda, MD.

American Psychiatric Association. 1987. **Diagnostic and Statistical Manual of Mental Disorders (Third Edition — Revised).** Washington, DC.

American Psychiatric Association. 1994. **Diagnostic and Statistical Manual of Mental Disorders Fourth Edition.** Washington, DC.

Armstrong, Missy and Sarah Lauzen. 1994. **Community Integration Program, 2nd Edition,** Idyll Arbor, Inc., Ravensdale, WA.

Ayres, A. Jean. 1971. **Sensory Integration And Learning Disorders.** Western Psychological Services, Los Angeles, CA.

Blackman, J. A. 1990. **Medical Aspects of Developmental Disabilities in Children Birth to Three.** Aspen Publications, Gaithersburg, MD.

Bond-Howard, Barbara. 1993. **Introduction To Stroke.** Idyll Arbor, Inc., Ravensdale, WA.

Bowlby, Carol. 1993. **Therapeutic Activities with Person's Disables by Alzheimer's Disease and Related Disorders.** Aspen Publishers, Gaithersburg, MD.

Bradford, Leland P. 1976. **Making Meetings Work: A Guide for Leaders and Group Members.** University Associates, La Jolla, CA.

burlingame, j. and T. M. Blaschko. 1990. **Assessment Tools for Recreational Therapy.** Idyll Arbor, Inc., Ravensdale, WA.

burlingame, j. and T. M. Blaschko. 1991. **Therapy in Intermediate Care Facilities for the Mentally Retarded.** Idyll Arbor, Inc., Ravensdale, WA.

Burnside, Irene Mortenson. 1978. **Working with the Elderly: Group Process and Techniques.** Duxbury Press, Belmont, CA.

Campanelli, Linda and Dan Leviton. "Intergenerational health promotion and rehabilitation: the adult health and development program model," **Topics in Geriatric Rehab** 1989; 4(3) 61-69. Aspen Publishing, Inc., Gaithersburg, MD.

Campbell, Joseph with Moyer, Bill. 1988. **The Power of Myth.** Doubleday, New York, NY.

Cunninghis, Richelle. 1995. **Reality Activities: A How To Manual for Increasing Orientation, Second Edition.** Idyll Arbor, Inc., Ravensdale, WA.

Cunninghis, Richelle and Elizabeth Best Martini. 1996. **Quality Assurance for Activity Programs, Second Edition.** Idyll Arbor, Inc., Ravensdale, WA.

D'Antonio-Nocera, Anne, Nancy DeBolt and Nadine Touhey, Eds. 1996. **The Professional Activity Manager and Consultant.** Idyll Arbor, Inc., Ravensdale, WA.

Erikson, Erik H., Joan M. Erikson, Helen Q. Kivnick. **Vital Involvement in Old Age.** WW Norton, New York, NY.

Feil, Naomi. 1993. **The Validation Breakthrough.** Health Professions Press, Baltimore, MD.

Hall, Beth A., CTRS and Michele M. Nolte, CTRS, ACC. 1996. **The Activity Care Planning Cookbook 2.0: An "MDS 2.0" Based Guide to Building Better Resident Care Plans.** Recreation Therapy Consultants, San Diego, CA.

Harris Lord, Janice. 1988. **Beyond Sympathy: What to Say and Do for Someone Suffering an Injury, Illness or Loss.** Pathfinder Publishing.

Health Care Financing Administration. **RAI Training Manual.** US Department of Commerce National Technical Information Service. Springfield, VA.

Health Care Financing Administration. 1990. **Resident Assessment System For Long Term Care Facilities.** US Department of Commerce National Technical Information Service. Springfield, VA.

Health Care Financing Administration. 1995. **State Operations Manual Provider Certification.** US Department of Commerce National Technical Information Service. Springfield, VA.

Hopkins, H. L. and H. D. Smith. 1983. **Willard and Spackman's Occupational Therapy, Sixth Edition.** J. B. Lippincott Company, New York, NY.

Karam, C. 1989. **A Practical Guide to Cardiac Rehabilitation.** Aspen Publications, Gaithersburg, MD.

Kemp, B., K. Brummel-Smith and J. W. Ramsdell. 1990. **Geriatric Rehabilitation.** College Hill Publications, Boston, MA.

Kisner, C. and Colby, L. A. 1990. **Therapeutic Exercise: Foundations and Techniques, Second Edition.** F. A. Davis, Philadelphia, PA.

Krames Communications, 1898. "Risk Management: Your Role in Providing Quality Care." Krames Communication. Daly City, CA.

Kübler-Ross, E. 1969 **On Death and Dying.** Macmillan Publishing Co., Inc., New York, NY.

Lewis, C. B., 1989 **Improving Mobility in Older Persons: A Manual for Geriatric Specialists.** Aspen Publication, Gaithersburg, MD.

Lewis, C. S. 1961. **A Grief Observed.** Bantam Books.

Lightner, Candy and Nancy Hathaway. 1990. **Giving Sorrow Words: How to Cope with Grief and Get on With Your Life.** Warner Books.

MacNeil, Richard D. and Michael L. Teague. 1987. **Aging and Leisure Vitality in Later Life.** Prentice Hall, Englewood Cliffs, NJ.

Manning, Doug. 1985. **Comforting Those Who Grieve: A Guide for Helping Others.** Harper and Row.

McKay, Davis, Fanning. 1983. **Messages: The Communication Skills Book.** New Harbinger Publications, Oakland. CA.

Parker, Sandra and Carol Will. 1993. **Activities for the Elderly Volume 2, A Guide to Working with Residents with Significant Physical and Cognitive Disabilities.** Idyll Arbor, Ravensdale, WA.

Peabody, Larry. 1982. **Deskbook on Writing.** Writing Services, Olympia, WA.

Randall-David, E. 1989. **Strategies for Working With Culturally Diverse Communities and Clients.** Association for the Care of Children's Health, Bethesda, MD.

Reber, A. S. 1985. **Dictionary of Psychology.** Penguin Books, New York, NY.

Richardson-Brown, C and G. Payton. 1993. **CompuPlan Guide.** Med America Corporation, Indianapolis, IN.

Rodman, G. P., C. McEwen and S. L. Wallace. 1973. *Primer on the Rheumatic Diseases.* Reprinted from **The Journal of the American Medical Association** 224, no. 5 (April 30, 1973) (Supplement).

Ross, Mildred, OTR and Dona Burdick, CTRS. 1981. **Sensory Integration.** Slack, Inc., Thorofare, NJ.

US Department of Health and Human Services. 1983. **CDC Guidelines for Isolation Precautions in Hospitals and CDC Guidelines for Infection Control in Hospital Personnel.** Centers for Disease Control, Atlanta. GA.

Uniak, Ann. 1996. **Documentation in a Snap for Activity Programs (with MDS Version 2.0).** SNAP, San Anselmo, CA.

Voelkl, J. E. 1988. **Risk Management in Therapeutic Recreation: A Component of Quality Assurance.** Venture Publishing, State College, PA.

Zoltan, Barbara, Ellen Siev and Brenda Freishtat. 1986. **The Adult Stroke Patient: A Manual for Evaluation and Treatment of Perceptual and Cognitive Dysfunction.** Slack, Thorofare, NJ.

Zoltan, Barbara. 1996. **Vision, Perception and Cognition: A Manual for Evaluation and Treatment of the Neurologically Impaired Adult, Third Edition.** Slack, Thorofare, NJ.

# Index

past lifestyle. *see previous lifestyle*
pathfinding, 208, 353
patients, 266
peer review, 310
penalties, 309
perception deficit, 353
perception-motor functioning, 149
perceptual accuracy, 149
peripheral vision, 365
perseveration, 353
personal space, 61
personality theory, 8, 9
pet therapy, 22, 26, 122, 126, 171, 295
phantom pain, 353
phobias, 34, 353
*photo release*, 297
physical abuse, 266, 353
physical needs, 302
physical restraints, 354
physical safety, 265
physical status, 301
physical therapist, 164
physician, 164, 166, 246, 275, 277, 281, 282, 286, 287
Pick's Disease, 354
plan of correction, 309
plaque, 354
playfulness, 354
policy, 294, 311, 354
policy and procedure manual, 294
poor judgment skills, 95
post traumatic stress response, 354
posterior, 354
postural drainage, 354
postural dysfunction, 355
postural fault, 355
potassium products, 316
potential, 355
powerlessness, 355
precipitating factors, 355
predictor, 355
prescription, 355
pressure release, 355
pressure sores, 261, 265, 269, 324, 355
pressure ulcer. *see pressure sores*
previous lifestyle, 76, 77, 184
primary care, 175
privacy, 66, 296, 298, 303
problem solving, 91, 355
problem, need, strength statement, 205
procedure, 294, 355
processing deficits, 356
professional standards, 175, 265
professionalism, 51, 356
prognosis, 19, 356
program levels, **69**
program review, 76
programs, **69–82**

progress notes, 180, 217, 306, 356. *see also quarterly progress notes*
progressive relaxation, 27, 356
proof of care, 176
proprioceptive, 96, 97, 119, 120, 148, 356
provider, 267
pseudodementia, 32, 34, 356
psychiatric diagnosis, 31
psychiatric seclusion, 356
psychiatrist, 287
psychoactive medications, 218, 281, 283, 316, 325, 356
psychological abuse, 267
psychologist, 164, 287
psychosis, 34
psychosocial needs, 302
psychosocial plan, 243
psychosocial well-being, 302, 303, 357, 382
psychotic disorders, 33
psychotropic medications. *see psychoactive medications*
Public Health Service, 266
punishment, 266
purchase order, 293

—Q—

quality assurance, 176, **245–56**, 357
quality assurance committee, 306
quality of care, 2, 305
quality of life, 2, 8, 9, 19, 51, 55, 61, 77, 84, 100, 205, 238, 243, 299, 357
quarterly care conferences, 218
quarterly progress notes, 181, 182, 218, 220, 357. *see also progress notes*
quarterly review form, 193

—R—

RAI. *see Resident Assessment Instrument*
range of motion, 22, 26, 29, 90, 91, 273, 357
    active, 357
    passive, 357
RAPs. *see Resident Assessment Protocols*
reaction time, 322
reactions to illness, 10
reading skills, 165
reality awareness, 21, 65, 186
reality orientation, 56, 185, 357
reasoning, 357
receptive communication, 331
receptor, 357
recognition, 358
records, 297
recreation needs, 83
recreational therapist, 164, 358
referral, 358
refusal, 297
refusing activities, 74

## —T—

# About The Authors

## *Elizabeth Best Martini*

Elizabeth Best Martini has been a Recreational Therapist Certified (RTC) in California since 1978. She is a nationally Certified Therapeutic Recreation Specialist (CTRS) and also is an Activity Consultant Certified with NAAP (ACC). She received her Master of Science degree in Therapeutic Recreation and Leisure Studies from San Francisco State University. For the next four years, she held the position of Recreational Therapist/Activity Coordinator/Social Service Coordinator for a 99-bed nursing facility.

In 1983, Elizabeth began her private practice under the name of Recreation Consultation. This consulting company provides consultation to long term care settings and other agencies throughout Northern California.

She is a qualified instructor for both the NAAP Basic Education and Advanced Management Courses. She currently teaches the BEC Course in three college settings in Northern California. In addition she teaches two Living History classes for elderly clients weekly.

Elizabeth currently consults in Northern California in both nursing homes and state hospital settings. She is a board member of the national LITA Association. LITA is a volunteer organization which provides one-on-one friends to nursing home residents without family or visitors.

She and her husband live in Marin County, California, with their two pygmy goats, who also visit in long term care settings and appear at National Park Service Visitor Centers.

## *Mary Anne Weeks*

Mary Anne Weeks has worked as a Social Worker (SSC) in nursing facilities since November of 1982. At that time, few facilities in California had yet realized a need for such a discipline so there were no "rules." Fortunately, Mary Anne had long ago, in 1965, worked as a summer intern in a prototype retirement home in Rochester, New York. Her past experience in this setting with various levels of care made the environment in nursing settings more familiar to her.

In the meantime, she had also received an undergraduate degree from the State University of New York, Genesee and pursued graduate work at University of California, Berkeley where she completed her Master Degree in Public Health.

Mary Anne lives in Sonoma, California, with her husband and two children. She is the Social Service Coordinator in an nursing facility, provides consultation in the specialty area of social services and is a lecturer at the community college level.

## *Priscilla Wirth*

Priscilla Wirth is a Health Information Consultant for long term care facilities. She is a Registered Records Administrator, receiving her degree from Seattle University. She has been in the health information profession since 1980.

Her Bachelor of Science degree and Master of Library Sciences were received from Northern Illinois University. Priscilla is currently practicing in Sonoma County, California and is a member of the American Medical Record Association, the California Health Information Association and the Network of Health Record Consultants. She is a lecturer at the community college level.